What We See through Cardiac Imaging

What We See through Cardiac Imaging

Guest Editors

Valeria Pergola
Martina Perazzolo Marra

MDPI

Basel • Beijing • Wuhan • Barcelona • Belgrade • Novi Sad • Cluj • Manchester

Guest Editors

Valeria Pergola
Department of Cardiac,
Thoracic, Vascular Sciences
and Public Health
University of Padua
Medical School
Padua
Italy

Martina Perazzolo Marra
Department of Cardiac,
Thoracic, Vascular Sciences
and Public Health
University of Padua
Medical School
Padua
Italy

Editorial Office
MDPI AG
Grosspeteranlage 5
4052 Basel, Switzerland

This is a reprint of the Special Issue, published open access by the journal *Journal of Clinical Medicine* (ISSN 2077-0383), freely accessible at: https://www.mdpi.com/journal/jcm/special_issues/W671RHP67F.

For citation purposes, cite each article independently as indicated on the article page online and as indicated below:

Lastname, A.A.; Lastname, B.B. Article Title. *Journal Name* **Year**, *Volume Number*, Page Range.

ISBN 978-3-7258-5811-8 (Hbk)
ISBN 978-3-7258-5812-5 (PDF)
https://doi.org/10.3390/books978-3-7258-5812-5

Contents

About the Editors

Valeria Pergola

Valeria Pergola, MD, is a senior consultant cardiologist and adjunct professor of cardiac imaging at Padua University Hospital. Previously, she led the cardiac imaging service at Croydon University Hospital and served as an honorary consultant at the Royal Brompton and King's College Hospitals in London between 2016 and 2019. Earlier appointments include imaging consultant at the King Faisal Specialist Hospital in Riyadh (2012–2016) and consultant cardiologist at the Azienda Ospedaliera dei Colli in Naples, where she was Director of the Outpatient Clinic Service. She holds level 3 certifications in transthoracic and transoesophageal echocardiography and qualifications in cardiovascular CT, and she is a Fellow of both the European Society of Cardiology and the European Association of Cardiovascular Imaging. She practices multimodality cardiac imaging—advanced echocardiography and cardiac CT. Her work spans clinical practice, research, and teaching, with interests in stress echocardiography, structural heart disease, infective endocarditis, and advanced heart failure.

Martina Perazzolo Marra

Martina Perazzolo Marra, MD, PhD, is an associate professor in the Department of Cardiac, Thoracic and Vascular Sciences and Public Health at the University of Padua. Since 2020, she has held the role of director and quality referent of the University's School of Specialization in Cardiovascular Diseases, a four-year postgraduate program for physicians specializing in cardiology. She teaches courses on echocardiography and cardiac magnetic resonance, focusing on methods and practical applications for students of medicine and cardiovascular medicine. In addition to her teaching, she practices multimodality cardiac imaging—including echocardiography and cardiac MRI—to diagnose and manage cardiomyopathies and other structural heart diseases. Her research and professional activities within the European Association of Cardiovascular Imaging emphasize the integration of advanced imaging techniques into clinical care and the mentoring of future cardiovascular imagers.

Preface

We are delighted to present this Reprint, curated by Guest Editors Valeria Pergola and Martina Perazzolo Marra, which distills the central themes of the Special Issue "What We See through Cardiac Imaging." Cardiac imaging has evolved from an anatomical descriptor to a predictive, therapeutic shaping tool. The assembled articles cover congenital and acquired heart disease, coronary anatomy, heart failure, and surgical interventions, highlighting how structural, functional, and dynamic insights from multimodality imaging now underpin diagnosis, risk stratification, and therapeutic planning. This Reprint is intended for clinicians, researchers, and trainees who wish to deepen their understanding of state-of-the-art echocardiography, cardiac magnetic resonance, computed tomography, and emerging biomarkers. By sharing these innovations and emphasizing the need for standardized protocols and multicentre validation, we hope to inspire thoughtful application of imaging and to foster collaboration across disciplines, ultimately improving patient care.

Valeria Pergola and Martina Perazzolo Marra
Guest Editors

Journal of
Clinical Medicine

MDPI

Editorial

Editorial: What We See Through Cardiac Imaging

Valeria Pergola * and Martina Perazzolo Marra

Cardiology Unit, Cardio-Thoracic-Vascular, and Public Health Department, Padova University Hospital, 35128 Padova, Italy; martina.perazzolomarra@unipd.it
* Correspondence: valeria.pergola@unipd.it

The evolving landscape of cardiac imaging continues to redefine our ability to diagnose, stratify risk, and monitor cardiomyopathies. In both congenital and acquired conditions, structural, functional, and dynamic myocardial insights are no longer ancillary; they are foundational. This Special Issue, "What We See through Cardiac Imaging", assembles diverse contributions reflecting the growing role of multimodality imaging (MMI) as both a diagnostic and prognostic cornerstone.

In patients with systemic right ventricle (sRV) physiology, such as those with transposition of the great arteries (TGA), post-atrial switch, or congenitally corrected TGA (ccTGA), subpulmonary left ventricular (LV) function has historically received limited attention. Piana et al. [1] demonstrate that LV global longitudinal strain (GLS), measured by cardiac magnetic resonance feature tracking (CMR-FT), predicts adverse outcomes in this group, confirming the prognostic significance of this neglected chamber. While the intra-vendor reproducibility of the strain is good [2], inter-vendor variability remains a significant barrier to widespread adoption. Standardization of acquisition, post-processing, and threshold values is essential to ensure reliable surveillance. A related challenge is addressed in patients with repaired aortic coarctation [3]. This supports earlier observations [4] that anatomical severity alone does not predict functional limitation. Integration of exercise testing with cross-sectional imaging and longitudinal outcomes will help define intervention thresholds with greater precision.

Coronary artery anatomy shows considerable variability, ranging from benign variants to anomalies causing hemodynamic compromise or sudden cardiac death (SCD). Baz [5] provides a structured review of coronary artery anomalies (CAAs) and emphasizes CT coronary angiography (CTCA) as the reference non-invasive modality for detailed anatomical assessment. Recent advances in cardiac CT technology have enabled high-quality imaging without ECG synchronization, improving efficiency and reducing patient burden. These early results suggest a promising diagnostic tool, though its applicability may be limited in patients with arrhythmias or very high heart rates, warranting further investigation [6]. Hardware innovations in computed tomography are already enabling shorter and simpler diagnostic workflows. On the other hand, the convergence of artificial intelligence and the metaverse opens scenarios in which the patient becomes an active participant in the diagnostic experience. The near-perfect accuracy achieved by the ICA-based algorithm, further discussed in immersive VR environments, suggests that the future is not only about streamlining procedures but also about reshaping the doctor–patient relationship in a participatory and interactive way [7].

Galzerano et al. [8] highlight the integration of three-dimensional echocardiography, myocardial strain, and vortex dynamics as a promising approach for heart failure assessment, with the potential to uncover subtle ventricular dysfunction before clinical decline. In this context, vortex analysis has also been applied to the athlete's heart, where it complements morphological remodeling by demonstrating higher energetic parameters in highly trained individuals, thereby reflecting the effects of training intensity and energy consumption [9]. While promising, its prognostic and therapeutic impact remains to be established in longitudinal studies.

Postoperative paradoxical septum (POPS) is a frequent but usually benign finding after cardiac surgery, characterized by preserved LV function, normal perfusion, and absence of injury. Di Virgilio et al. [10] review fifty years of hypotheses, culminating in a heuristic model in which POPS arises from the geometric realignment of ventricular anchor points rather than myocardial damage. This reframes POPS as a functional adaptation rather than pathology. Historical work by Weyman et al. [11] links paradoxical septal motion to RV volume overload, but Di Virgilio et al. [10] integrate past and present evidence into a unified geometric-shift model. While compelling, it remains unproven; prospective, quantitative imaging studies—particularly using 3D deformation analysis—are needed to validate its diagnostic and prognostic relevance.

An extensive review of the Ross procedure by Galzerano et al. [12] underscores its growing recognition, despite a current class IIb guideline status, for offering superior survival, fewer valve-related complications, and better quality of life compared with conventional prostheses in young patients. Consistently, analysis of over 2000 adolescents and young adults from the ECCDB demonstrated excellent outcomes with the Ross procedure, showing the lowest mortality rate (0.4%) and reinforcing its value as a durable and safe option in this challenging population [13]. While the Ross procedure appears to be a compelling option for carefully selected patients, questions remain over long-term (>20 year) autograft durability and optimal homograft preservation. Coordinated, prospective multicenter studies with standardized imaging follow-up are essential to define candidacy and refine guidelines.

Pergola et al. [14] argue for moving beyond a simple ejection-fraction–based classification of heart failure, advocating instead for an integrated multimodality approach that reflects the dynamic and patient-specific nature of the condition. In line with this perspective, a recent comprehensive review of early-stage HFpEF emphasizes the challenges of timely diagnosis, the importance of advanced imaging, and the need for early intervention to reduce progression to overt and advanced disease [15]. MMI is pivotal for candidate selection, surgical planning, and complication detection, including RV failure, thrombosis, valvular dysfunction, and device malposition. While MMI clearly enhances peri- and post-operative assessment, prospective multicenter trials and standardized imaging protocols are needed to confirm survival and quality-of-life benefits [16].

Moving to CTCA, Napoli et al. [17] highlight epicardial and pericoronary adipose tissue (EAT/PCAT) as active contributors to coronary inflammation, plaque vulnerability, and acute coronary syndromes. They position PCAT-CT attenuation as a non-invasive biomarker of coronary inflammation with prognostic potential in CAD. Previous studies [18] showed that in angiographically non-obstructive coronary syndromes, PCAT demonstrates a transient but measurable inflammatory phenotype on CCTA via the pericoronary fat attenuation index (pFAI). Consistently, the large ORFAN study demonstrated that the perivascular fat attenuation index (FAI) robustly predicts cardiac mortality and MACE independently of traditional risk factors and CAD burden, with AI-enhanced risk stratification further refining prognostic accuracy, particularly in patients without obstructive disease [19]. These findings support a paradigm shift toward inflammation-based risk assessment. Still, validation in larger, diverse cohorts and trials linking PCAT modulation to outcome improvements are needed before clinical integration.

Finally, Sonaglioni et al. [20] report a rare, isolated RV thrombosis post-cardiac surgery, initially misdiagnosed as tumor. The case illustrates the diagnostic pitfalls of intracardiac masses and the value of multimodality imaging—and particularly echocardiography—in guiding timely intervention. Extending this diagnostic framework, pulsed-wave tissue Doppler imaging has been proposed for distinguishing pathological right atrial masses from benign pseudomasses such as a prominent crista terminalis or the Chiari network [21]. While promising for embolic risk stratification, its clinical adoption is limited by scarce validation. Multicenter studies are needed to determine its sensitivity, specificity, and reproducibility.

Taken together, the contributions in this Special Issue reinforce the central message: Cardiac imaging has moved beyond anatomy to become a predictive, therapeutic-shaping tool. Across congenital, structural, coronary, and heart failure domains, MMI enables earlier disease detection, sharper risk stratification, and tailored interventions. The challenge ahead is to translate these promising approaches into standardized, evidence-based protocols, validated by robust multicenter trials, to ensure that they benefit the broad patient populations who stand to gain from them.

Author Contributions: Conceptualization: V.P. and M.P.M., Writing original article: V.P., Writing review: M.P.M., Project administration: V.P., Funding acquisition: M.P.M. All authors have read and agreed to the published version of the manuscript.

Conflicts of Interest: The authors declare no conflict of interest.

References

1. Piana, S.; Pozza, A.; Cavaliere, A.; Molinaroli, A.; Cattapan, I.; Fumanelli, J.; Avesani, M.; Reffo, E.; Di Salvo, G. The Sub-Pulmonary Left Ventricle in Patients with Systemic Right Ventricle, the Paradoxical Neglected Chamber: A Cardiac Magnetic Resonance Feature Tracking Study. *J. Clin. Med.* **2024**, *13*, 6033. [CrossRef] [PubMed] [PubMed Central]
2. Colquitt, J.L.; Wilkinson, J.C.; Liu, A.M.; Pignatelli, R.H.; Loar, R.W. Single systemic right ventricle longitudinal strain: Intravendor reproducibility and intervendor agreement in children. *Echocardiography* **2021**, *38*, 402–409. [CrossRef] [PubMed]
3. Di Salvo, G.; Fumanelli, J.; Graziano, S.; Pozza, A.; Cattapan, I.; Moscatelli, S.; Castaldi, B.; Galzerano, D. Stress Echocardiography in the Follow-Up of Young Patients with Repaired Aortic Coarctation. *J. Clin. Med.* **2024**, *13*, 5587. [CrossRef] [PubMed] [PubMed Central]
4. Ramachandran, A.; Talmor, N.; Saric, M.; Feinberg, J.; Small, A.J.; Halpern, D.G. Anatomical/Physiological Correlates of Functional Capacity in Adults With Repaired and Nonsevere Coarctation of the Aorta. *JACC Adv.* **2023**, *2*, 100672. [CrossRef] [PubMed] [PubMed Central]
5. Baz, R.O.; Refi, D.; Scheau, C.; Savulescu-Fiedler, I.; Baz, R.A.; Niscoveanu, C. Coronary Artery Anomalies: A Computed Tomography Angiography Pictorial Review. *J. Clin. Med.* **2024**, *13*, 3920. [CrossRef]
6. Mochizuki, J.; Suzuki, M.; Misawa, S.; Matsumi, H.; Hata, Y. Advances in Cardiac Computed Tomography: Highlighting the Diagnostic Potential of Nonelectrocardiography-Synchronized Imaging. *JACC Case Rep.* **2025**, *30*, 104026. [CrossRef] [PubMed]
7. Sivaranjani, T.; Sasikumar, B.; Sugitha, G. Metaverse-based deep learning framework for coronary artery stenosis classification using Monte Carlo Dropout-based ResNet-152. *Comput. Biol. Med.* **2025**, *196*, 110720. [CrossRef] [PubMed]
8. Galzerano, D.; Savo, M.T.; Castaldi, B.; Kholaif, N.; Khaliel, F.; Pozza, A.; Aljheish, S.; Cattapan, I.; Martini, M.; Lassandro, E.; et al. Transforming Heart Failure Management: The Power of Strain Imaging, 3D Imaging, and Vortex Analysis in Echocardiography. *J. Clin. Med.* **2024**, *13*, 5759. [CrossRef]
9. Corsi, M.; Falconi, E.; Palazzo, R.; Orlandi, M.; Mascherini, G.; Bini, V.; Stefani, L. An Independent Marker of Myocardial Function in Athlete's Heart: Role of Vortex Analysis in Triathlon. *J. Cardiovasc. Echogr.* **2025**, *35*, 37–42. [CrossRef] [PubMed] [PubMed Central]
10. Di Virgilio, E.; Basile, P.; Carella, M.C.; Monitillo, F.; Santoro, D.; Latorre, M.D.; D'alessandro, S.; Fusini, L.; Fazzari, F.; Pontone, G.; et al. The Postoperative Paradoxical Septum (POPS): A Comprehensive Review on Physio-Pathological Mechanisms. *J. Clin. Med.* **2024**, *13*, 2309. [CrossRef]
11. Weyman, A.; Wann, S.; Feigenbaum, H.; Dillon, J.C. Mechanism of abnormal septal motion in patients with right ventricular volume overload: A cross-sectional echocardiographic study. *Circulation* **1976**, *54*, 179–186. [CrossRef] [PubMed]
12. Galzerano, D.; Kholaif, N.; Al Amro, B.; Al Admawi, M.; Eltayeb, A.; Alshammari, A.; Di Salvo, G.; Al-Halees, Z.Y. The Ross Procedure: Imaging, Outcomes and Future Directions in Aortic Valve Replacement. *J. Clin. Med.* **2024**, *13*, 630. [CrossRef] [PubMed] [PubMed Central]

13. Guariento, A.; Cattapan, C.; Doulamis, I.P.; Tobota, Z.; Maruszewski, B.; Bleiweis, M.S.; Jacobs, J.P.; E Sarris, G.; Vida, V. Aortic valve surgery in adolescents and young adults: Analysis of early operative data from the European Congenital Heart Surgeons Association database. *Eur. J. Cardiothorac. Surg.* **2025**, *67*, ezaf101. [CrossRef] [PubMed] [PubMed Central]
14. Pergola, V.; Cameli, M.; Mattesi, G.; Mushtaq, S.; D'Andrea, A.; Guaricci, A.I.; Pastore, M.C.; Amato, F.; Dellino, C.M.; Motta, R.; et al. Multimodality Imaging in Advanced Heart Failure for Diagnosis, Management and Follow-Up: A Comprehensive Review. *J. Clin. Med.* **2023**, *12*, 7641. [CrossRef] [PubMed]
15. Yaku, H.; Shah, S.J. The Key Role of Diagnostic Imaging in Early HFpEF. *JACC Cardiovasc. Imaging* **2025**, S1936-878X(25)00306-7. [CrossRef] [PubMed]
16. McDonagh, T.A.; Metra, M.; Adamo, M.; Gardner, R.S.; Baumbach, A.; Böhm, M.; Burri, H.; Butler, J.; Čelutkienė, J.; Chioncel, O.; et al. 2023 Focused Update of the 2021 ESC Guidelines for the diagnosis and treatment of acute and chronic heart failure. *Eur. Heart J.* **2023**, *44*, 3627–3639; Erratum in *Eur. Heart J.* **2024**, *45*, 53. [CrossRef] [PubMed]
17. Napoli, G.; Pergola, V.; Basile, P.; De Feo, D.; Bertrandino, F.; Baggiano, A.; Mushtaq, S.; Fusini, L.; Fazzari, F.; Carrabba, N.; et al. Epicardial and Pericoronary Adipose Tissue, Coronary Inflammation, and Acute Coronary Syndromes. *J. Clin. Med.* **2023**, *12*, 7212. [CrossRef] [PubMed] [PubMed Central]
18. Pergola, V.; Previtero, M.; Cecere, A.; Storer, V.; Castiello, T.; Baritussio, A.; Cabrelle, G.; Mele, D.; Motta, R.; Caforio, A.P.; et al. Clinical Value and Time Course of Pericoronary Fat Inflammation in Patients with Angiographically Nonobstructive Coronaries: A Preliminary Report. *J. Clin. Med.* **2021**, *10*, 1786. [CrossRef] [PubMed] [PubMed Central]
19. Chan, K.; Wahome, E.; Tsiachristas, A.; Antonopoulos, A.S.; Patel, P.; Lyasheva, M.; Kingham, L.; West, H.; Oikonomou, E.K.; Volpe, L.; et al. Inflammatory risk and cardiovascular events in patients without obstructive coronary artery disease: The ORFAN multicentre, longitudinal cohort study. *Lancet* **2024**, *403*, 2606–2618. [CrossRef] [PubMed] [PubMed Central]
20. Sonaglioni, A.; Lucidi, A.; Luisi, F.; Caminati, A.; Nicolosi, G.L.; Rispoli, G.A.; Zompatori, M.; Lombardo, M.; Harari, S. A Dynamic Multimodality Imaging Assessment of Right Ventricular Thrombosis in a Middle-Aged Man with Lymphocytic Interstitial Pneumonia: The Additive Role of Tissue Doppler Imaging. *J. Clin. Med.* **2025**, *14*, 2035. [CrossRef] [PubMed] [PubMed Central]
21. Sonaglioni, A.; Nicolosi, G.L.; Lombardo, M.; Anzà, C.; Ambrosio, G. Prognostic Relevance of Left Ventricular Thrombus Motility: Assessment by Pulsed Wave Tissue Doppler Imaging. *Angiology* **2021**, *72*, 355–363. [CrossRef] [PubMed]

Journal of
Clinical Medicine

MDPI

Review

Epicardial and Pericoronary Adipose Tissue, Coronary Inflammation, and Acute Coronary Syndromes

Gianluigi Napoli [1,†], Valeria Pergola [2,†], Paolo Basile [1], Daniele De Feo [1], Fulvio Bertrandino [1], Andrea Baggiano [3], Saima Mushtaq [3], Laura Fusini [3], Fabio Fazzari [3], Nazario Carrabba [4], Mark G. Rabbat [5,6], Raffaella Motta [7], Marco Matteo Ciccone [1], Gianluca Pontone [3] and Andrea Igoren Guaricci [1,*]

1 University Cardiologic Unit, Interdisciplinary Department of Medicine, Polyclinic University Hospital, 70124 Bari, Italy; gianluiginapoli@gmail.com (G.N.); pabas2304@gmail.com (P.B.); daniele.df93@gmail.com (D.D.F.); fbertrandino@gmail.com (F.B.); marcomatteo.ciccone@uniba.it (M.M.C.)
2 Department of Cardiac, Thoracic and Vascular Sciences and Public Health, University of Padua, 35122 Padua, Italy; valeria.pergola@yahoo.it
3 Department of Perioperative Cardiology and Cardiovascular Imaging, Centro Cardiologico Monzino, IRCCS, 20138 Milan, Italy; andrea.baggiano@cardiologicomonzino.it (A.B.); saima.mushtaq@cardiologicomonzino.it (S.M.); laura.fusini@cardiologicomonzino.it (L.F.); fabio.fazzari@cardiologicomonzino.it (F.F.); gianluca.pontone@cardiologicomonzino.it (G.P.)
4 Department of Cardiothoracovascular Medicine, Azienda Ospedaliero Universitaria Careggi, 50134 Florence, Italy; n.carrabba@virgilio.it
5 Division of Cardiology, Loyola University of Chicago, Chicago, IL 60611, USA; mrabbat@lumc.edu
6 Edward Hines Jr. VA Hospital, Hines, IL 60141, USA
7 Radiology Unit, University Hospital of Padova, 35128 Padua, Italy; raffaella.motta@unipd.it
* Correspondence: andreaigoren.guaricci@uniba.it
† These authors contributed equally to this work.

Abstract: Vascular inflammation is recognized as the primary trigger of acute coronary syndrome (ACS). However, current noninvasive methods are not capable of accurately detecting coronary inflammation. Epicardial adipose tissue (EAT) and pericoronary adipose tissue (PCAT), in addition to their role as an energy reserve system, have been found to contribute to the development and progression of coronary artery calcification, inflammation, and plaque vulnerability. They also participate in the vascular response during ischemia, sympathetic stimuli, and arrhythmia. As a result, the evaluation of EAT and PCAT using imaging techniques such as computed tomography (CT), cardiac magnetic resonance (CMR), and nuclear imaging has gained significant attention. PCAT-CT attenuation, which measures the average CT attenuation in Hounsfield units (HU) of the adipose tissue, reflects adipocyte differentiation/size and leukocyte infiltration. It is emerging as a marker of tissue inflammation and has shown prognostic value in coronary artery disease (CAD), being associated with plaque development, vulnerability, and rupture. In patients with acute myocardial infarction (AMI), an inflammatory pericoronary microenvironment promoted by dysfunctional EAT/PCAT has been demonstrated, and more recently, it has been associated with plaque rupture in non-ST-segment elevation myocardial infarction (NSTEMI). Endothelial dysfunction, known for its detrimental effects on coronary vessels and its association with plaque progression, is bidirectionally linked to PCAT. PCAT modulates the secretory profile of endothelial cells in response to inflammation and also plays a crucial role in regulating vascular tone in the coronary district. Consequently, dysregulated PCAT has been hypothesized to contribute to type 2 myocardial infarction with non-obstructive coronary arteries (MINOCA) and coronary vasculitis. Recently, quantitative measures of EAT derived from coronary CT angiography (CCTA) have been included in artificial intelligence (AI) models for cardiovascular risk stratification. These models have shown incremental utility in predicting major adverse cardiovascular events (MACEs) compared to plaque characteristics alone. Therefore, the analysis of PCAT and EAT, particularly through PCAT-CT attenuation, appears to be a safe, valuable, and sufficiently specific noninvasive method for accurately identifying coronary inflammation and subsequent high-risk plaque. These findings are supported by biopsy and in vivo evidence. Although speculative, these pieces of evidence open the door for a fascinating new strategy in cardiovascular risk stratification. The incorporation of PCAT and EAT analysis, mainly through

PCAT-CT attenuation, could potentially lead to improved risk stratification and guide early targeted primary prevention and intensive secondary prevention in patients at higher risk of cardiac events.

Keywords: epicardial adipose tissue; pericoronary adipose tissue; coronary inflammation; acute coronary syndromes

1. Introduction

The burden of acute coronary syndrome (ACS) and its associated mortality have consistently increased over time [1,2]. Recent advancements in diagnostics and treatment have partially mitigated this upward trend. Coronary computed tomography angiography (CCTA) provides various tools with which to assess coronary artery disease, ranging from calcium scoring to coronary plaque analysis. These tools are utilized as comprehensive prognostic indicators (based on scores) [3–17].

Epicardial adipose tissue (EAT) and pericoronary adipose tissue (PCAT) contribute to cardiovascular risk in different ways. They have been shown to have a prognostic role in coronary artery disease (CAD) [18,19], to contribute to the development and progression of coronary artery calcification (CAC) and coronary plaque vulnerability [20–22], and to impact the inflammatory damage observed in coronary arteritis and myocardial infarction with non-obstructive coronary arteries (MINOCA) [23,24].

Emerging evidence suggests that the paracrine activity of EAT and PCAT is associated with coronary plaque instability [25,26]. It is clear that EAT and PCAT exhibit distinct biological properties which manifest differently under various circumstances. This review focuses on the emerging role of EAT in coronary inflammation, CAD development, plaque vulnerability, and ACS, with particular emphasis on its endocrine properties and the imaging modalities currently employed for its evaluation.

2. Imaging Evaluation of EAT and PCAT

EAT and PCAT, as well as thoracic fat, are commonly assessed using non-contrast computed tomography (CT) or cardiac magnetic resonance (CMR). Echocardiographic evaluation of EAT has also been described. Transthoracic echocardiography (TTE) is a readily available and user-friendly imaging modality for measuring EAT thickness. Typically, EAT is visualized in parasternal long-axis views as the hypoechoic space between the free wall of the right ventricle and the visceral layer of the pericardium during end-systole. Previous reports have indicated a median thickness of 7 mm [27,28]. However, the use of TTE for EAT evaluation is limited due to operator dependence, frequent poor acoustic windows, and poor correlation with CT-derived volume.

CMR can quantify EAT volume using black blood T1-weighted diastolic single-shot spin echo sequences [29] CMR allows for excellent visualization of the visceral and parietal pericardium, making EAT visualization straightforward, without the need for radiation exposure or contrast agents. However, the high cost, incompatibility with implanted devices, and claustrophobia in some patients are important limitations of this method.

Currently, the epidemiological evidence on the role of EAT as a biomarker and predictor of cardiovascular disease (CVD) is mainly derived from CT imaging. In CT scan protocols, adipose tissue is identified by voxels with attenuation values between −30 and −190 Hounsfield Units (HU), depending on its normal or inflamed condition. The CT attenuation of PCAT represents the average attenuation, in HU, of the adipose tissue within the defined volume of interest. It reflects the balance between lipid and aqueous phases, with a well-established association between signal attenuation and adipocyte differentiation and size, primarily driven by intracellular lipid accumulation. Generally, a gradient from higher to lower attenuation has been observed from PCAT to EAT [18,30–33] (Figures 1 and 2 and Table 1).

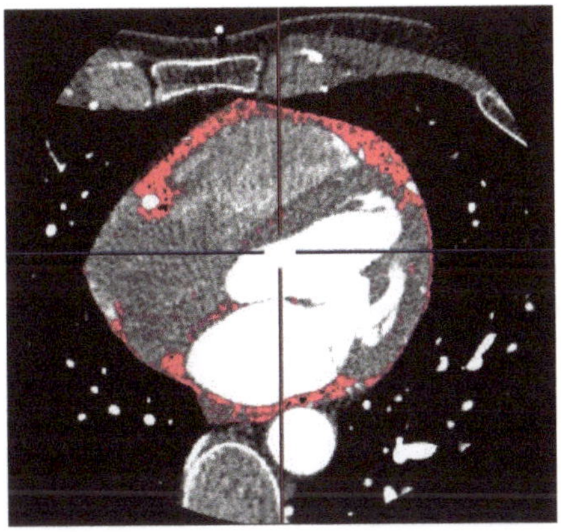

Figure 1. CT scan of a 49-year-old male patient depicting the epicardial adipose tissue (red) immediately internal to the pericardium.

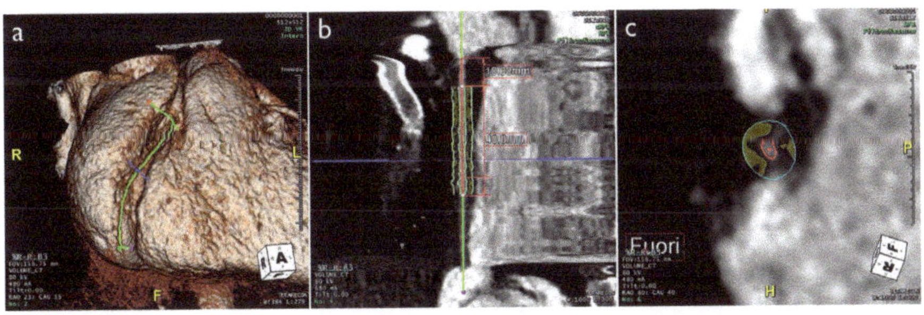

Figure 2. CT scan of a 39-year-old female patient. (**a**) 3D reconstruction of the heart, focusing on the middle segment of RCA. (**b**,**c**) PCAT distribution around RCA in longitudinal and ortogonal view, respectively (yellow spots). CT, computed tomography; PCAT, pericoronary adipose tissue; RCA, right coronary artery.

Table 1. Imaging modalities by which to assess adipose tissue.

	TTE	**CCTA**	**CMR**
Availability	●●●	●●○	●○○
Cost	●○○	●●○	●●●
Lack of iodine contrast use	✓	⊗	✓
Lack of ionizing radiation exposure	✓	⊗	✓
Reproducibility	●○○	●●●	●●●
Spatial resolution	●○○	●●●	●●○
3D volume data	⊗	✓	✓
AT thickness	✓	✓	✓
AT area	⊗	✓	✓
AT volume	⊗	✓	✓
AT attenuation	⊗	✓	⊗
AT radiomic profile	⊗	✓	⊗

AT, adipose tissue; CCTA, coronary computed tomography angiography; CMR, cardiac magnetic resonance; TTE, transthoracic echocardiography. ●●●, high; ●●○, medium; ●○○, low; ✓, condition satisfied/measure allowed; ⊗, N/A.

3. Pathophysiologic Role of EAT and PCAT

It is widely recognized that approximately 20% of the total ventricular mass is comprised of adipocytes [29,34–36]. EAT is situated in the atrioventricular and interventricular sulcus, surrounding the two appendages and the free walls of the atria. It maintains a consistent fat/muscle ratio even during hypertrophic changes [37–39]. EAT and PCAT, which originate from brown adipose tissue, share a close spatial and metabolic relationship with myocardial cells. Their role in immunological, inflammatory, metabolic, and vascular modulation of the heart has gained significant attention.

Under normal conditions, EAT exhibits various cardioprotective and metabolic properties. These include the release of free fatty acids (FFAs) as an energy source for the myocardium during periods of increased metabolic demand, the expression of the thermogenic protein UCP-1 in response to cold exposure, and the production of cardioprotective factors such as adrenomedullin. Adrenomedullin is a potent vasodilator and antioxidative peptide with anti-inflammatory and anti-atherogenic properties [40,41]. EAT also acts in a paracrine manner as a key regulator of vascular response during ischemia, sympathetic stimuli, and arrhythmia [42–44].

Firstly, EAT plays a role in initiating inflammatory signals in response to regional ischemia, leading to the release of interleukin (IL)-1β, IL-6, IL-6 soluble receptor, and tumor necrosis factor-α (TNFα), as well as a decrease in the secretion of adiponectin, an adipokine with anti-inflammatory and antiatherogenic properties [45,46]. Potential mechanisms involve the release of adipokines from PCAT, which may traverse the coronary wall through paracrine diffusion or direct release into the vasa vasorum, subsequently passing into the arterial wall in a vasocrine manner [40].

Secondly, increased EAT volume in obesity can disrupt ion channel properties, creating an arrhythmogenic substrate for atrial fibrillation (AF) [43]. Additionally, EAT has demonstrated heightened adrenergic activity in heart failure, as evidenced by higher concentrations of norepinephrine compared to plasma and the expression of catecholamine biosynthetic enzymes. This establishes a negative feedback loop, ultimately leading to functional and anatomical denervation of the heart [44].

4. Correlation between EAT, Coronary Inflammation, Coronary Flow Reserve, and Cardiovascular Risk

EAT consists of adipocytes, pre-adipocytes, ganglia, interconnecting nerves, immune cells, and inflammatory infiltrate, primarily macrophages [42,47]. The imbalance between pro-inflammatory M1 and anti-inflammatory M2 macrophages is observed in patients with CAD [48]. EAT, which is in close proximity to myocardiocytes, can release pro-inflammatory and pro-atherogenic substances directly into the coronary lumen under pathological conditions. The transcriptome of EAT encodes inflammatory cytokines, affecting its pro-atherogenic characteristics, especially in unfavorable metabolic conditions like diabetes [49–54]. Radiographic fat density correlates with adipocyte enlargement, while CT attenuation is inversely related to adipocyte size. Higher CT attenuation in EAT indicates the presence of enlarged adipocytes and infiltration of pro-inflammatory M1 macrophages, indicating inflammation [48]. CT attenuation of the surrounding PCAT has prognostic significance in CAD, as elevated attenuation is associated with reduced coronary flow reserve [18,19,32], while a pericoronary fat attenuation index (pFAI) exceeding a specific threshold is predictive of both all-cause and cardiac mortality [55]. Utilizing the pFAI could potentially improve risk assessment and guide targeted prevention strategies for individuals at higher risk [56].

PCAT has shown a positive association with the presence, amount, and progression of CAC, independent of total body fat [20–22] Even after considering conventional cardiovascular risk factors and inflammatory markers, the volume of EAT remains a significant predictor of CAC burden [21]. This may be attributed to the development of an inflammatory micro-environment, lower levels of anti-atherogenic cytokines, and the secretion of inflammatory substances such as ILs and monocyte chemoattractant protein-1 (MCP-1).

Consequently, dysfunctional EAT/PCAT promotes inflammatory infiltration, leading to tissue changes that are reflected in the attenuation observed through CT imaging (Figure 3).

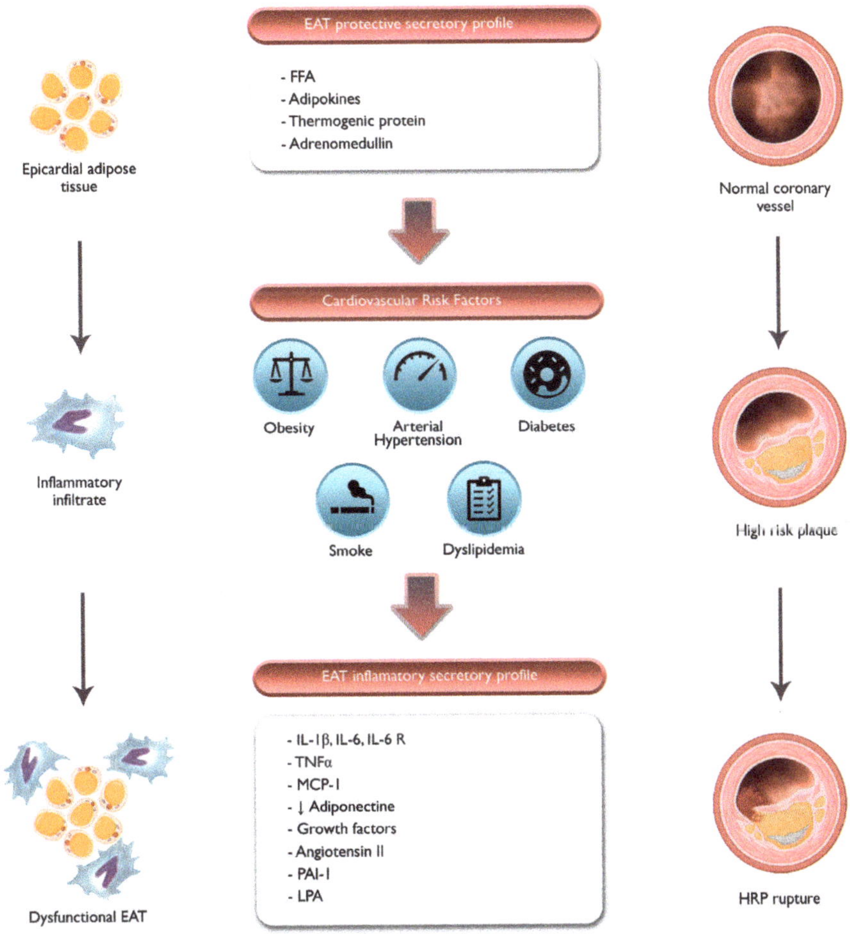

Figure 3. Interaction between EAT, PCAT, and atherogenesis. EAT, epicardial adipose tissue; FFA, free fatty acid; HRP, high-risk plaque; IL, interleukin; LPA, lysophosphatidic acid; MCP, monocyte chemoattractant protein; PAI, plasminogen activator inhibitor; TNF, tumor necrosis factor. EAT, located around the coronary arteries, secretes various bioactive molecules such as adipokines, cytokines, and FFAs. In the presence of cardiovascular risk factors, EAT undergoes inflammation, which is characterized by increased infiltration of immune cells. Dysfunction of PCAT and its effects on the coronary arteries can contribute to the initiation and progression of atherosclerosis, leading to the development of HRP.

Moreover, EAT volume has previously been associated with an increased CVD risk profile in a directly proportional manner [57–59]. However, in advanced heart failure (HF), reductions in EAT mass have been observed due to the lipolytic activity induced by natriuretic peptides. In end-stage HF, lower EAT volume predicts a poorer prognosis [60]. This suggests a U-shaped association between EAT volume and CVD risk across the entire spectrum of ejection fraction. Furthermore, a recent meta-analysis has confirmed the prognostic role of EAT/PCAT volume, demonstrating positive associations with obstructive CAD and major adverse cardiovascular events (MACE) [57].

5. EAT/PCAT Activity Overcomes Systemic Inflammatory Markers in ACS

Various biomarkers, including microRNA (miRNA), IL-6, B-type natriuretic peptide (BNP), cardiac troponin I (c-TnI), adiponectin, adipocyte fatty acid-binding protein (A-FABP), high-sensitivity C-reactive protein (hs-CRP), and lipocalin-2, have been associated with coronary inflammation and ACS. However, their lack of specificity limits their clinical utility [61]. Standard non-invasive approaches fail to accurately identify coronary inflammation, endothelial dysfunction, and high-risk coronary plaques (HRP) [62,63].

C-TnI is released from myocardiocytes following cardiac injury, not only in the case of myocardial infarction but also in other pathological conditions such as HF, myocarditis, sepsis, pulmonary embolism, and renal failure [64,65]. BNP, primarily a marker of ventricular stretch, increases in response to ventricular hypertrophy and myocardial infarction, playing a role in volume homeostasis and ventricular remodeling in HF [66–69]. Adiponectin, an anti-inflammatory and anti-atherogenic adipokine, has been inversely associated with endothelial dysfunction and obstructive CAD, but its plasma level is influenced differently by factors such as body mass, insulin resistance, and triglycerides [67]. A-FABP, expressed in adipocytes and macrophages, is involved in glucose and lipid metabolism and has been linked to the severity of coronary atherosclerosis, although its expression is similarly influenced by insulin resistance, hypertension, and HF [70,71]. Lipocalin-2, an inflammatory marker found in various tissues, including adipose tissue, has been associated with atherosclerosis development and CAD severity, and its levels increase in response to factors such as body mass, type 2 diabetes mellitus (T2DM), and insulin resistance [67,72,73]. Elevated levels of circulating hs-CRP and IL-6 in patients with stable angina have been correlated with HRP, MACE, and hospitalization for HF [74–76], with higher CRP levels observed in patients with acute myocardial infarction (AMI) compared to those with stable CAD [77,78]. However, while these biomarkers can detect both systemic and coronary inflammation, they lack specificity and do not provide information regarding the localization of coronary plaques.

On the other hand, CT imaging of PCAT inflammation can specifically identify HRP, with progressively higher attenuation observed from stable CAD to ACS [79,80]. PCAT CT attenuation does not correlate with standard circulating inflammatory biomarkers, as shown in a post hoc analysis of the SCOT-HEART study. This suggests that CT attenuation can identify coronary inflammatory status and active plaques that cannot be traced by systemic markers [81]. Furthermore, studies indicate that mean PCAT attenuation is higher in patients with myocardial infarction compared to those with stable CAD, suggesting phenotypic changes in the entire coronary tree during ACS, which is consistent with findings from intracoronary imaging [79,80,82].

6. Correlation between PCAT, Plaque Vulnerability, and ACS

EAT plays a role in plaque instability and ACS through its paracrine regulation of coronary vessels. HRP are prone to rupture and exhibit positive remodeling without significant lumen narrowing. Standard imaging methods may not accurately assess non-obstructive, but high-risk, plaques [83]. However, innovative approaches using 18F-sodium fluoride (18F-NaF) positron emission tomography (PET) uptake and PCAT attenuation on CT have shown promise [84–86].

PCAT may contribute to atherogenesis, plaque instability, and ACS (Figure 3) [25,26,87]. Studies have demonstrated that increased PCAT CT attenuation is associated with atherosclerotic coronary segments and plaque rupture in non-ST elevation myocardial infarction (NSTEMI). Moreover, EAT attenuation has been shown to be directly proportional to the probability of future AMI [88]. PCAT CT attenuation is higher in culprit lesions compared to non-culprit lesions and stable CAD controls. Indeed, it has emerged as an independent predictor of culprit lesions in patients with multivessel CAD.

The exact mechanisms underlying the relationship between PCAT and HRP development are not fully understood. It remains unclear whether inflammatory signals from coronary vessels with HRP influence PCAT or whether PCAT exerts vasocrine regulation through inflammatory pathways. PCAT, which is closer to the coronary arteries than EAT, has a greater number of small pre-adipocytes, with a higher adipogenic gene expression profile than mature adipocytes as result of the paracrine actions of the inflammatory environment implicated in CAD [31]. Whereas EAT catches both paracrine and autocrine signals, PCAT is primarily impacted by paracrine signaling from the blood vessels. Proposed mechanisms include the release of growth factors by adipocytes, secretion of angiotensin II and plasminogen activator inhibitor-1 by EAT, and the release of lysophosphatidic acid (LPA) promoting smooth muscle cell proliferation (Figure 3) [89,90].

Further research is needed in order to fully comprehend the complex interactions between PCAT, coronary inflammation, and plaque vulnerability. These findings highlight the potential of PCAT attenuation for CT and 18F-NaF PET uptake as non-invasive markers of coronary inflammation and plaque instability [86].

Increased myocardial oxidative stress leads to the release of oxidation messenger products, which can affect the secretory profile of EAT and its role in heart disease [91]. EAT, in response to oxidative stress, releases adiponectin, an adipokine with antioxidant properties, to protect the myocardiocytes and endothelium from oxidative stress. Thus, the phenotype of PCAT could be the result, rather than the cause, of underlying heart disease [91].

Regardless of the underlying mechanism, these findings suggest that PCAT can be used as a non-invasive tool to detect HRP, enhancing the identification of high-risk patients who could benefit from aggressive primary prevention strategies.

Autoptic Evaluation of EAT and Risk of Sudden Cardiac Death

PCAT attenuation on CT is emerging as a highly sensitive method to evaluate coronary inflammation, with biopsy-proven results supporting its validity [91]. In an autoptic study of 139 cross-sections of the left anterior descending (LAD) artery obtained from 16 patients, the ratio between plaque volume and media thickness was directly proportional to EAT volume and macrophage infiltration of PCAT. PCAT volume was also proportionate to the extension of a lipid core and to the inflammatory infiltration of atherosclerotic plaque [92].

In a post mortem comparison of CT data vs. autoptic findings in 116 human hearts, patients with significant CAD showed higher extension of EAT and PCAT. Moreover, both the thickness and volume of EAT significantly correlated with the grade of epicardial coronary artery obstruction, even after adjusting for confounding factors [93].

Sudden cardiac death (SCD) describes a natural death, usually occurring within an hour of the beginning of symptoms after rapid loss of consciousness if appropriate resuscitation techniques are not performed promptly [94]. It has a multifaceted etiology in which a preexisting cardiovascular disease, usually undetected, culminates in cardiac rhythm abnormalities and cardiac arrest. Since visceral adipose tissue as a CVR factor in SCD has sparked interest, EAT has been investigated as marker of coronary atherosclerosis. In a forensic, retrospective case–control study, EAT was an independent predictor of SCD [95]. Moreover, in a retrospective analysis of 321 autopsy cases, Hogea et al. demonstrated that patients with silent myocardial infarction (SMI) had higher prevalence of EAT at the left circumflex artery and the LAD artery, which were found to be independent predictors of SMI upon multivariate analysis [96].

7. Correlation between PCAT and Coronary Arteritis

Perivascular adipose tissue (PVAT) is located at the outermost boundary of the arterial wall and has been suggested to play a role in the pathogenesis of vasculitis. Studies have hypothesized that PVAT may play a triggering role in the development of vasculitis, and isolated peri-adventitial inflammation has been associated with an increased likelihood of developing giant cell arteritis. This suggests a primary role of PVAT in the pathogenesis of systemic vasculitis [23].

In Takayasu arteritis (TAK), a type of inflammatory arteritis affecting the aorta and its branches, the density of periaortic adipose tissue (PAAT) and PCAT has been quantified. Patients with TAK showed higher PAAT and PCAT density compared to patients with CAD or controls, independently of other factors. PAAT and PCAT density were closely related to markers of disease activity in TAK, indicating a potential role of PAAT and PCAT in the pathogenesis of TAK. PCAT density was also identified as an independent predictor of coronary inflammation, as visualized by 68Ga-DOT PET imaging [24].

Kawasaki disease (KD), a type of acute inflammatory vasculitis primarily affecting medium-sized elastic arteries, particularly the coronary arteries, is a major cause of acquired heart disease in children. Coronary artery aneurysms and inflammatory cell infiltration have been observed in KD, and adipokines have been suggested to play a central role in its pathogenesis. A meta-analysis showed that resistin and adiponectin levels were significantly elevated in KD patients with coronary artery lesions compared to those without coronary involvement [97–99].

While further research is needed in order to fully understand the relationship between PCAT and arteritis, it is reasonable to assume that the inflammatory microenvironment surrounding coronary vessels, including the contribution of PCAT through paracrine secretion, plays a causative role in the development and progression of coronary damage. Future studies are needed to investigate the role of PCAT in regulating vessel inflammation and to explore potential therapeutic approaches in this field.

8. Correlation between PCAT and MINOCA

MINOCA is diagnosed when invasive coronary angiography reveals a patent coronary tree in a patient with AMI [100]. The prevalence of MINOCA is 1–13% of all patients with a clinical diagnosis of AMI, and several potential etiologies exist. After initial negative angiography, MINOCA may be reclassified as type 1 or type 2 AMI due to mechanisms of myocardial ischemia; the first represents a plaque-induced event where plaque rupture or erosion with superimposed thrombus develops spontaneous recanalization. On the contrary, type 2 AMI arises from non-plaque-induced conditions due to reduced blood supply and oxygen imbalance, such as spontaneous coronary artery dissection (SCAD), embolism, vasospasm, and microvascular disease [101]. Mechanisms causally connecting plaque rupture/erosion with PCAT, as well as endothelial dysfunction and EAT, have been described previously in this document. Furthermore, emerging evidence currently exists regarding the contributory role of EAT in other type-2 MINOCA [102].

8.1. Spontaneous Coronary Artery Dissection

SCAD is defined as a non-traumatic, non-atherosclerotic separation of the layers of the arterial wall, resulting in the creation of a false lumen. The role of inflammatory infiltrate in the pathogenesis of SCAD is still debated, and a causative or healing role has not been conclusively determined. Some reports suggest a causative role of eosinophilic infiltrates in coronary wall injury, leading to the expansion of intramural hemorrhage through the release of cytotoxic products and stimulation of aberrant neovascularization [103,104]. On the other hand, a large pathology case series has suggested that periadventitial inflammation in SCAD is time-dependent and proportional to the time elapsed between symptom onset and death, indicating a healing response of the inflammatory infiltrate in SCAD [105].

Regardless of its contribution, an inflammatory environment is consistently present in SCAD, involving both the vessel wall and the PCAT bidirectionally [106]. In vivo detection of vascular inflammation would be useful, and several studies have evaluated the role of PCAT CT attenuation in this context. One study failed to show a significant difference in median PCAT attenuation between SCAD patients and controls, potentially due to the healing process and resolution of ACS with invasive or medical treatment [107]. However, another study demonstrated that elevated PCAT density on CT performed within 48 h of coronary angiography had a higher prevalence than the imaging of dissection identified by angiography [108]. Additionally, a cohort study showed a significant association between PCAT CT attenuation, wall motion abnormality, and initial elevated troponin levels in patients with high-degree stenosis due to SCAD or atherosclerosis [106].

While invasive coronary angiography is the first-line examination for patients presenting with ACS and suspected SCAD, CT may play a role, especially in those with early presentation and normal initial troponin levels. PCAT CT attenuation can provide valuable information, particularly when small dissections may not be detectable due to the spatial resolution limitations of CT [109].

8.2. Vasospastic Angina

The endothelium modulates vascular tone through the release of relaxing factors (mainly prostaglandins and nitric oxide) and hyperpolarizing factors. The former mediates the relaxation of large arteries (i.e., epicardial coronary arteries), while the latter plays a key role in regulating the resistances of small arteries by opening calcium-activated potassium channels and subsequently hyperpolarizing the membranes of vascular smooth muscle cells (VSMCs) [110]. Multiple studies have attempted to identify the mechanism behind coronary vasospasm, and different pathological reports have described extensive adventitial inflammation near the spastic coronary artery [111,112]. Such inflammatory environment seems to mediate VSMCs' hypercontraction by the influx of Ca^{2+} through L-type Ca-channel as an initial trigger, which is functionally up-regulated via PKC and a GTPase-Rho-dependent mechanism [110]. Moreover, Ohyama et al. recently demonstrated increased PCAT volume at the site of higher lumen reduction in spastic coronary segments, which suggests the involvement of PCAT in the inflammatory context leading to the spasm [113].

As previously described, 18F-FDG PET/CT is able to detect perivascular inflammation, with signal intensity directly proportional to macrophage density and microcalcifications [114]. As expected, ECG-gated 18F-FDG PET/CT recently showed significantly increased FDG uptake in patients with vasospastic angina, which significantly decreased during the follow-up period [115]. Numerous studies have suggested that PVAT regulates the vascular bed in a paracrine way, with opposite effects in the peripheral and coronary districts due to different proteomic responses secondary to local and systemic factors. Owen et al. previously demonstrated that biological factors are released from PCAT potentiate coronary vasoconstriction, with a directly proportional expression of RhoA (2.9-fold) and calpastatin (1.6-fold) to total fat volume, leading to increased function of VSMCs' Ca^{2+} channels, H_2O_2-sensitive K^+ channels, or mediators regulating these channels [116]. Notably, inhibition of Ca^{2+} channels with nifedipine or diltiazem is able to neutralize this effect.

These data suggest a key role of PCAT in regulating vascular tone in the coronary district beyond endothelial function and systemic mediators, highlighting the potential detrimental effects of dysregulated PCAT in type 2 MINOCA.

9. Future Perspectives: Application of Artificial Intelligence

The term artificial intelligence (AI) refers to the application of computing methods to tasks that ordinarily call for human intellect. AI subfields, such as machine learning (ML), are increasingly used in cardiovascular imaging; ML models can now be employed to merge clinical data with AI-derived information for personalized risk stratification [117]. CCTA-derived quantitative measures have previously been included in ML models, which have outperformed qualitative or quantitative high-risk plaque characteristics alone in terms of outcome prediction [118,119].

Deep learning (DL), a subset of ML, generates assumptions directly from input data through multilayered artificial neural networks. Recently, Driessen et al. applied DL to CT-derived fractional flow reserve (CT-FFR) software (HeartFlow FFR_{CT} version 2.7, Redwood City, CA, USA) to aid in identifying the coronary lumen border and generating analyses of hybrid computational fluid dynamics, demonstrating the greater diagnostic performance of CT-FFR compared to CCTA for stenosis evaluation and PET for ischemia detection [120]. Moreover, the ML method demonstrated advantageous application in PET/TC as well, allowing for automated CAC scoring from low-dose CT-attenuation images routinely acquired during PET protocol, with outstanding results compared to the reference standard of manual quantification [117]. More recently, Commanduer at al. compared DL to manual analysis of EAT, finding a high level of accuracy with the automated analysis, which also performed better than human evaluation in terms of identifying non-calcified plaque. Additionally, DL took about 1.57 s per patient, compared to 15 min for professional readers [121]. A boost ensemble ML method has recently been evaluated to compare EAT volume and CFR in non-contrast CT and PET. The ML composite risk score significantly enhanced the risk reclassification of impaired myocardial flow reserve compared to EAT volume or CAC score alone [122]. Thus, AI-integrated approaches are now not only feasible, but have been proven to enhance CVR assessment without additional radiation exposure, greatly reducing the time needed for manual measurements.

Interestingly, radiomics, a new frontier of imaging evaluation through data-characterization algorithms, has recently been applied in PCAT analysis with interesting results [123]. Oikonomou et al. used PCAT radiomic features to train a random forest ML model to create a patient-level "fat radiomic profile." This indicator demonstrated incremental utility for MACE prediction beyond traditional CCTA-based risk categorization when assessed in 1575 SCOT-HEART study participants [124]. Therefore, the texture and geometry-based parameters of PCAT may outperform PCAT CT attenuation in terms of discriminating high-risk plaque, even though the lack of standardized methodology in the radiomic workflow, complex manual delineation, and the need for highly experienced staff are important limitations to its widespread adoption [125]. However, the combination of radiomics and PCAT CT attenuation could further enhance the identification of patients at risk of acute coronary events.

10. Conclusions

Vascular inflammation is the main driver of ACS, but standard noninvasive approaches such as exercise treadmill testing (ETT) and perfusion imaging have failed to precisely identify coronary inflammation and subsequent endothelial dysfunction. Existing noninvasive methods, like 18F-NaF-PET, which is well standardized in terms of identifying coronary inflammation, require complex imaging protocols and processing. Additionally, circulating biomarkers that are widely used lack adequate specificity. As a result, the noninvasive detection of HRP and the dysfunctional endothelium remains challenging.

PCAT undeniably plays a key role in coronary inflammation and the development of HRP due to the bidirectional interconnection between epicardial fat and the coronary vessels. PCAT evaluation through CT attenuation has emerged as a promising method for predicting MACE, with demonstrated relationships between PCAT volume/density and coronary flow reserve (CFR), CAC, and cardiovascular risk. Furthermore, PCAT attenuation has recently shown the ability to predict plaque rupture in AMI and accurately identify culprit lesions in patients with multivessel CAD. Given its proximity to the vascular wall, PCAT has also been hypothesized to play a triggering role in coronary vasculitis and MINOCA.

AI has been progressively applied in cardiovascular risk stratification, and ML models incorporating CCTA-derived quantitative measures have demonstrated incremental utility in predicting MACE compared to plaque characteristics alone. Therefore, the evaluation of PCAT appears to be a safe, valuable, and sufficiently specific noninvasive method for accurately identifying coronary inflammation and subsequent HRP, with its results having been proven both via biopsy and in vivo.

While speculative, these pieces of evidence pave the way for a fascinating future strategy for cardiovascular risk stratification. It is conceivable that the assessment of EAT status may be incorporated into risk stratification tools, enabling early targeted primary prevention and intensive secondary prevention in patients at higher risk of cardiac and all-cause mortality.

Author Contributions: Conceptualization, G.N. and V.P.; methodology, A.I.G.; software, P.B. and M.G.R.; validation, G.P., A.I.G. and M.M.C.; formal analysis, G.N.; investigation, D.D.F. and L.F.; resources, F.B. and F.F.; data curation, A.B., N.C. and R.M.; writing—original draft preparation, G.N.; writing—review and editing, V.P.; visualization, S.M.; supervision, A.I.G.; project administration, G.P. All authors have read and agreed to the published version of the manuscript.

Funding: This research received no external funding.

Institutional Review Board Statement: Not applicable.

Informed Consent Statement: Not applicable.

Data Availability Statement: Not applicable.

Conflicts of Interest: The authors declare no conflict of interest.

Abbreviations

A-FAB	adipocyte fatty-acid-binding protein
ACS	acute coronary syndrome
AF	atrial fibrillation
AI	artificial intelligence
AMI	acute myocardial infarction
BNP	B-type natriuretic peptide
C-TnI	cardiac troponin I
CAC	coronary artery calcification
CAD	coronary artery disease
CCTA	coronary CT angiography
CFR	coronary flow reserve
CMR	cardiac magnetic resonance
CVD	cardiovascular disease
CT	computed tomography
CT-FFR	CT-derived fractional flow reserve
DL	deep learning
EAT	epicardial adipose tissue
ETT	exercise treadmill testing
FFAs	free fatty acids
HF	heart failure
HRP	high-risk coronary plaques
hs-CRP	high-sensitivity C-reactive protein
HU	Hounsfield units
IL	interleukin
KD	Kawasaki disease
LAD	left anterior descending
LPA	lysophosphatidic acid
MACE	major adverse cardiovascular events
ML	machine learning
MCP-1	monocyte chemoattractant protein-1
MINOCA	myocardial infarction with non-obstructive coronary arteries
MiRNA	microRNA
NSTEMI	non-ST-segment elevation myocardial infarction
PAAT	periaortic adipose tissue
PCAT	pericoronary adipose tissue
PET	positron emission tomography
pFAI	pericoronary fat attenuation index
PVAT	perivascular adipose tissue
SCAD	spontaneous coronary artery dissection

SCD	sudden cardiac death
SMI	silent myocardial infarction
T2DM	type 2 diabetes mellitus
TAK	Takayasu arteritis
TNFα	tumor necrosis factor-α
TTE	transthoracic echocardiography
VSMCs	vascular smooth muscle cells
18F-NaF	18F-sodium fluoride

References

1. Bueno, H. Epidemiology of acute coronary syndromes. In *The ESC Textbook of Cardiovascular Medicine*; James, S., Camm, A.J., Lüscher, T.F., Maurer, G., Serruys, P.W., Eds.; Oxford University Press: Oxford, UK, 2018; pp. 1214–1218.
2. Yao, H.; Ekou, A.; Brou, I.; Niamkey, T.; Koffi, F.; Tano, S.; Kouamé, I.; N'Guetta, R. Evolution of epidemiology and management of acute coronary syndromes in Abidjan: A cross-sectional study of 1011 patients. *Ann. Cardiol. Angeiol.* **2022**, *71*, 130–135. [CrossRef]
3. Maffei, E.; Seitun, S.; Martini, C.; Palumbo, A.; Tarantini, G.; Berti, E.; Grilli, R.; Tedeschi, C.; Messalli, G.; Guaricci, A.; et al. CT coronary angiography and exercise ECG in a population with chest pain and low-to-intermediate pre-test likelihood of coronary artery disease. *Heart* **2010**, *96*, 1973–1979. [CrossRef]
4. Maffei, E.; Seitun, S.; Martini, C.; Aldrovandi, A.; Cervellin, G.; Tedeschi, C.; Guaricci, A.; Messalli, G.; Catalano, O.; Cademartiri, F. Prognostic value of computed tomography coronary angiography in patients with chest pain of suspected cardiac origin. *Radiol. Med.* **2011**, *116*, 690–705. [CrossRef]
5. Guaricci, A.I.; Arcadi, T.; Brunetti, N.D.; Maffei, E.; Montrone, D.; Martini, C.; De Luca, M.; De Rosa, F.; Cocco, D.; Midiri, M.; et al. Carotid intima media thickness and coronary atherosclerosis linkage in symptomatic intermediate risk patients evaluated by coronary computed tomography angiography. *Int. J. Cardiol.* **2014**, *176*, 988–993. [CrossRef]
6. Guaricci, A.I.; Maffei, E.; Brunetti, N.D.; Montrone, D.; Di Biase, L.; Tedeschi, C.; Gentile, G.; Macarini, L.; Midiri, M.; Cademartiri, F.; et al. Heart rate control with oral ivabradine in computed tomography coronary angiography: A randomized comparison of 7.5 mg vs 5 mg regimen. *Int. J. Cardiol.* **2013**, *168*, 362–368. [CrossRef]
7. Narula, J.; Achenbach, S. Napkin-ring necrotic cores: Defining circumferential extent of necrotic cores in unstable plaques. *JACC Cardiovasc. Imaging* **2009**, *2*, 1436–1438. [CrossRef]
8. Dodd, J.D.; Rieber, J.; Pomerantsev, E.; Chaithiraphan, V.; Achenbach, S.; Moreiras, J.M.; Abbara, S.; Hoffmann, U.; Brady, T.J.; Cury, R.C. Quantification of nonculprit coronary lesions: Comparison of cardiac 64-MDCT and invasive coronary angiography. *AJR Am. J. Roentgenol.* **2008**, *191*, 432–438. [CrossRef]
9. Si, N.; Shi, K.; Li, N.; Dong, X.; Zhu, C.; Guo, Y.; Hu, J.; Cui, J.; Yang, F.; Zhang, T. Identification of patients with acute myocardial infarction based on coronary CT angiography: The value of pericoronary adipose tissue radiomics. *Eur. Radiol.* **2022**, *32*, 6868–6877. [CrossRef]
10. Pergola, V.; Cabrelle, G.; Mattesi, G.; Cattarin, S.; Furlan, A.; Dellino, C.M.; Continisio, S.; Montonati, C.; Giorgino, A.; Giraudo, C.; et al. Added Value of CCTA-Derived Features to Predict MACEs in Stable Patients Undergoing Coronary Computed Tomography. *Diagnostics* **2022**, *12*, 1446. [CrossRef]
11. Paul, J.F.; Rohnean, A.; Giroussens, H.; Pressat-Laffouilhere, T.; Wong, T. Evaluation of a deep learning model on coronary CT angiography for automatic stenosis detection. *Diagn. Interv. Imaging* **2022**, *103*, 316–323. [CrossRef]
12. Pontone, G.; Andreini, D.; Bertella, E.; Baggiano, A.; Mushtaq, S.; Loguercio, M.; Segurini, C.; Conte, E.; Beltrama, V.; Annoni, A.; et al. Impact of an intra-cycle motion correction algorithm on overall evaluability and diagnostic accuracy of computed tomography coronary angiography. *Eur. Radiol.* **2016**, *26*, 147–156. [CrossRef]
13. Baggiano, A.; Fusini, L.; Del Torto, A.; Vivona, P.; Guglielmo, M.; Muscogiuri, G.; Soldi, M.; Martini, C.; Fraschini, E.; Rabbat, M.G.; et al. Sequential Strategy Including FFR(CT) Plus Stress-CTP Impacts on Management of Patients with Stable Chest Pain: The Stress-CTP RIPCORD Study. *J. Clin. Med.* **2020**, *9*, 2147. [CrossRef]
14. Esposito, A.; Francone, M.; Andreini, D.; Buffa, V.; Cademartiri, F.; Carbone, I.; Clemente, A.; Guaricci, A.I.; Guglielmo, M.; Indolfi, C.; et al. SIRM-SIC appropriateness criteria for the use of Cardiac Computed Tomography. Part 1: Congenital heart diseases, primary prevention, risk assessment before surgery, suspected CAD in symptomatic patients, plaque and epicardial adipose tissue characterization, and functional assessment of stenosis. *Radiol. Med.* **2021**, *126*, 1236–1248. [CrossRef]
15. Neglia, D.; Liga, R.; Gimelli, A.; Podlesnikar, T.; Cvijić, M.; Pontone, G.; Miglioranza, M.H.; Guaricci, A.I.; Seitun, S.; Clemente, A.; et al. Use of cardiac imaging in chronic coronary syndromes: The EURECA Imaging registry. *Eur. Heart J.* **2022**, *44*, 142–158. [CrossRef]
16. Pontone, G.; Baggiano, A.; Andreini, D.; Guaricci, A.I.; Guglielmo, M.; Muscogiuri, G.; Fusini, L.; Soldi, M.; Del Torto, A.; Mushtaq, S.; et al. Diagnostic accuracy of simultaneous evaluation of coronary arteries and myocardial perfusion with single stress cardiac computed tomography acquisition compared to invasive coronary angiography plus invasive fractional flow reserve. *Int. J. Cardiol.* **2018**, *273*, 263–268. [CrossRef]

17. Pontone, G.; Andreini, D.; Guaricci, A.I.; Guglielmo, M.; Baggiano, A.; Muscogiuri, G.; Fusini, L.; Soldi, M.; Fazzari, F.; Berzovini, C.; et al. Quantitative vs. qualitative evaluation of static stress computed tomography perfusion to detect haemodynamically significant coronary artery disease. *Eur. Heart. J. Cardiovasc. Imaging* **2018**, *19*, 1244–1252. [CrossRef]
18. Antonopoulos, A.S.; Sanna, F.; Sabharwal, N.; Thomas, S.; Oikonomou, E.K.; Herdman, L.; Margaritis, M.; Shirodaria, C.; Kampoli, A.M.; Akoumianakis, I.; et al. Detecting human coronary inflammation by imaging perivascular fat. *Sci. Transl. Med.* **2017**, *9*, eaal2658. [CrossRef]
19. Goeller, M.; Rahman Ihdayhid, A.; Cadet, S.; Lin, A.; Adams, D.; Thakur, U.; Yap, G.; Marwan, M.; Achenbach, S.; Dey, D.; et al. Pericoronary adipose tissue and quantitative global non-calcified plaque characteristics from CT angiography do not differ in matched South Asian, East Asian and European-origin Caucasian patients with stable chest pain. *Eur. J. Radiol.* **2020**, *125*, 108874. [CrossRef]
20. Cosson, E.; Nguyen, M.T.; Rezgani, I.; Tatulashvili, S.; Sal, M.; Berkane, N.; Allard, L.; Brillet, P.-Y.; Bihan, H. Epicardial adipose tissue volume and coronary calcification among people living with diabetes: A cross-sectional study. *Cardiovasc. Diabetol.* **2021**, *20*, 35. [CrossRef]
21. Yerramasu, A.; Dey, D.; Venuraju, S.; Anand, D.V.; Atwal, S.; Corder, R.; Berman, D.S.; Lahiri, A. Increased volume of epicardial fat is an independent risk factor for accelerated progression of sub-clinical coronary atherosclerosis. *Atherosclerosis* **2012**, *220*, 223–230. [CrossRef]
22. Vancheri, F.; Longo, G.; Vancheri, S.; Danial, J.S.H.; Henein, M.Y. Coronary Artery Microcalcification: Imaging and Clinical Implications. *Diagnostics* **2019**, *9*, 125. [CrossRef]
23. Galli, E.; Muratore, F.; Boiardi, L.; Restuccia, G.; Cavazza, A.; Catanoso, M.; Macchioni, P.; Spaggiari, L.; Casali, M.; Pipitone, N.; et al. Significance of inflammation restricted to adventitial/periadventitial tissue on temporal artery biopsy. *Semin. Arthritis Rheum.* **2020**, *50*, 1064–1072. [CrossRef]
24. Wall, C.; Huang, Y.; Le, E.P.V.; Ćorović, A.; Uy, C.P.; Gopalan, D.; Ma, C.; Manavaki, R.; Fryer, T.D.; Aloj, L.; et al. Pericoronary and periaortic adipose tissue density are associated with inflammatory disease activity in Takayasu arteritis and atherosclerosis. *Eur. Heart. J. Open* **2021**, *1*, oeab019. [CrossRef]
25. Marwan, M.; Hell, M.; Schuhbäck, A.; Gauss, S.; Bittner, D.; Pflederer, T.; Achenbach, S. CT Attenuation of Pericoronary Adipose Tissue in Normal Versus Atherosclerotic Coronary Segments as Defined by Intravascular Ultrasound. *J. Comput. Assist. Tomogr.* **2017**, *41*, 762–767. [CrossRef]
26. Nakajima, A.; Sugiyama, T.; Araki, M.; Seegers, L.M.; Dey, D.; McNulty, I.; Lee, H.; Yonetsu, T.; Yasui, Y.; Teng, Y.; et al. Plaque Rupture, Compared with Plaque Erosion, Is Associated with a Higher Level of Pancoronary Inflammation. *JACC Cardiovasc. Imaging* **2022**, *15*, 828–839. [CrossRef]
27. Iacobellis, G.; Willens, H.J. Echocardiographic Epicardial Fat: A Review of Research and Clinical Applications. *J. Am. Soc. Echocardiogr.* **2009**, *22*, 1311–1319. [CrossRef]
28. Natale, F.; Tedesco, M.A.; Mocerino, R.; de Simone, V.; Di Marco, G.M.; Aronne, L.; Credendino, M.; Siniscalchi, C.; Calabrò, P.; Cotrufo, M.; et al. Visceral adiposity and arterial stiffness: Echocardiographic epicardial fat thickness reflects, better than waist circumference, carotid arterial stiffness in a large population of hypertensives. *Eur. J. Echocardiogr.* **2009**, *10*, 549–555. [CrossRef]
29. Guglielmo, M.; Lin, A.; Dey, D.; Baggiano, A.; Fusini, L.; Muscogiuri, G.; Pontone, G. Epicardial fat and coronary artery disease: Role of cardiac imaging. *Atherosclerosis* **2021**, *321*, 30–38. [CrossRef]
30. Hell, M.M.; Achenbach, S.; Schuhbaeck, A.; Klinghammer, L.; May, M.S.; Marwan, M. CT-based analysis of pericoronary adipose tissue density: Relation to cardiovascular risk factors and epicardial adipose tissue volume. *J. Cardiovasc. Comput. Tomogr.* **2016**, *10*, 52–60. [CrossRef]
31. Ma, R.; Fari, R.; van der Harst, P.; De Cecco, C.N.; Stillman, A.E.; Vliegenthart, R.; van Assen, M. Evaluation of pericoronary adipose tissue attenuation on CT. *Br. J. Radiol.* **2023**, *96*, 20220885. [CrossRef]
32. Duncker, H.; Achenbach, S.; Moshage, M.; Dey, D.; Bittner, D.O.; Ammon, F.; Marwan, M.; Goeller, M. Computed Tomography-derived Characterization of Pericoronary, Epicardial, and Paracardial Adipose Tissue and Its Association with Myocardial Ischemia as Assessed by Computed Fractional Flow Reserve. *J. Thorac. Imaging* **2023**, *38*, 46–53. [CrossRef]
33. Yuvaraj, J.; Cheng, K.; Lin, A.; Psaltis, P.J.; Nicholls, S.J.; Wong, D.T.L. The Emerging Role of CT-Based Imaging in Adipose Tissue and Coronary Inflammation. *Cells* **2021**, *10*, 1196. [CrossRef]
34. Toemen, L.; Santos, S.; Roest, A.A.; Jelic, G.; van der Lugt, A.; Felix, J.F.; Helbing, W.A.; Gaillard, R.; Jaddoe, V.W.V. Body Fat Distribution, Overweight, and Cardiac Structures in School-Age Children: A Population-Based Cardiac Magnetic Resonance Imaging Study. *J. Am. Heart Assoc.* **2020**, *9*, e014933. [CrossRef]
35. Marciniak, M.; van Deutekom, A.W.; Toemen, L.; Lewandowski, A.J.; Gaillard, R.; Young, A.A.; Jaddoe, V.W.V.; Lamata, P. A three-dimensional atlas of child's cardiac anatomy and the unique morphological alterations associated with obesity. *Eur. Heart J. Cardiovasc. Imaging* **2022**, *23*, 1645–1653. [CrossRef]
36. Wong, C.; Marwick, T.H. Obesity cardiomyopathy: Pathogenesis and pathophysiology. *Nat. Clin. Pract. Cardiovasc. Med.* **2007**, *4*, 436–443. [CrossRef]
37. Corradi, D.; Maestri, R.; Callegari, S.; Pastori, P.; Goldoni, M.; Luong, T.V.; Bordi, C. The ventricular epicardial fat is related to the myocardial mass in normal, ischemic and hypertrophic hearts. *Cardiovasc. Pathol.* **2004**, *13*, 313–316. [CrossRef]
38. Iacobellis, G.; Ribaudo, M.C.; Zappaterreno, A.; Iannucci, C.V.; Leonetti, F. Relation between epicardial adipose tissue and left ventricular mass. *Am. J. Cardiol.* **2004**, *94*, 1084–1087. [CrossRef]

39. Marchington, J.M.; Mattacks, C.A.; Pond, C.M. Adipose tissue in the mammalian heart and pericardium: Structure, foetal development and biochemical properties. *Comp. Biochem. Physiol. B* **1989**, *94*, 225–232. [CrossRef]
40. Iacobellis, G.; Bianco, A.C. Epicardial adipose tissue: Emerging physiological, pathophysiological and clinical features. *Trends Endocrinol. Metab.* **2011**, *22*, 450–457. [CrossRef]
41. Silaghi, A.; Achard, V.; Paulmyer-Lacroix, O.; Scridon, T.; Tassistro, V.; Duncea, I.; Clément, K.; Dutour, A.; Grino, M. Expression of adrenomedullin in human epicardial adipose tissue: Role of coronary status. *Am. J. Physiol. Endocrinol. Metab.* **2007**, *293*, E1443–E1450. [CrossRef]
42. Iacobellis, G.; Corradi, D.; Sharma, A.M. Epicardial adipose tissue: Anatomic, biomolecular and clinical relationships with the heart. *Nat. Clin. Pract. Cardiovasc. Med.* **2005**, *2*, 536–543. [CrossRef]
43. Lin, Y.-K.; Chen, Y.-C.; Chen, J.-H.; Chen, S.-A.; Chen, Y.-J. Adipocytes modulate the electrophysiology of atrial myocytes: Implications in obesity-induced atrial fibrillation. *Basic Res. Cardiol.* **2012**, *107*, 293. [CrossRef]
44. Parisi, V.; Rengo, G.; Perrone-Filardi, P.; Pagano, G.; Femminella, G.D.; Paolillo, S.; Petraglia, L.; Gambino, G.; Caruso, A.; Grimaldi, M.G.; et al. Increased Epicardial Adipose Tissue Volume Correlates with Cardiac Sympathetic Denervation in Patients with Heart Failure. *Circ. Res.* **2016**, *118*, 1244–1253. [CrossRef]
45. Mazurek, T.; Zhang, L.; Zalewski, A.; Mannion, J.D.; Diehl, J.T.; Arafat, H.; Sarov-Blat, L.; O'Brien, S.; Keiper, E.A.; Johnson, A.G.; et al. Human epicardial adipose tissue is a source of inflammatory mediators. *Circulation* **2003**, *108*, 2460–2466. [CrossRef]
46. Iacobellis, G.; Pistilli, D.; Gucciardo, M.; Leonetti, F.; Miraldi, F.; Brancaccio, G.; Gallo, P.; di Gioia, C.R. Adiponectin expression in human epicardial adipose tissue in vivo is lower in patients with coronary artery disease. *Cytokine* **2005**, *29*, 251–255. [CrossRef]
47. McAninch, E.A.; Fonseca, T.L.; Poggioli, R.; Panos, A.L.; Salerno, T.A.; Deng, Y.; Li, Y.; Bianco, A.C.; Iacobellis, G. Epicardial adipose tissue has a unique transcriptome modified in severe coronary artery disease. *Obesity* **2015**, *23*, 1267–1278. [CrossRef]
48. Hirata, Y.; Tabata, M.; Kurobe, H.; Motoki, T.; Akaike, M.; Nishio, C.; Higashida, M.; Mikasa, H.; Nakaya, Y.; Takanashi, S.; et al. Coronary Atherosclerosis Is Associated with Macrophage Polarization in Epicardial Adipose Tissue. *J. Am. Coll. Cardiol.* **2011**, *58*, 248–255. [CrossRef]
49. Iacobellis, G.; Mahabadi, A.A. Is epicardial fat attenuation a novel marker of coronary inflammation? *Atherosclerosis* **2019**, *284*, 212–213. [CrossRef]
50. Christensen, R.H.; von Scholten, B.J.; Hansen, C.S.; Jensen, M.T.; Vilsbøll, T.; Rossing, P.; Jørgensen, P.G. Epicardial adipose tissue predicts incident cardiovascular disease and mortality in patients with type 2 diabetes. *Cardiovasc. Diabetol.* **2019**, *18*, 114. [CrossRef]
51. Yang, X.; Feng, C.; Feng, J. Epicardial Adipose Tissue and Diabetic Cardiomyopathy. *J. Cardiovasc. Pharmacol. Ther.* **2023**, *28*, 10742484231151820. [CrossRef]
52. Maffei, E.; Seitun, S.; Nieman, K.; Martini, C.; Guaricci, A.I.; Tedeschi, C.; Weustink, A.C.; Mollet, N.R.; Berti, E.; Grilli, R.; et al. Assessment of coronary artery disease and calcified coronary plaque burden by computed tomography in patients with and without diabetes mellitus. *Eur. Radiol.* **2011**, *21*, 944–953. [CrossRef]
53. Guaricci, A.I.; Lorenzoni, V.; Guglielmo, M.; Mushtaq, S.; Muscogiuri, G.; Cademartiri, F.; Rabbat, M.; Andreini, D.; Serviddio, G.; Gaibazzi, N.; et al. Prognostic relevance of subclinical coronary and carotid atherosclerosis in a diabetic and nondiabetic asymptomatic population. *Clin. Cardiol.* **2018**, *41*, 769–777. [CrossRef]
54. Basile, P.; Guaricci, A.I.; Piazzolla, G.; Volpe, S.; Vozza, A.; Benedetto, M.; Carella, M.C.; Santoro, D.; Monitillo, F.; Baggiano, A.; et al. Improvement of Left Ventricular Global Longitudinal Strain after 6-Month Therapy with GLP-1RAs Semaglutide and Dulaglutide in Type 2 Diabetes Mellitus: A Pilot Study. *J. Clin. Med.* **2023**, *12*, 1586. [CrossRef]
55. Nomura, C.H.; Assuncao-Jr, A.N.; Guimarães, P.O.; Liberato, G.; Morais, T.C.; Fahel, M.G.; Giorgi, M.C.P.; Meneghetti, J.C.; Parga, J.R.; Dantas-Jr, R.N.; et al. Association between perivascular inflammation and downstream myocardial perfusion in patients with suspected coronary artery disease. *Eur. Heart J. Cardiovasc. Imaging* **2020**, *21*, 599–605. [CrossRef]
56. Oikonomou, E.K.; Marwan, M.; Desai, M.Y.; Mancio, J.; Alashi, A.; Hutt Centeno, E.; Thomas, S.; Herdman, L.; Kotanidis, C.P.; Thomas, K.E.; et al. Non-invasive detection of coronary inflammation using computed tomography and prediction of residual cardiovascular risk (the CRISP CT study): A post-hoc analysis of prospective outcome data. *Lancet* **2018**, *392*, 929–939. [CrossRef]
57. Mancio, J.; Azevedo, D.; Saraiva, F.; Azevedo, A.I.; Pires-Morais, G.; Leite-Moreira, A.; Falcao-Pires, I.; Lunet, N.; Bettencourt, N. Epicardial adipose tissue volume assessed by computed tomography and coronary artery disease: A systematic review and meta-analysis. *Eur. Heart J.—Cardiovasc. Imaging* **2017**, *19*, 490–497. [CrossRef]
58. Rajani, R.; Shmilovich, H.; Nakazato, R.; Nakanishi, R.; Otaki, Y.; Cheng, V.Y.; Hayes, S.W.; Thomson, L.E.; Friedman, J.D.; Slomka, P.J.; et al. Relationship of epicardial fat volume to coronary plaque, severe coronary stenosis, and high-risk coronary plaque features assessed by coronary CT angiography. *J. Cardiovasc. Comput. Tomogr.* **2013**, *7*, 125–132. [CrossRef]
59. Bo, X.; Ma, L.; Fan, J.; Jiang, Z.; Zhou, Y.; Zhang, L.; Li, W. Epicardial fat volume is correlated with coronary lesion and its severity. *Int. J. Clin. Exp. Med.* **2015**, *8*, 4328–4334.
60. Antonopoulos, A.S.; Tousoulis, D. The molecular mechanisms of obesity paradox. *Cardiovasc. Res.* **2017**, *113*, 1074–1086. [CrossRef]
61. Guaricci, A.I.; Pontone, G.; Fusini, L.; De Luca, M.; Cafarelli, F.P.; Guglielmo, M.; Baggiano, A.; Beltrama, V.; Muscogiuri, G.; Mushtaq, S.; et al. Additional value of inflammatory biomarkers and carotid artery disease in prediction of significant coronary artery disease as assessed by coronary computed tomography angiography. *Eur. Heart J. Cardiovasc. Imaging* **2017**, *18*, 1049–1056. [CrossRef]

62. Hansson, G.K.; Libby, P.; Tabas, I. Inflammation and plaque vulnerability. *J. Intern. Med.* **2015**, *278*, 483–493. [CrossRef]
63. Sarwar, N.; Butterworth, A.S.; Freitag, D.F.; Gregson, J.; Willeit, P.; Gorman, D.N.; Gao, P.; Saleheen, D.; Rendon, A.; Nelson, C.P.; et al. Interleukin-6 receptor pathways in coronary heart disease: A collaborative meta-analysis of 82 studies. *Lancet* **2012**, *379*, 1205–1213. [CrossRef]
64. Roongsritong, C.; Warraich, I.; Bradley, C. Common causes of troponin elevations in the absence of acute myocardial infarction: Incidence and clinical significance. *Chest* **2004**, *125*, 1877–1884. [CrossRef]
65. Guaricci, A.I.; Masci, P.G.; Muscogiuri, G.; Guglielmo, M.; Baggiano, A.; Fusini, L.; Lorenzoni, V.; Martini, C.; Andreini, D.; Pavon, A.G.; et al. CarDiac magnEtic Resonance for prophylactic Implantable-cardioVerter defibrillAtor ThErapy in Non-Ischaemic dilated CardioMyopathy: An international Registry. *Europace* **2021**, *23*, 1072–1083. [CrossRef]
66. Morita, E.; Yasue, H.; Yoshimura, M.; Ogawa, H.; Jougasaki, M.; Matsumura, T.; Mukoyama, M.; Nakao, K. Increased plasma levels of brain natriuretic peptide in patients with acute myocardial infarction. *Circulation* **1993**, *88*, 82–91. [CrossRef]
67. Wong, Y.-K.; Tse, H.-F. Circulating Biomarkers for Cardiovascular Disease Risk Prediction in Patients with Cardiovascular Disease. *Front. Cardiovasc. Med.* **2021**, *8*, 713191. [CrossRef]
68. Guaricci, A.I.; Santoro, F.; Paoletti Perini, A.; Ioffredo, L.; Trivedi, C.; Pontone, G.; Di Biase, M.; Brunetti, N.D. Correlations between NT-proBNP, outcome and haemodynamics in patients with septic shock. *Acta Cardiol.* **2015**, *70*, 545–552. [CrossRef]
69. Guaricci, A.I.; Bulzis, G.; Pontone, G.; Scicchitano, P.; Carbonara, R.; Rabbat, M.; De Santis, D.; Ciccone, M.M. Current interpretation of myocardial stunning. *Trends Cardiovasc. Med.* **2018**, *28*, 263–271. [CrossRef]
70. Hsu, B.G.; Chen, Y.C.; Lee, R.P.; Lee, C.C.; Lee, C.J.; Wang, J.H. Fasting serum level of fatty-acid-binding protein 4 positively correlates with metabolic syndrome in patients with coronary artery disease. *Circ. J.* **2010**, *74*, 327–331. [CrossRef]
71. Bao, Y.; Lu, Z.; Zhou, M.; Li, H.; Wang, Y.; Gao, M.; Wei, M.; Jia, W. Serum levels of adipocyte fatty acid-binding protein are associated with the severity of coronary artery disease in Chinese women. *PLoS ONE* **2011**, *6*, e19115. [CrossRef]
72. Zografos, T.; Haliassos, A.; Korovesis, S.; Giazitzoglou, E.; Voridis, E.; Katritsis, D. Association of neutrophil gelatinase-associated lipocalin with the severity of coronary artery disease. *Am. J. Cardiol.* **2009**, *104*, 917–920. [CrossRef]
73. Elkhidir, A.E.; Eltaher, H.B.; Mohamed, A.O. Association of lipocalin-2 level, glycemic status and obesity in type 2 diabetes mellitus. *BMC Res. Notes* **2017**, *10*, 285. [CrossRef]
74. Caselli, C.; Rovai, D.; Lorenzoni, V.; Carpeggiani, C.; Teresinska, A.; Aguade, S.; Todiere, G.; Gimelli, A.; Schroeder, S.; Casolo, G.; et al. A New Integrated Clinical-Biohumoral Model to Predict Functionally Significant Coronary Artery Disease in Patients with Chronic Chest Pain. *Can. J. Cardiol.* **2015**, *31*, 709–716. [CrossRef]
75. Caselli, C.; De Graaf, M.A.; Lorenzoni, V.; Rovai, D.; Marinelli, M.; Del Ry, S.; Giannessi, D.; Bax, J.J.; Neglia, D.; Scholte, A.J. HDL cholesterol, leptin and interleukin-6 predict high risk coronary anatomy assessed by CT angiography in patients with stable chest pain. *Atherosclerosis* **2015**, *241*, 55–61. [CrossRef]
76. Pepe, M.; Napoli, G.; Biondi-Zoccai, G.; Giordano, A. Anti-Inflammatory Therapy for Acute Coronary Syndromes: Is It Time for a Shift in the Treatment Paradigm? *J. Cardiovasc. Pharmacol.* **2022**, *80*, 633–635. [CrossRef]
77. Held, C.; White, H.D.; Stewart, R.A.H.; Budaj, A.; Cannon, C.P.; Hochman, J.S.; Koenig, W.; Siegbahn, A.; Steg, P.G.; Soffer, J.; et al. Inflammatory Biomarkers Interleukin-6 and C-Reactive Protein and Outcomes in Stable Coronary Heart Disease: Experiences from the STABILITY (Stabilization of Atherosclerotic Plaque by Initiation of Darapladib Therapy) Trial. *J. Am. Heart Assoc.* **2017**, *6*, e005077. [CrossRef]
78. Zebrack, J.S.; Anderson, J.L.; Maycock, C.A.; Horne, B.D.; Bair, T.L.; Muhlestein, J.B. Usefulness of high-sensitivity C-reactive protein in predicting long-term risk of death or acute myocardial infarction in patients with unstable or stable angina pectoris or acute myocardial infarction. *Am. J. Cardiol.* **2002**, *89*, 145–149. [CrossRef]
79. Lin, A.; Nerlekar, N.; Yuvaraj, J.; Fernandes, K.; Jiang, C.; Nicholls, S.J.; Dey, D.; Wong, D.T.L. Pericoronary adipose tissue computed tomography attenuation distinguishes different stages of coronary artery disease: A cross-sectional study. *Eur. Heart J. Cardiovasc. Imaging* **2021**, *22*, 298–306. [CrossRef]
80. Araki, M.; Sugiyama, T.; Nakajima, A.; Yonetsu, T.; Seegers, L.M.; Dey, D.; Lee, H.; McNulty, I.; Yasui, Y.; Teng, Y.; et al. Level of Vascular Inflammation Is Higher in Acute Coronary Syndromes Compared with Chronic Coronary Disease. *Circ. Cardiovasc. Imaging* **2022**, *15*, e014191. [CrossRef]
81. Tzolos, E.; Williams, M.C.; McElhinney, P.; Lin, A.; Grodecki, K.; Flores Tomasino, G.; Cadet, S.; Kwiecinski, J.; Doris, M.; Adamson, P.D.; et al. Pericoronary Adipose Tissue Attenuation, Low-Attenuation Plaque Burden, and 5-Year Risk of Myocardial Infarction. *JACC Cardiovasc. Imaging* **2022**, *15*, 1078–1088. [CrossRef]
82. Kubo, T.; Imanishi, T.; Kashiwagi, M.; Ikejima, H.; Tsujioka, H.; Kuroi, A.; Ishibashi, K.; Komukai, K.; Tanimoto, T.; Ino, Y.; et al. Multiple coronary lesion instability in patients with acute myocardial infarction as determined by optical coherence tomography. *Am. J. Cardiol.* **2010**, *105*, 318–322. [CrossRef]
83. Dawson, L.P.; Layland, J. High-Risk Coronary Plaque Features: A Narrative Review. *Cardiol. Ther.* **2022**, *11*, 319–335. [CrossRef]
84. Nerlekar, N.; Ha, F.J.; Cheshire, C.; Rashid, H.; Cameron, J.D.; Wong, D.T.; Seneviratne, S.; Brown, A.J. Computed Tomographic Coronary Angiography-Derived Plaque Characteristics Predict Major Adverse Cardiovascular Events: A Systematic Review and Meta-Analysis. *Circ. Cardiovasc. Imaging* **2018**, *11*, e006973. [CrossRef]
85. Narula, J.; Nakano, M.; Virmani, R.; Kolodgie, F.D.; Petersen, R.; Newcomb, R.; Malik, S.; Fuster, V.; Finn, A.V. Histopathologic characteristics of atherosclerotic coronary disease and implications of the findings for the invasive and noninvasive detection of vulnerable plaques. *J. Am. Coll. Cardiol.* **2013**, *61*, 1041–1051. [CrossRef]

86. Joshi, N.V.; Vesey, A.T.; Williams, M.C.; Shah, A.S.; Calvert, P.A.; Craighead, F.H.; Yeoh, S.E.; Wallace, W.; Salter, D.; Fletcher, A.M.; et al. 18F-fluoride positron emission tomography for identification of ruptured and high-risk coronary atherosclerotic plaques: A prospective clinical trial. *Lancet* **2014**, *383*, 705–713. [CrossRef]
87. Goeller, M.; Achenbach, S.; Cadet, S.; Kwan, A.C.; Commandeur, F.; Slomka, P.J.; Gransar, H.; Albrecht, M.H.; Tamarappoo, B.K.; Berman, D.S.; et al. Pericoronary Adipose Tissue Computed Tomography Attenuation and High-Risk Plaque Characteristics in Acute Coronary Syndrome Compared with Stable Coronary Artery Disease. *JAMA Cardiol.* **2018**, *3*, 858–863. [CrossRef]
88. Mahabadi, A.A.; Balcer, B.; Dykun, I.; Forsting, M.; Schlosser, T.; Heusch, G.; Rassaf, T. Cardiac computed tomography-derived epicardial fat volume and attenuation independently distinguish patients with and without myocardial infarction. *PLoS ONE* **2017**, *12*, e0183514. [CrossRef]
89. Barandier, C.; Montani, J.-P.; Yang, Z. Mature adipocytes and perivascular adipose tissue stimulate vascular smooth muscle cell proliferation: Effects of aging and obesity. *Am. J. Physiol.-Heart Circ. Physiol.* **2005**, *289*, H1807–H1813. [CrossRef]
90. Gennero, I.; Xuereb, J.M.; Simon, M.F.; Girolami, J.P.; Bascands, J.L.; Chap, H.; Boneu, B.; Sié, P. Effects of lysophosphatidic acid on proliferation and cytosolic Ca++ of human adult vascular smooth muscle cells in culture. *Thromb. Res.* **1999**, *94*, 317–326. [CrossRef]
91. Antonopoulos, A.S.; Margaritis, M.; Verheule, S.; Recalde, A.; Sanna, F.; Herdman, L.; Psarros, C.; Nasrallah, H.; Coutinho, P.; Akoumianakis, I.; et al. Mutual Regulation of Epicardial Adipose Tissue and Myocardial Redox State by PPAR-γ/Adiponectin Signalling. *Circ. Res.* **2016**, *118*, 842–855. [CrossRef]
92. Verhagen, S.N.; Vink, A.; van der Graaf, Y.; Visseren, F.L. Coronary perivascular adipose tissue characteristics are related to atherosclerotic plaque size and composition. A post-mortem study. *Atherosclerosis* **2012**, *225*, 99–104. [CrossRef]
93. Sequeira, D.I.; Ebert, L.C.; Flach, P.M.; Ruder, T.D.; Thali, M.J.; Ampanozi, G. The correlation of epicardial adipose tissue on postmortem CT with coronary artery stenosis as determined by autopsy. *Forensic Sci. Med. Pathol.* **2015**, *11*, 186–192. [CrossRef]
94. Kelly, K.L.; Lin, P.T.; Basso, C.; Bois, M.; Buja, L.M.; Cohle, S.D.; d'Amati, G.; Duncanson, E.; Fallon, J.T.; Firchau, D.; et al. Sudden cardiac death in the young: A consensus statement on recommended practices for cardiac examination by pathologists from the Society for Cardiovascular Pathology. *Cardiovasc. Pathol.* **2023**, *63*, 107497. [CrossRef]
95. Hogea, T.; Noemi, N.; Suciu, B.A.; Brinzaniuc, K.; Chinezu, L.; Arbănași, E.M.; Kaller, R.; Carașca, C.; Arbănași, E.M.; Vunvulea, V.; et al. Increased Epicardial Adipose Tissue and Heart Characteristics Are Correlated with BMI and Predict Silent Myocardial Infarction in Sudden Cardiac Death Subjects: An Autopsy Study. *Diagnostics* **2023**, *13*, 2157. [CrossRef]
96. Hogea, T.; Suciu, B.A.; Ivănescu, A.D.; Carașca, C.; Chinezu, L.; Arbănași, E.M.; Russu, E.; Kaller, R.; Arbănași, E.M.; Mureșan, A.V.; et al. Increased Epicardial Adipose Tissue (EAT), Left Coronary Artery Plaque Morphology, and Valvular Atherosclerosis as Risks Factors for Sudden Cardiac Death from a Forensic Perspective. *Diagnostics* **2023**, *13*, 142. [CrossRef]
97. Harnden, A.; Takahashi, M.; Burgner, D. Kawasaki disease. *BMJ* **2009**, *338*, b1514. [CrossRef]
98. Shi, H.; Wu, H.; Winkler, M.A.; Belin de Chantemèle, E.J.; Lee, R.; Kim, H.W.; Weintraub, N.L. Perivascular adipose tissue in autoimmune rheumatic diseases. *Pharmacol. Res.* **2022**, *182*, 106354. [CrossRef]
99. Cai, X.; Zhu, Q.; Wu, T.; Zhu, B.; Liu, S.; Liu, S.; Aierken, X.; Ahmat, A.; Li, N. Association of circulating resistin and adiponectin levels with Kawasaki disease: A meta-analysis. *Exp. Ther. Med.* **2020**, *19*, 1033–1041. [CrossRef]
100. Agewall, S.; Beltrame, J.F.; Reynolds, H.R.; Niessner, A.; Rosano, G.; Caforio, A.L.P.; De Caterina, R.; Zimarino, M.; Roffi, M.; Kjeldsen, K.; et al. ESC working group position paper on myocardial infarction with non-obstructive coronary arteries. *Eur. Heart J.* **2016**, *38*, 143–153. [CrossRef]
101. Occhipinti, G.; Bucciarelli-Ducci, C.; Capodanno, D. Diagnostic pathways in myocardial infarction with non-obstructive coronary artery disease (MINOCA). *Eur. Heart J. Acute Cardiovasc. Care* **2021**, *10*, 813–822. [CrossRef]
102. Pergola, V.; Previtero, M.; Cecere, A.; Storer, V.; Castiello, T.; Baritussio, A.; Cabrelle, G.; Mele, D.; Motta, R.; Caforio, A.P.; et al. Clinical Value and Time Course of Pericoronary Fat Inflammation in Patients with Angiographically Nonobstructive Coronaries: A Preliminary Report. *J. Clin. Med.* **2021**, *10*, 1786. [CrossRef]
103. Robinowitz, M.; Virmani, R.; McAllister, H.A.J. Spontaneous coronary artery dissection and eosinophilic inflammation: A cause and effect relationship? *Am. J. Med.* **1982**, *72*, 923–928. [CrossRef]
104. Pitliya, A.; Datta, S.; Kalayci, A.; Kahe, F.; Sharfaei, S.; Jafarizade, M.; Goudarzi, S.; Chi, G. Eosinophilic inflammation in spontaneous coronary artery dissection: A potential therapeutic target? *Med. Hypotheses* **2018**, *121*, 91–94. [CrossRef]
105. Margaritis, M.; Sheppard, M.; Parsons, S.; Robertus, J.L.; Vink, A.; Samani, N.; Adlam, D. Abstract 15829: Periadvential Inflammation in Spontaneous Coronary Artery Dissection: Causal Role or Response to Injury? *Circulation* **2018**, *138*, A15829.
106. Hedgire, S.; Baliyan, V.; Zucker, E.J.; Bittner, D.O.; Staziaki, P.V.; Takx, R.A.P.; Scholtz, J.E.; Meyersohn, N.; Hoffmann, U.; Ghoshhajra, B. Perivascular Epicardial Fat Stranding at Coronary CT Angiography: A Marker of Acute Plaque Rupture and Spontaneous Coronary Artery Dissection. *Radiology* **2018**, *287*, 808–815. [CrossRef]
107. Yuvaraj, J.; Lin, A.; Nerlekar, N.; Rashid, H.; Cameron, J.D.; Seneviratne, S.; Nicholls, S.; Psaltis, P.J.; Wong, D.T.L. Is spontaneous coronary artery dissection (SCAD) related to vascular inflammation and epicardial fat? -insights from computed tomography coronary angiography. *Cardiovasc. Diagn. Ther.* **2020**, *10*, 239–241. [CrossRef]
108. Tweet, M.S.; Akhtar, N.J.; Hayes, S.N.; Best, P.J.; Gulati, R.; Araoz, P.A. Spontaneous coronary artery dissection: Acute findings on coronary computed tomography angiography. *Eur. Heart J. Acute Cardiovasc. Care* **2019**, *8*, 467–475. [CrossRef]

109. Pergola, V.; Continisio, S.; Mantovani, F.; Motta, R.; Mattesi, G.; Marrazzo, G.; Dellino, C.M.; Montonati, C.; De Conti, G.; Galzerano, D.; et al. Spontaneous coronary artery dissection: The emerging role of coronary computed tomography. *Eur. Heart J. Cardiovasc. Imaging* **2023**, *24*, 839–850. [CrossRef]
110. Shimokawa, H. 2014 Williams Harvey Lecture: Importance of coronary vasomotion abnormalities—From bench to bedside. *Eur. Heart J.* **2014**, *35*, 3180–3193. [CrossRef]
111. Forman, M.B.; Oates, J.A.; Robertson, D.; Robertson, R.M.; Roberts, L.J., 2nd; Virmani, R. Increased adventitial mast cells in a patient with coronary spasm. *N. Engl. J. Med.* **1985**, *313*, 1138–1141. [CrossRef]
112. Lange, R.A.; Cigarroa, R.G.; Yancy, C.W., Jr.; Willard, J.E.; Popma, J.J.; Sills, M.N.; McBride, W.; Kim, A.S.; Hillis, L.D. Cocaine-induced coronary-artery vasoconstriction. *N. Engl. J. Med.* **1989**, *321*, 1557–1562. [CrossRef]
113. Ohyama, K.; Matsumoto, Y.; Nishimiya, K.; Hao, K.; Tsuburaya, R.; Ota, H.; Amamizu, H.; Uzuka, H.; Takahashi, J.; Ito, K.; et al. Increased Coronary Perivascular Adipose Tissue Volume in Patients with Vasospastic Angina. *Circ. J.* **2016**, *80*, 1653–1656. [CrossRef]
114. Ohyama, K.; Matsumoto, Y.; Amamizu, H.; Uzuka, H.; Nishimiya, K.; Morosawa, S.; Hirano, M.; Watabe, H.; Funaki, Y.; Miyata, S.; et al. Association of Coronary Perivascular Adipose Tissue Inflammation and Drug-Eluting Stent-Induced Coronary Hyperconstricting Responses in Pigs: (18)F-Fluorodeoxyglucose Positron Emission Tomography Imaging Study. *Arterioscler. Thromb. Vasc. Biol.* **2017**, *37*, 1757–1764. [CrossRef]
115. Ohyama, K.; Matsumoto, Y.; Takanami, K.; Ota, H.; Nishimiya, K.; Sugisawa, J.; Tsuchiya, S.; Amamizu, H.; Uzuka, H.; Suda, A.; et al. Coronary Adventitial and Perivascular Adipose Tissue Inflammation in Patients with Vasospastic Angina. *J. Am. Coll. Cardiol.* **2018**, *71*, 414–425. [CrossRef]
116. Owen, M.K.; Witzmann, F.A.; McKenney, M.L.; Lai, X.; Berwick, Z.C.; Moberly, S.P.; Alloosh, M.; Sturek, M.; Tune, J.D. Perivascular adipose tissue potentiates contraction of coronary vascular smooth muscle: Influence of obesity. *Circulation* **2013**, *128*, 9–18. [CrossRef]
117. Lin, A.; Kolossváry, M.; Motwani, M.; Išgum, I.; Maurovich-Horvat, P.; Slomka, P.J.; Dey, D. Artificial Intelligence in Cardiovascular Imaging for Risk Stratification in Coronary Artery Disease. *Radiol. Cardiothorac. Imaging* **2021**, *3*, e200512. [CrossRef]
118. Al'Aref, S.J.; Singh, G.; Choi, J.W.; Xu, Z.; Maliakal, G.; van Rosendael, A.R.; Lee, B.C.; Fatima, Z.; Andreini, D.; Bax, J.J.; et al. A Boosted Ensemble Algorithm for Determination of Plaque Stability in High-Risk Patients on Coronary CTA. *JACC Cardiovasc. Imaging* **2020**, *13*, 2162–2173. [CrossRef]
119. Dey, D.; Gaur, S.; Ovrehus, K.A.; Slomka, P.J.; Betancur, J.; Goeller, M.; Hell, M.M.; Gransar, H.; Berman, D.S.; Achenbach, S.; et al. Integrated prediction of lesion-specific ischaemia from quantitative coronary CT angiography using machine learning: A multicentre study. *Eur. Radiol.* **2018**, *28*, 2655–2664. [CrossRef]
120. Driessen, R.S.; Danad, I.; Stuijfzand, W.J.; Raijmakers, P.G.; Schumacher, S.P.; van Diemen, P.A.; Leipsic, J.A.; Knuuti, J.; Underwood, S.R.; van de Ven, P.M.; et al. Comparison of Coronary Computed Tomography Angiography, Fractional Flow Reserve, and Perfusion Imaging for Ischemia Diagnosis. *J. Am. Coll. Cardiol.* **2019**, *73*, 161–173. [CrossRef]
121. Commandeur, F.; Goeller, M.; Razipour, A.; Cadet, S.; Hell, M.M.; Kwiecinski, J.; Chen, X.; Chang, H.-J.; Marwan, M.; Achenbach, S.; et al. Fully Automated CT Quantification of Epicardial Adipose Tissue by Deep Learning: A Multicenter Study. *Radiol. Artif. Intell.* **2019**, *1*, e190045. [CrossRef]
122. Otaki, Y.; Hell, M.; Slomka, P.J.; Schuhbaeck, A.; Gransar, H.; Huber, B.; Nakazato, R.; Germano, G.; Hayes, S.W.; Thomson, L.E.; et al. Relationship of epicardial fat volume from noncontrast CT with impaired myocardial flow reserve by positron emission tomography. *J. Cardiovasc. Comput. Tomogr.* **2015**, *9*, 303–309. [CrossRef]
123. Muscogiuri, G.; Chiesa, M.; Baggiano, A.; Spadafora, P.; De Santis, R.; Guglielmo, M.; Scafuri, S.; Fusini, L.; Mushtaq, S.; Conte, E.; et al. Diagnostic performance of deep learning algorithm for analysis of computed tomography myocardial perfusion. *Eur. J. Nucl. Med. Mol. Imaging* **2022**, *49*, 3119–3128. [CrossRef]
124. Oikonomou, E.K.; Williams, M.C.; Kotanidis, C.P.; Desai, M.Y.; Marwan, M.; Antonopoulos, A.S.; Thomas, K.E.; Thomas, S.; Akoumianakis, I.; Fan, L.M.; et al. A novel machine learning-derived radiotranscriptomic signature of perivascular fat improves cardiac risk prediction using coronary CT angiography. *Eur. Heart J.* **2019**, *40*, 3529–3543. [CrossRef]
125. Lin, A.; Kolossváry, M.; Yuvaraj, J.; Cadet, S.; McElhinney, P.A.; Jiang, C.; Nerlekar, N.; Nicholls, S.J.; Slomka, P.J.; Maurovich-Horvat, P.; et al. Myocardial Infarction Associates with a Distinct Pericoronary Adipose Tissue Radiomic Phenotype: A Prospective Case-Control Study. *JACC Cardiovasc. Imaging* **2020**, *13*, 2371–2383. [CrossRef]

Journal of
Clinical Medicine

MDPI

Review

Multimodality Imaging in Advanced Heart Failure for Diagnosis, Management and Follow-Up: A Comprehensive Review

Valeria Pergola [1,*], Matteo Cameli [2], Giulia Mattesi [1], Saima Mushtaq [3], Antonello D'Andrea [4], Andrea Igoren Guaricci [5], Maria Concetta Pastore [2], Filippo Amato [1], Carlo Maria Dellino [3], Raffaella Motta [6], Martina Perazzolo Marra [1], Santo Dellegrottaglie [7], Roberto Pedrinelli [8], Sabino Iliceto [1], Savina Nodari [9], Pasquale Perrone Filardi [10], Gianluca Pontone [3,11] and on behalf of the Cluster Imaging of Italian Society of Cardiology (SIC)

1 Department of Cardiac, Thoracic and Vascular Sciences and Public Health, University of Padua, Via Giustiniani 2, 35128 Padova, Italy; giulia.mattesi@aopd.veneto.it (G.M.); filippo.amato@studenti.unipd.it (F.A.); martina.perazzolomarra@unipd.it (M.P.M.); sabino.iliceto@unipd.it (S.I.)
2 Department of Cardiovascular Diseases, University of Sienna, 53100 Siena, Italy; matteo.cameli@unisi.it (M.C.); mariaconce.pastore@unisi.it (M.C.P.)
3 Department of Perioperative Cardiology and Cardiovascular Imaging, Centro Cardiologico Monzino IRCCS, 20138 Milan, Italy; saima.mushtaq@cardiologicomonzino.it (S.M.); carlo.dellino@humanitas.it (C.M.D.); gianluca.pontone@unimi.it (G.P.)
4 Cardiology Unit, Umberto I Hospital, 84014 Nocera Inferiore, Italy; antonellodandrea@libero.it
5 University Cardiology Unit, Interdisciplinary Department of Medicine, Policlinic University Hospital, 70121 Bari, Italy; andreaigoren.guaricci@uniba.it
6 Unit of Radiology, Department of Medicine, Medical School, University of Padua, 35122 Padua, Italy; raffaella.motta@unipd.it
7 Division of Cardiology, Ospedale Medico-Chirurgico Accreditato Villa dei Fiori, 80011 Acerra, Italy; sandel74@hotmail.com
8 Cardiac, Thoracic and Vascular Department, University of Pisa, 56126 Pisa, Italy; roberto.pedrinelli@unipi.it
9 Department of Medical and Surgical Specialties, Radiological Sciences, and Public Health, Institute of Cardiology, University of Brescia, 25123 Brescia, Italy; savina.nodari@unibs.it
10 Department of Advanced Biomedical Sciences, Federico II University of Naples, 80138 Naples, Italy; pasquale.perrone@unina.it
11 Department of Biomedical, Surgical and Sciences, University of Milan, 20122 Milan, Italy
* Correspondence: valeria.pergola@aopd.veneto.it

Abstract: Advanced heart failure (AHF) presents a complex landscape with challenges spanning diagnosis, management, and patient outcomes. In response, the integration of multimodality imaging techniques has emerged as a pivotal approach. This comprehensive review delves into the profound significance of these imaging strategies within AHF scenarios. Multimodality imaging, encompassing echocardiography, cardiac magnetic resonance imaging (CMR), nuclear imaging and cardiac computed tomography (CCT), stands as a cornerstone in the care of patients with both short- and long-term mechanical support devices. These techniques facilitate precise device selection, placement, and vigilant monitoring, ensuring patient safety and optimal device functionality. In the context of orthotopic cardiac transplant (OTC), the role of multimodality imaging remains indispensable. Echocardiography offers invaluable insights into allograft function and potential complications. Advanced methods, like speckle tracking echocardiography (STE), empower the detection of acute cell rejection. Nuclear imaging, CMR and CCT further enhance diagnostic precision, especially concerning allograft rejection and cardiac allograft vasculopathy. This comprehensive imaging approach goes beyond diagnosis, shaping treatment strategies and risk assessment. By harmonizing diverse imaging modalities, clinicians gain a panoramic understanding of each patient's unique condition, facilitating well-informed decisions. The aim is to highlight the novelty and unique aspects of recently published papers in the field. Thus, this review underscores the irreplaceable role of multimodality imaging in elevating patient outcomes, refining treatment precision, and propelling advancements in the evolving landscape of advanced heart failure management.

Keywords: multimodality imaging; advanced heart failure; extracorporeal cardiac support; cardiac transplant

1. Introduction

According to the European Society of Cardiology (ESC) and the American College of Cardiology (ACC)/American Heart Association (AHA)/Heart Failure Society of America (HFSA) Guidelines, advanced heart failure (AHF) is recognized as a clinical syndrome characterized by signs and symptoms of volume overload and inadequate blood perfusion despite maximal therapy, resulting in recurrent hospitalizations and high mortality [1,2]. AHF is further defined by marked symptoms significantly impacting daily life, leading to recurrent hospitalizations despite attempts to optimize guideline-directed medical therapy [2]. The prevalence of AHF is on the rise due to an aging population, improved treatment, and increased survival from HF [3].

Despite medical advancements, patients with AHF still face a poor prognosis, with 1-year mortality rates ranging from 25% to 75% [1]. Additionally, they suffer recurrent episodes of pulmonary or systemic congestion, low cardiac output, and malignant arrhythmias, leading to at least one unplanned hospitalization per year [4].

AHF patients typically exhibit severe exercise intolerance, as evidenced by parameters such as a 6-min walking test distance of <300 m or peak oxygen consumption (pVO2) <12 mL/kg/min or <50% of the predicted value [5]. Furthermore, recent evidence highlights that a significant proportion of patients with AHF exhibit mildly reduced or preserved left-ventricular ejection fraction (LVmrEF and LVpEF, respectively), and their survival outcomes are poor irrespective of EF [6,7]. The challenge in comprehending AHF lies in the absence of a singular diagnostic criterion, thereby complicating the establishment of a universally applicable case definition within diverse populations.

Patients at this stage of HF often exhibit poor responses to conventional therapies, including optimal medical management, cardiac resynchronization therapy (CRT), and various percutaneous and surgical interventions aimed at addressing valvular and coronary artery issues. The clinical spectrum of AHF ranges from progressive refractory deterioration to cardiogenic shock [1]. While inotropic agents can provide temporary relief, their use is limited due to the risk of myocardial ischemia and tachyarrhythmias [8]. As per the latest guidelines from the European Society of Cardiology (ESC) for heart failure [1], treatment options may include adding sacubitril-valsartan or sodium-glucose co-transporter-2 (SGLT2) inhibitors, doubling the dose of loop diuretics, or combining them with thiazide-type diuretics such as metolazone. In cases of refractory diuretic treatment, renal replacement therapy should be considered [1].

The Interagency Registry for Mechanically Assisted Circulatory Support (INTERMACS) classification system plays a crucial role in assessing the severity of HF, ranging from class III NYHA (New York Heart Association) to critical cardiogenic shock, despite escalating therapeutic support [9]. For patients classified as INTERMACS 1 or 2, short-term mechanical circulatory support (MCS) devices are the preferred choice [10]. Therefore, when patients fail to stabilize with medical therapies alone, they become eligible for MCS devices, whether in acute or chronic settings. A variety of short- and long-term MCS devices are available to clinicians [10,11].

MCS devices can serve as a bridge to decision (BTD), bridge to recovery (BTR), bridge to other bridge therapies (BTB), such as long-term MCS, or as a bridge to urgent cardiac transplant (BTT) [11]. These devices encompass intra-aortic balloon pumps (IABP), mpella, veno-arterial extracorporeal membrane oxygenation (ECMO), and left-ventricular assist devices (LVADs). Regular imaging assessments, particularly echocardiography, are essential for monitoring device function, detecting complications, and optimizing patient outcomes. Imaging helps assess ventricular function, valve function, and the presence of any thrombus or device-related issues, ensuring timely intervention when necessary [1].

LVADs can be used as a BTT, a bridge to candidacy (BTC), or as permanent treatment, such as "destination therapy" (DT) (refractory HF, no transplant candidate), in order to overcome the shortage of heart donors [12]. In this setting, RV assessment is crucial since the RV supports the cardiac output and RV failure occurs in up to 50% of cases following LVAD implantation, resulting in high perioperative mortality and morbidity rates [13,14]. A biventricular assist device (BiVAD) is an implantable pump designed to help the heart function better when both the right and left pumping chambers of the heart are failing. However, BiVAD recipients have greater mortality and morbidity than LVAD recipients [15]. Therefore, MCS with BiVAD and total artificial heart (TAH) options remain challenging.

Orthotopic cardiac transplant (OCT) stands as the gold standard of care for eligible patients with advanced, refractory HF. OCT has demonstrated the ability to improve both the quality of life and overall survival [16]. However, the limited availability of suitable donor organs and the presence of numerous contraindications restrict the applicability of this option to a select group of patients [1]. Cardiac imaging is vital in the evaluation of transplant candidates. Echocardiography is the first-line imaging modality to assess the suitability of the donor's heart. It also helps detect any potential contraindications such as valvular abnormalities, or ventricular dysfunction, which may influence the decision to proceed with transplantation [17].

Cardiac imaging modalities play a pivotal role in the assessment and management of AHF patients. They provide crucial insights into myocardial function and assist in identifying potential candidates for advanced therapies, selecting the most appropriate mechanical cardiac support (MCS) device, and optimizing its settings for individual patients [1,18].

Evaluating AHF through echocardiography has seen considerable growth, with an emphasis on hemodynamic and strain assessments. Nuclear techniques have also evolved, with innovations like positron emission tomography/computed tomography (PET/CT) and single-photon emission-computed tomography positron-emission tomography (SPECT), enhancing both diagnostic precision and the ability to assess myocardial blood flow (MBF) and viability. Meanwhile, cardiac computed tomography (CCT) imaging, already established for coronary disease evaluation, is increasingly valuable for characterizing myopathic conditions. Furthermore, cardiac magnetic resonance (CMR) is expanding its role in tissue characterization, now encompassing a broader range of diseases [18].

The purpose of this review is to provide a multimodality imaging approach for patients with AHF. Clinical decisions about HF management are frequently based on measurements of LV function, relying mainly on transthoracic and transesophageal echocardiographic (TTE and TEE) measurements. These tools are almost always available in primary care; this means that AHF clinical diagnosis and decision-making can take weeks, even months, of in-hospital stay and costly frequent visits to HF outpatient clinics. As a result, the opportunity for early detection of AHF is often lost. Currently, the availability of other imaging modalities, such as CCT, nuclear imaging, and CMR, in tertiary centers is of utmost importance in the assessment of complex scenarios, and this may have an impact on the survival of AHF patients. The aim of this review is to emphasize the novelty and unique aspects of recently published papers in the field, distinguishing it from previous reviews on this topic.

2. Multimodal Approach to Advanced Heart Failure

2.1. Transthoracic Echocardiography in AHF

The echocardiographic parameters used to evaluate in patients with AHF are:

1. Left-ventricular ejection fraction (LVEF). LVEF is a crucial indicator in assessing heart failure. In individuals with AHF, approximately 50% of patients may exhibit a reduced LVEF [1]. It is noteworthy, however, that half of AHF cases present with mildly reduced or preserved EF, with poor survival rates irrespective of EF values [6,7]. The accurate measurement of LVEF is essential and can be achieved through the Simpson' biplane method or 3D imaging. In instances of poor acoustic window quality, the use of ultrasound-enhancing agents (UEAs) is recommended to enhance the visualization

of the endocardial borders [19]. According to the 2022 AHA/ACC/HFSA Guideline, the diagnosis of HF with an LVEF exceeding 40% necessitates a demonstration of increased filling pressures. While increased cardiac filling pressure is presumed for HFrEF, individuals with HFmrEF or HFpEF require evidence demonstrating spontaneously or provokable increased LV filling pressures for a confirmed diagnosis of HF. Such supporting evidence can be obtained through noninvasive methods such as natriuretic peptide assessment or imaging for diastolic function [2]. Patients who initially had HFrEF and subsequently, at follow-up, show an LVEF surpassing 40%, are classified as having heart failure with improved EF (HFimpEF) [2].

2. Presence of regional wall motion abnormalities (RWMA). In AHF, the presence of RWMA serves as a significant clinical indicator, which may be caused by factors such as ischemia, scar tissue formation, or underlying structural heart disease. These abnormalities contribute to the overall dysfunction of the heart and can further compromise its pumping capacity [1,2].
3. Ventricular diameters and volumes: LV end-diastolic diameter (EDD) upper cut-off normal values are >52.2 mm in females and >58.4 mm in males. LV end-diastolic volume (EDV) upper cut-off values are >61 mm/m^2 in the female sex and >74 mm/m^2 in the male sex. Three-dimensional (3D) echocardiography is currently the most accurate technique in determining LV volume and function. It correlates with cardiac magnetic resonance, reducing the need for geometric assumptions. However, it has some limitations, such as lower spatial and temporal resolution [20]. In a retrospective study on 443 patients initially diagnosed with HFrEF, those with persistent EF $\leq$ 40% (HFprEF) at the 1 year follow-up had a poorer prognosis compared to those with HFimpEF. Notably, LV end-systolic diameter (LVESD) at discharge emerged as a significant predictor, with an LVESD $\geq$ 55 mm associated with a higher incidence of persistent HFrEF, suggesting its potential value for risk stratification in patients with advanced HF refractory for guideline-directed medical therapy [21]
4. Stroke volume (SV): the SV through the aortic valve is calculated as the product of the cross-sectional area times the integral of the velocity/time curve of flow through that area. The lower cut-off for indexed SV value is <35 mL/m^2 [22]. Monitoring changes in indexed SV over time can provide insights into the progression or improvement of heart failure, guiding adjustments to therapeutic interventions.
5. LV global longitudinal strain (GLS). The normal value is strictly variable depending on sex and age, with a mean normal value of -22.5 ± 2.7 and a confidence interval = -17.2 to -27.7 [23]. In patients with HF with reduced LVEF, GLS is an accurate noninvasive measure of myocardial fibrosis and a better predictor of all causes of mortality than other echocardiographic parameters, especially in males and in sinus rhythm [24]. A GLS <16% has been proposed as a lower value for LV systolic dysfunction [2].
6. Mitral and tricuspidal regurgitation. TTE using quantitative parameters allows for the quantification of the seriousness of these valvular heart diseases, also being able to provide indications on the need for a possible percutaneous treatment. There are qualitative, semiquantitative, and quantitative parameters (Pisa radium, regurgitant volume (RV) and effective regurgitant orifice area (EROA)). For mitral regurgitation, the presence of EROA > 40 mm^2 and Rvol > 60 mL is indicative of severity, while the severity cut-off for tricuspid regurgitation is: EROA > 40 mm, Rvol > 45 mL and Pisa radium > 9 mm [25];
7. Diastolic function. The E/E′ ratio > 14 and average e′ velocity < 9 cm/s identify an increase in LV filling pressure. During diastole, blood flows through the mitral valve when the LV relaxes, causing an early diastolic mitral velocity (E), and then additional blood is pumped through the valve when the left atrium contracts during late diastole (A). The E/A ratio can be altered as diastolic dysfunction progresses (with an initial decline (E/A < 1); then, there is a pseudonormalization (E/A $\geq$ 1) and, finally, a restrictive filling pattern (E/A $\geq$ 2) appears [26]. Tissue Doppler imaging is

an echocardiographic technique that measures the velocity of the mitral annulus. This velocity has been shown to be an important marker of early myocardial dysfunction. With abnormal active relaxation, mitral annulus velocity during early diastole (e′) is decreased while mitral annulus velocity during late diastole (a′) is increased, resulting in a lowered e′/a′ ratio [27] and a higher E/e′ ratio. Indicators of increased filling pressures include an average E/e′ ≥15, a septal e′ velocity less than 7 cm/s, a lateral e′ velocity less than 10 cm/s, a tricuspid regurgitation (TR) velocity greater than 2.8 m/s, and an estimated systolic pulmonary artery pressure (sPAP) exceeding 35 mmHg [2].

8. LV mass and wall thickness (WT). The quantification of the myocardial mass and the measurement of the thickness allows for the identification of pathological hypertrophy. An example is hypertrophic cardiomyopathy, in which there is asymmetric LV hypertrophy with septal thicknesses above 15 mm. There are two main patterns of hypertrophy: concentric and eccentric. Concentric hypertrophy occurs in cases of chronic pressure overload such as in aortic stenosis or poorly controlled arterial hypertension. Eccentric hypertrophy is typical of volume overload—typical, for example, of aortic insufficiency or cases of dilated heart disease; the latter type of hypertrophy usually belongs to dysfunctional ventricles and therefore is a negative prognostic marker [25]. The proposed criteria for detecting structural heart disease are an LV indexed mass greater than 116/95 g/m^2, a relative WT exceeding 0.42, and an LV wall thickness > 12 mm [2].
9. Left atrial (LA) function. LA enlargement predicts cardiovascular risk, and an alteration of LA deformation property (strain) is a marker of negative outcomes such as cardiovascular morbidity and mortality [28]. Following the 2022 AHA/ACC/HFSA Guideline, a left atrial volume index (LAVI) equal to or exceeding 34 mL/m^2 is proposed as indicative of elevated filling pressures [2].
10. Advanced echocardiography. RV global longitudinal strain (RVGLS) and free-wall right-ventricular longitudinal strain (RVFWS) are two important parameters for evaluating RV function. The normal values are >−17.5% for RVGLS and >−15.3% for RVFWS. RVFWS is a more sensitive indicator of RV function since RVGLS, involving interventricular septum deformation analysis, can be influenced by LV dysfunction [29].

2.1.1. Novel Approaches in TTE Evaluation for AHF

TTE is the foremost imaging modality for investigating the etiology of AHF and guiding associated therapeutic interventions [30]. Employing a "Focus Cardiac Ultrasound" (FoCUS) is recommended in the acute setting to assess LV global systolic and diastolic function, regional wall abnormalities, valvular heart conditions, and pericardial disease. Furthermore, the evaluation of right-heart structure and function, along with pulmonary pressures, carries significant prognostic implications in AHF patients [31]

Recently, lung ultrasound (LUS) has emerged as a valuable, cost-effective, portable, real-time, and radiation-free modality for detecting and monitoring pulmonary congestion in AHF patients. It surpasses the diagnostic accuracy of chest radiographs in identifying pleural and lung effusion, utilizing B-lines. The number of B-lines correlates with the severity of congestion, offering 85% sensitivity and 92% specificity for identifying cardiogenic dyspnea. The persistence of the B profile in clinically stable outpatients predicts HF-related events or mortality, providing a dynamic assessment of pulmonary congestion and response to treatment [32].

Moreover, abdominal ultrasound (AUS) has proved to be valuable in assessing inferior vena cava (IVC) diameter as an indirect measure of right atrial pressures, aiding in the early detection of abnormal intravascular volume. Additionally, AUS can identify ascites and abdominal aortic aneurysms in HF patients. Recent implementations of ultrasound techniques to assess renal blood flow offer further insights into the hemodynamic status of AHF patients [33]. Novel approaches include systemic venous ultrasonography for prognostication in AHF patients. The Venous Excess Ultrasound System (VExUS) score, incorporating IVC dilatation and the pulsed-wave Doppler morphology of hepatic, portal, intra-renal, and femoral veins, provides a comprehensive assessment of systemic congestion. Notably, an intra-renal monophasic pattern, portal pulsatility > 50%, and a VExUS score of 3 (indicating severe congestion) have demonstrated predictive value for adverse outcomes in AHF patients. The integration of these ultrasonographic findings into early and multidisciplinary follow-up visits enhances the prognostic evaluation of AHF, offering a holistic and dynamic approach to patient care [34].

2.1.2. Role of Cardiac Magnetic Resonance Imaging in AHF

CMR imaging plays a fundamental role in AHF due to its high sensitivity in identifying the underlying etiology [35]. Late gadolinium enhancement (LGE) patterns help distinguish between ischemic cardiomyopathy (ICM) and non-ischemic cardiomyopathy (NICM) [36].

In ICM, LGE is transmural or subendocardial, while in a certain proportion of NICM cases, the presence of intramural or subepicardial LGE is detected. Notably, the absence of LGE does not completely exclude ICM in the case of hibernating myocardium [22]. In ICM, an important role of CMR is the assessment of myocardial viability. The presence of scars extending more than 75% of the myocardial wall indicates a low probability of recovery after revascularization. On the other hand, the presence of scars affecting less than 25% of the myocardial wall indicates a good chance of recovery [37]. In NICM, LGE has important prognostic implications in terms of site and distribution, as its extent correlates to a major number of cardiovascular events. Examples of CMR findings are shown in Figure 1.

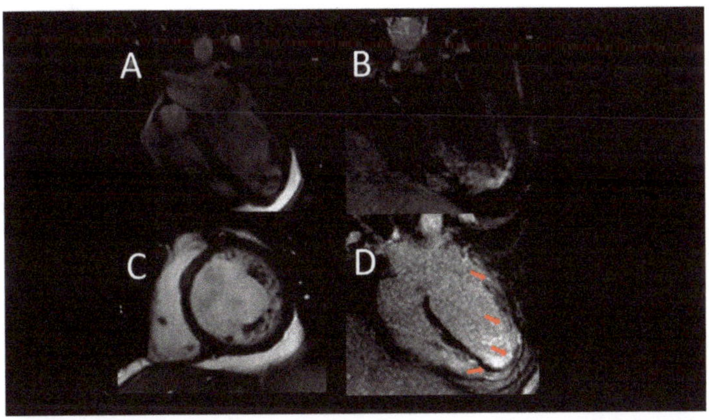

Figure 1. Representative case of use of cardiac magnetic resonance (CMR) in acute heart failure. **(A)** **(B)** acute heart failure, CMR images showing severe LV (left ventricle) dilatation, associated with hypertrabeculation. **(C)** T2-weight images exclude edema. **(D)** a diffuse endocardial late enhancement (red arrows) was detected, compatible with endomyocardial disease.

CMR is crucial for assessing and diagnosing myocardial infiltrative diseases, such as amyloidosis, iron overload and Anderson–Fabry disease, also including rare conditions like hemochromatosis and sarcoidosis. The variability in the progression and severity of HF among individuals depends on factors such as disease subtype, organ involvement, and promptness of diagnosis and treatment [38]. While echocardiography is typically the initial imaging method for patients with HF, the utilization of CMR has grown in cases of infiltrative diseases due to its ability to reveal hypertrophy, visualize infiltration, quantify its burden, and offer potential prognostic value, with characteristic features becoming more evident in advanced stages [39]. Within cardiac amyloidosis (CA) patients, CMR holds the potential to differentiate between light chain immunoglobulin (AL) and transthyretin amyloidosis (ATTR), revealing asymmetrical LV hypertrophy (LVH) as the prevalent morphology in ATTR, often manifesting as sigmoid septum or reverse septal contour; while in AL-CA, symmetrical and concentric LVH predominates, necessitating careful differentiation from hypertrophic cardiomyopathy (HCM) or hypertensive heart disease. CMR possesses the ability to differentiate tissue properties by evaluating LGE images and quantifying cardiac amyloid burden using T1 mapping and extracellular volume (ECV) measurement [40]. CMR with LGE is also considered the preferred diagnostic method for detecting cardiac sarcoidosis involvement, revealing scar tissue and potential inflammation-related extracellular expansion. It also enables the identification of morphological abnormalities (scars and aneurisms) and the assessment of cardiac chamber function [41].

CMR stands as a pivotal diagnostic tool in guiding revascularization decisions, particularly in cases of ischemic cardiomyopathy. The degree of myocardial hyperenhancement, as detected by CMR, demonstrates a noteworthy inverse correlation with the subsequent improvement in myocardial contractility following either surgical or percutaneous revascularization procedures [42].

The great spatial resolution of CMR plays a critical role in providing precise quantification of both the extent and transmurality of myocardial scar tissue, as well as identifying viable myocardium. Notably, if the transmurality of late gadolinium enhancement (LGE) in a myocardial segment exceeds 50%, it signifies a non-viable myocardium (NVM). This serves as a crucial indicator pointing towards inadequate contractile recovery post-revascularization [43].

2.1.3. Role of Cardiac Computed Tomography in AHF

In patients with AHF, CCT can be used to assess ventricular function when echocardiographic windows are suboptimal and CMR is contraindicated (i.e., for the presence of devices, which are particularly frequent in such patients). CCT provides a true volumetric method to assess both LV and RV size and systolic function at high spatial resolution. It can also identify typical characteristics of non-compact LV, hypertrophic cardiopathy, and arrhythmogenic RV cardiomyopathy (RV dilation and dysfunction, adipose infiltration) [44,45]. According to the 2010 Appropriate Use Criteria for Cardiac Computed Tomography, CCT angiography is considered appropriate for evaluating coronary artery disease (CAD) in patients with HF with reduced ejection fraction (HFrEF) who present a low to intermediate probability of CAD [46].

Furthermore, CCT acquisition has the potential to identify myocardial fibrosis in specific LV regions without the need for extra contrast agents or increased radiation exposure [47].

Recent validation studies have shown that CCT is capable of accurately assessing extracellular volume (ECV) in cases of cardiac amyloidosis, demonstrating good concordance with results obtained through CMR [48]. Additionally, the estimation of ECV using a single-source, single-energy CT scanner for the entire heart has proven to be both feasible and accurate. This integration of ECV measurement into a comprehensive CCT evaluation for individuals newly diagnosed with dilated cardiomyopathy can be accomplished with only a marginal rise in overall radiation exposure [49].

2.1.4. Role of Nuclear Imaging in AHF

Various noninvasive imaging modalities are available for assessing biventricular function, including contrast-enhanced echocardiography, three-dimensional echocardiography (3DE), and gated heart-pool scan (GHPS) [50]. Studies exploring the concordance among these modalities in measuring LVEF and RVEF within the same patient cohort reveal discrepancies, with Pearson's correlation coefficients ranging from 0.64 to 0.91 for LVEF and 0.27 to 0.86 for RVEF measurements [50]. This highlights the need for careful consideration in clinical management and sequential patient follow-up.

Multgated acquisition nuclear imaging (MUGA), also known as radionucleotide ventriculography (RVG) and gated equilibrium radionucleotide angiography (ERNA), emerges as a valuable third-line option when echocardiography and CMR are unavailable for LVEF assessment [51,52]. Despite its high reproducibility and minimal variability, concerns persist about radiation exposure, particularly in young patients [51,52].

Automated gated blood-pool scintigraphy (GBPS) presents itself as a potential alternative for assessing ventricular function, especially in dilated cardiomyopathy (DCM) patients. A prospective evaluation comparing GBPS with first-pass radionuclide ventriculography (FPRNV) and planar MUGA demonstrated notable correlations for LVEF values between MUGA, GBPS, and echocardiography. Strong correlations were also observed for RVEF values between GBPS and FPRNV, suggesting the routine use of automated GBPS in evaluating cardiac function in DCM patients as an alternative to traditional approaches like FPRNV [53].

Ongoing research, including modalities like MUGA, contributes to refining our understanding of their comparative utility and guides their optimal integration into cardiovascular care [50–53]. Additionally, the inclusion of modalities like MUGA enhances the cardiovascular imaging landscape, providing valuable insights for comprehensive patient care and management [54]. Stress nuclear imaging plays a crucial role in the comprehensive assessment of HF patients, providing valuable insights into cardiac function and perfusion under physiological stress. [50–53].

In HF patients, stress nuclear imaging, often performed using single-photon emission computed tomography (SPECT) or positron emission tomography (PET), helps unmask potential myocardial ischemia, assess the response of the LV under increased workload, and identify regions of impaired perfusion.

The evaluation of myocardial perfusion during stress is crucial in HF patients, where compromised blood supply can worsen existing cardiac dysfunction. Additionally, stress nuclear imaging plays a pivotal role in determining the extent of the viable myocardium, providing valuable information for informed decision-making about revascularization procedures and guiding optimal therapeutic strategies [50–53]. Furthermore, stress nuclear imaging contributes significantly to risk stratification and prognosis assessment in HF. The identification of areas with reversible ischemia and an assessment of overall cardiac performance during stress predict the likelihood of adverse cardiovascular events [50–53].

Additionally, stress nuclear myocardial perfusion imaging (SNMPI) demonstrates high sensitivity (86%) for detecting single-vessel disease, making it effective in identifying coronary artery abnormalities. It is considered the best option for patients with left bundle branch block or pacemakers causing abnormal septal motion, where other modalities might yield suboptimal results [55]

However, SNMPI involves radiation exposure, with radioactivity persisting for 3 to 4 days post-procedure. Diagnostic accuracy can be compromised by arrhythmias and soft-tissue attenuation, potentially leading to false results [55,56].

Stress is induced through exercise or pharmacologically using regadenoson. SPECT and PET scans offer perfusion information, with PET providing more quantitative measures and a better identification of perfusion defect location and severity. Isotope options include thallium-201 (Tl-201), technetium-99 sestamibi (Tc-99m), or technetium-99 tetrofosmin. Images are obtained at rest and after stress (Figure 2), typically taking about 20 min for each scan [55,56].

Table 1 describes the advantages, limitations, specific indications and prognostic role of different imaging modalities in AHF.

Table 1. Advantages, limitations, specific indications and prognostic role of different imaging modalities in advanced heart failure (AHF).

Imaging Modality	Advantages	Limitations	Specific Indications	Prognostic Role
Echocardiography	• Real-time, noninvasive • Comprehensive assessment of heart function • Various modalities (TTE, FoCUS, LUS, AUS) • Dynamic assessment of pulmonary congestion	• Acoustic window limitations • Operator-dependent • Limited in patients with poor acoustic window • Limited by patient factors (obesity, COPD)	• Assessment of LV/RV function, valvular conditions • Detection of regional wall abnormalities • Evaluation of LV mass, wall thickness • Novel approaches (LUS, AUS, VExUS) for prognostication	• LVGLS as predictor of mortality in HF with reduced EF • Diastolic parameters for evaluating filling pressures. • LA enlargement predicts cardiovascular risk
Cardiac MRI	• High sensitivity in identifying etiology. • Quantification of cardiac amyloid burden • Visualize hypertrophy, infiltration, • Comprehensive evaluation without contrast agent	• Contraindications (claustrophobia, pacemakers) • Limited availability in some settings • Longer acquisition time. • Limited spatial resolution	• Differentiation of ICM and NICM, myocardial viability • Detection of scars and inflammation in cardiac sarcoidosis • Assessment of LV and RV size and systolic function • Estimation of ECV for cardiac amyloidosis	• Assessment of myocardial infiltrative diseases • Differentiation between AL-CA and ATTR in CA patients • Prognostic value in infiltrative diseases
Cardiac CT	• True volumetric assessment • Assessment of myocardial fibrosis • High spatial resolution	• Radiation exposure (but improving) • Limited by device presence (pacemakers) • Suboptimal for infiltrative diseases	• Evaluation of LV and RV size and systolic function • Identification of coronary artery disease in HFrEF patients • Assessment of myocardial fibrosis	• Identification of non-compact LV, hypertrophic cardiopathy • Estimation of ECV for cardiac amyloidosis
Nuclear Imaging	• Different modalities (MUGA, MPI with SPECT/PET) • Reproducibility in LVEF assessment • Potential alternatives (GBPS, SNMPI)	• Radiation exposure (concerns in young patients) • Limited by arrhythmias, soft-tissue attenuation • Compromised diagnostic accuracy	• Assessment of LVEF when echo or CMR not available • Detection of myocardial ischemia, viable myocardium • Assessment of cardiac function in DCM patients	• Risk stratification and prognosis assessment in HF • Identification of coronary artery abnormalities • High sensitivity for detecting single-vessel disease

TTE = transthoracic echocardiography, LUS = lung ultrasound, AUS = abdominal ultrasound, COPD = chronic obstructive pulmonary disease, LV = left ventricle, RV = right ventricle, HF = heart failure, EF = ejection fraction, ICM = ischemic cardiomyopathy, NICM = non-ischemic cardiomyopathy, ECV = extracellular volume, VExUS = venous excess ultrasound system, CA = cardiac amyloidosis, ATTR = Transthyretin Amyloidosis, MUGA = multigated acquisition, MPI = myocardial perfusion imaging, SPECT = single-photon emission computed tomography, PET = positron emission tomography, GBPS = gated blood-pool scintigraphy, SNMPI = stress nuclear myocardial perfusion imaging, DCM = dilated cardiomyopathy.

2.2. Short-Term Mechanical Support

2.2.1. The Intra-Aortic Balloon Pump

The intra-aortic balloon pump (IABP) consists of a percutaneously placed device that inflates in diastole, thus increasing blood flow to the coronary arteries, and deflates in systole, thus decreasing afterload. The two actions combined reduce myocardial oxygen demand and increase myocardial oxygen supply [57].

The IABP is typically placed in the cardiac catheterization laboratory under fluoroscopic guidance. However, TEE can be used to guide positioning in intubated patients in the intra-operative setting. The ideal positioning of the balloon tip is 1–2 cm distal to the left subclavian artery. This position can be confirmed by visualizing the descending aorta and then withdrawing the TEE probe until the left subclavian artery and aortic arch are visualized. Once the balloon pump is activated, the gas-filled balloon will cause shadowing and reverberation artifacts, which can be used as confirmation of the device functioning properly. In the absence of these artifacts or if bubbles are visualized in the aorta, the rupture of the IABP should be suspected. After IABP placement, although not supported by current guidelines, TTE can be used in clinical practice to monitor LV function and guide the weaning of IABP support. It can also visualize any new or worsening aortic regurgitation [58].

CCT may play a role in detecting possible complications of IABP. First, it can highlight a fearful complication—aortic dissection. Moreover, it can show the displacement of the aortic balloon or arterial embolization and organ parenchyma infarct-related soft tissue enhancement/attenuation. CMR is not indicated in monitoring possible complications. Table 2 depicts the indications and timing of echocardiographic and CCT evaluation.

Table 2. Timing and role of TTE (transthoracic echocardiography), TEE (transesophageal echocardiography) and CCT (cardiac computed tomography) in IAPB (intra-aortic balloon pump).

	TTE	TEE	CCT
Role	Monitor LV function. Guide the weaning of IABP support.	Guide positioning.	Indicated in the suspicion of complications.
Timing	Post-procedural.	Intra-procedural.	Post-procedural.
Identification of complications	New or worsening aortic regurgitations.		Aortic dissection. Displacement of aortic balloon. Arterial embolizations infarct-related soft tissue enhancement/attenuation

TTE = transthoracic echocardiography, TEE = transesophageal echocardiography, CCT = cardiac computed tomography.

2.2.2. The Impella

The Impella is a rotary micro axial pump with insertion into the femoral artery and retrograde advancement up to the LV across the aortic valve: blood is aspirated from the LV and pushed into the ascending aorta. This system allows for a reduction in LV preload and an improvement in cardiac output [59]. TTE evaluation is crucial to determine if a patient is eligible for the Impella placement. The presence of severe aortic stenosis and mechanical aortic valves represent contraindications to Impella placement, whereas the presence of aortic regurgitation does not contraindicate the Impella positioning, but it should be known that regurgitation can worsen after its placement [60]. The existence of LV thrombosis represents an additional contraindication due to the potential risk of systemic embolization. Furthermore, it is essential to report the presence of conditions such as patent foramen ovale and atrial or interventricular defects, as the placement of the Impella device could potentially exacerbate a pre-existing right-to-left shunt. [61].

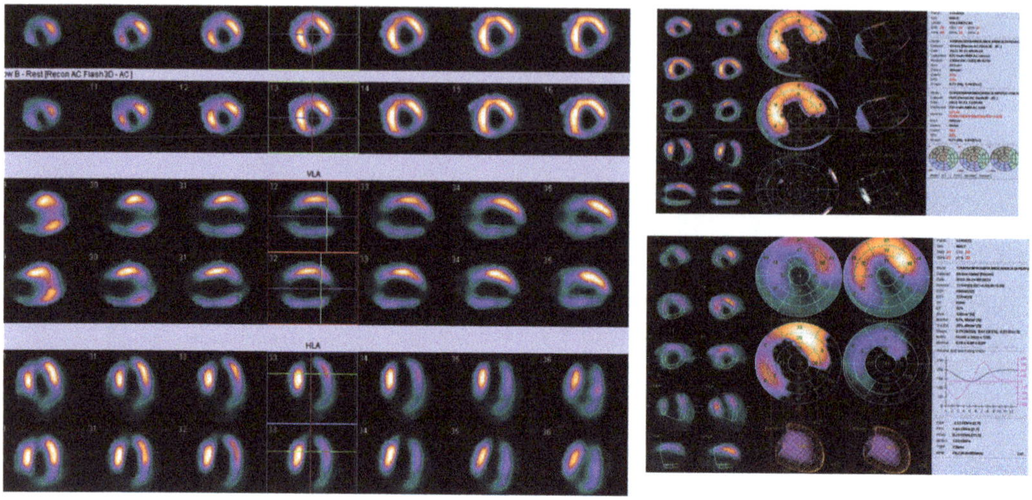

Figure 2. Stress/rest myocardial scintigraphy revealed the absence of myocardial ischemia but necrotic areas in the apical, inferior, and lateral walls were detected. The ejection fraction was measured at 32% after stress, and significant alterations were noted in wall motion and wall thickening in the same regions.

As for IABP, Impella devices are commonly placed under fluoroscopic guidance, but in patients with refractory shock, preventing transportation of the patient to the cardiac catheterization laboratory, TEE can help with bedside positioning of the device [62]. One single-center study demonstrated no difference in Impella-related complications when comparing TEE-alone guided placement with the fluoroscopic guided cohort [63]. The mid-esophageal long-axis and four-chamber views can be used to visualize the guidewire crossing the aortic valve. The catheter should be oriented towards the ventricular apex. TEE can also confirm the absence of iatrogenic aortic dissection from the procedure [62]. Both TTE and TEE are helpful in identifying the correct positioning of the Impella device (Figure 3).

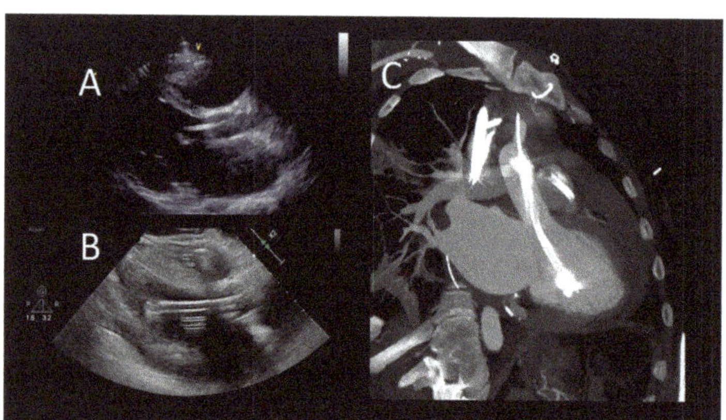

Figure 3. Transthoracic echocardiographic evaluation after Impella implantation (**A**) device's correct position; (**B**) incorrect position (towards the left ventricle apex), (**C**) cardiac computed tomography showing incorrect, apical position.

The distance from the aortic valve to the Impella inlet should be 3.5–5 cm, while the Impella outlet should be 1.5–2 cm above the sinuses of Valsalva [62]. Color-flow Doppler shows a mosaic pattern at the Impella inlet and outlet, further confirming its proper position. Of note, the Impella devices can migrate: in this case, the mosaic pattern will be visualized on the same side of the aortic valve [62]. Three-dimensional echocardiography can help visualize Impella positioning in comparison to other anatomical structures [64]. After placement, additional complications of the Impella placement such as damage to the mitral or aortic valve, pericardial effusion, and rupture of LV free wall must be excluded. The ideal position of the septum is median during the diastole, and displacements may indicate the presence of a right dysfunction or the need to change the speed of the Impella device. Finally, echocardiographic data can be used in conjunction with hemodynamic data to guide the weaning of the Impella by evaluating the response of the LV to progressive reduction in the support provided by the Impella (the P level). CCT plays an important role in confirming endoventricular thrombi before Impella implantation [65]. We know that the most common complications after Impella placement are hemolysis, vascular complications, bleeding, and limb ischemia. A CCT scan can identify complications such as damage to the mitral and aortic valve systems and the positioning of the device. CMR is not indicated in monitoring after Impella implantation (see Table 3).

Table 3. Timing and role of TTE (transthoracic echocardiography), TEE (transesophageal echocardiography), and CCT (cardiac computed tomography) in Impella patients.

	TTE	TEE	CCT
Role	Selection of candidates. Guide the placement	Selection of candidates. Guide the placement	To exclude complications.
Timing	Pre-procedural. Post-operative.	Pre-procedural. Intra-operative. Post-operative.	Post-procedural.
Identification of complications	Mitral and aortic regurgitations. Pericardial effusion. Rupture of LV free wall.	Exclude iatrogenic aortic dissection. Damage of mitralic and aortic valve.	Aortic dissection. Damage of mitral and aortic valve system.

TTE = transthoracic echocardiography, TEE = transesophageal echocardiography, CCT = cardiac computed tomography, LV = left ventricular.

2.2.3. The Veno-Arterial Extracorporeal Membrane Oxygenation

The veno-arterial extracorporeal membrane oxygenation (V-A ECMO) system is a percutaneous system that takes over the heart and lungs. It consists of a system of inflow and outflow cannulas, a centrifugal pump, and an oxygenating membrane [66]. The ECMO provides a blood flow rate greater than 4.5 L. The effect is a noticeable reduction in LV preload increasing the afterload [67].

An echocardiographic evaluation should be performed prior to ECMO cannulation [68]. First, reversible causes of cardiovascular collapse, such as cardiac tamponade and acute valve pathology, must be excluded. The presence of an aortic dissection is a relative contraindication to ECMO positioning as it can cause an extension of the dissecting flap. The presence of aortic stenosis or mitral regurgitation should be also evaluated as they may worsen due to increased afterload due to ECMO [69]. The ECMO can be placed under fluoroscopic, TTE or TEE guidance. Usually, the venous cannula is placed in the right atrium. The mid-oesophageal bi-caval view at the TEE can easily show complications such as the passage of the cannula through the atrial septum. The arterial cannula is typically positioned within the descending aorta; TEE can confirm this location. Moreover, TEE can prevent atheromatous plaque embolization from this procedural step by referring its presence in the aorta to the operator [70].

Echocardiography also plays an essential role in assessing cardiac function when supported by the ECMO system [70]. It is important to ascertain that the aortic valve opens during systole since the high afterload due to the arterial cannula can reduce the valve opening frequency, increasing the risk of LV and aortic valve thrombosis.

Finally, echocardiography can guide ECMO weaning [71]. Echocardiographic parameters that are predictors of successful weaning are LVEF >20–25%, aortic velocity time integral (VTI) >10 cm, and lateral mitral annular systolic wave velocity (S′) >6 cm/s [71].

The CCT scan plays a role in the identification of complications related to the placement of the ECMO. The presence of opacification defects of the arterial system is indicative of pseudo-lesion with emergent surgical indication. CCT can also be used to evaluate other complications such as cannula malposition, hematoma formation, and hemothorax (Figure 4).

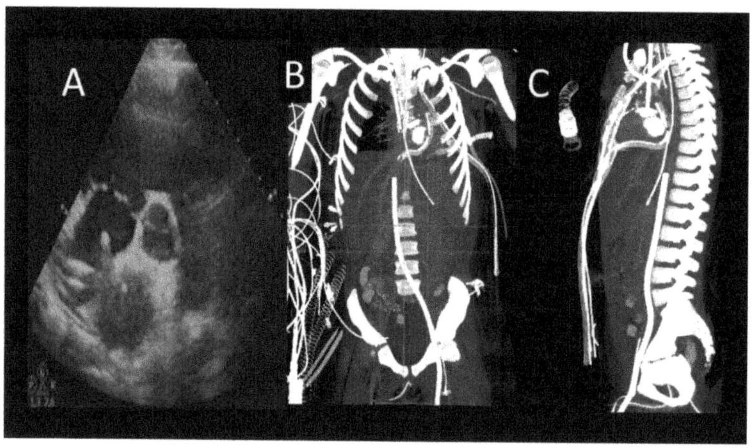

Figure 4. Evaluation after veno-arterial extracorporeal membrane oxygenation (VA ECMO) implantation. (**A**) Transthoracic echocardiography showing the correct position of the right atrial (RA) cannula. (**B**) Cardiac computed tomography (CCT) scan showing correct position of RA and femoral vein ECMO cannulas (**C**) Sagittal CCT showing correct position of RA and femoral vein ECMO cannulas.

An important complication of ECMO is thrombosis of the arterial system, in particular of the ascending aorta proximal to the insertion of the arterial cannula; this is mainly linked to the low flow that determines blood stasis and therefore leads to the formation of thrombi [72].

In patients with impaired RV function, there is also a predisposition to the development of pulmonary embolism [72]. Pulmonary circulation evaluation in these patients can be difficult since the contrast injected at the venous level is captured by the venous cannula before an adequate opacification of the pulmonary circulation. As a solution, the revs of the ECMO can be reduced to 500 / min for 15–25 s during contrast injection [72].

Table 4 shows the timing and role of different imaging modalities.

2.3. Long-Term Mechanical Circulatory Support

LVADs consist of a pump that holds the LV by receiving blood from it by means of an inflow cannula and pushing it to the level of the aorta by means of an outflow cannula. The device is placed in the mediastinum and is powered by a cable that extends abdominally to connect to a controller and a power source. There are two main types of FDA-approved LVADs: pulsatile and non-pulsatile. Those of the older generation were characterized by a pulsatile flow with a high risk of device malfunction and low survival. Heartware and Heart Mate III are characterized by a centrifugal flow; the pump is intrapericardial. Heart Mate II is characterized by an axial flow; the pump is in a pocket [73].

Table 4. Timing and role of TTE (transthoracic echocardiography), TEE (transesophageal echocardiography), and CCT (cardiac computed tomography) in veno-arterial extracorporeal membrane oxygenation.

	TTE	TEE	CT
Role	• Selection of candidates. • Identification of complications. • Weaning.	• Guide the placement. • Identification of complications.	• Identification of complications.
Timing	• Pre-procedural. • Post-procedural.	• Intra-procedural. • Post-procedural.	• Post-procedural.
Identification of complications	• Aortic dissections. • Mitral and aortic regurgitations.	• Cannula malposition. • Plaque embolizations. • Aortic dissections. • Mitral and aortic regurgitations.	• Defect of opacification of arterial system. • Cannula malposition. • Hematoma. • Hemothorax. • Thrombosis of arterial system.

TTE = transthoracic echocardiography, TEE = transesophageal echocardiography, CCT = cardiac computed tomography, LV = left ventricular.

2.3.1. Selection of LVAD Potential Candidates

TTE has a central role in the selection of the optimal candidate for LVAD implants, since it allows for evaluating (see also Table 5) [73]:

1. LVEF (particularly the demonstration of an LVEF < 25%), ventricular size and cardiac output. It may be difficult to implant patients with small LV size, especially with increased LV trabeculation.
2. The presence of intracardiac thrombi; this is not an absolute contraindication to LVAD implants, but it increases the risk of stroke during the LV cannulation procedure.
3. RV function. It is essential to evaluate the presence of signs of RV dysfunction (such as TAPSE < 18 mm, $s' < 9.5$ cm/s, FAC < 35%), RV dilation, dilation of inferior vena cava, and moderate or greater tricuspid regurgitation. The presence of preoperative severe RV dysfunction may suggest the use of a biventricular MCS.
4. Valve diseases. Before LVAD implantation, it is important to detect and quantify valvular regurgitation, valvular stenosis, and prosthetic valve dysfunction. The presence of moderate to severe mitral stenosis can prevent LV cannula inflow. The presence of aortic stenosis of any severity does not affect LVAD function. In fact, LVAD bypasses the native LVOT. It is important to exclude significant aortic regurgitation (AR) before LVAD implantation because it can create a vicious cycle in which blood pumped into the aorta regurgitates into the LV. Of note, in patients with advanced HF and severe stroke volume reduction, it may be difficult to quantify aortic regurgitation. The presence of pre-operatory severe mitral regurgitation is often markedly improved after the initiation of LVAD support because of reduced LV size, reduced filling pressure and improved coaptation of MV leaflets; for these reasons, any grade of mitral regurgitation is not a contraindication to LVAD implantation. Conversely, the presence of pre-operative moderate or severe tricuspid regurgitation may indicate RV dysfunction. In patients with AV mechanical valve prostheses, reduced blood flow through the prosthesis after an LVAD implant may increase the risk of thrombosis; therefore, biological valve replacement may be considered. Finally, it is also important to exclude moderate or severe pulmonary regurgitation and pulmonary stenosis.
5. Congenital heart diseases. Some congenital common anomalies require correction before LVAD implantation. The presence of ventricular septal defects should be also excluded [73].

Table 5. Parameters to be evaluated in LVAD candidates and their influence on LVAD placement.

Parameter	Influence on LVAD Placement
EF (Ejection Fraction)	<25% indicates consideration for LVAD placement
LV Size	An adequate volume is essential to LVAD placement.
Intra-cardiac Thrombi	Exclude LVAD placement.
RV Function	Severe RV dysfunction may suggest biventricular support.
Valve Abnormalities	Significant aortic regurgitation, moderate to severe mitral stenosis, and moderate to severe tricuspid regurgitation exclude LVAD.
Congenital Heart Disease	Shunt lesions exclude LVAD placement.

LVAD = left-ventricular assist device, EF = ejection fraction, LV = left ventricle, RV = right ventricle.

2.3.2. LVAD Surveillance Echocardiography

Periodic standard TTE exams are recommended after an LVAD implant [59]. The first one is performed 2 weeks after the implant; then, they are conducted at 1, 3, 6, and 12 months post-implant and every 6 to 12 months thereafter. During the standard echocardiographic exam, it is important to evaluate and report [73]:

1. LV size and function. The most reproducible is the LV internal diameter end diastole (LVIDd) from the 2D parasternal long-axis image. The LVIDd might paradoxically be smaller than the LV internal diameter at the end of systole (LVIDs). This is a significant observation, as it is linked to excessive unloading of the LV supported by LVADs and/or severe RV dysfunction [73]. The evaluation of LVEF can demonstrate possible LV worsening or recovery. A possible complication to evaluate is LV suction with induced ventricular ectopy; this condition can be due to LV underfilling that causes the impact of inflow cannula with LV endocardium, and the solution may be speed turndown, or fluid administration in case of hypovolemia.
2. Position of interventricular septum (IVS) and cannulas. The end-diastolic IVS position may be neutral, leftward-shifted or rightward-shifted. A leftward shift can be due to elevated RV end-diastolic pressures, reduced LV preload, or LV over-decompression resulting from excessive LVAD speed. A rightward IVS shift is generally due to elevated LV end-diastolic pressures resulting from an inadequate LVAD speed setting, pump dysfunction, severe AR, or an increased LV afterload. The inflow cannula can be evaluated in the parasternal or apical TTE views. It is important to reveal the cannula's location and orientation in relation to IVS and other LV structures. The color Doppler interrogation should demonstrate a one-directional laminar flow from LV to inflow cannula without turbulence or regurgitation. At continuous Doppler interrogation, the flow should have a peak velocity between 1 and 2 m/s; a higher velocity may suggest inflow obstruction.
3. Aortic valve (AV) opening and AR severity. It is important to evaluate the presence and the degree of AV opening because it is determined by different parameters like LVAD speed, LV native function, volume status and peripheral vascular resistance. LVAD types differ in aortic valve opening pattern, especially for the intermittent low-speed phase (e.g., 9 s for Jarvick) [74]. It is recommended that LVAD speed is set to allow at least one intermittent opening of the AV. The AV opening is assessed with M-Mode. In patients with very depressed LVEF, AV opening may not occur. When the AV remains closed, the aortic root thrombus should also be excluded. Another risk in LVAD patients is the development of AR, which is not uncommon after LVAD implantation. The assessment of its severity is partly based on careful color Doppler analysis in the parasternal long-axis view.
4. RV size and function. During TTE follow-up, RV function must be carefully evaluated. The shift of the IVS to the left side by LVADs may reduce the IVS contribution to the RV contraction. Furthermore, increased venous return created by increased cardiac output from the LVAD may worsen the RV function. This increased workload is a

concern for worsening RV function that LVAD patients may already have. The classical criteria for RV dysfunction included the following parameters: TAPSE < 17 mm, tricuspid annulus systolic peak velocity (S′) velocity < 10 cm/s and RVFAC < 35% [22]. Nevertheless, the evaluation of RV function is also challenging because the correlation between RV systolic function and TAPSE and/or S′ should be considered weaker after cardiothoracic surgery.

5. Evidence of intracardiac thrombi. Recent studies on patients implanted with new-generation LVADs suggest that the LV may be a relevant site of local thrombosis and cardioembolism. Pump speed, AV opening, cannula location, and orientation are important determinants of LV flow that are drastically disrupted in LVAD patients, leading to blood stasis or abnormally large shear stresses (Figure 5) [73].

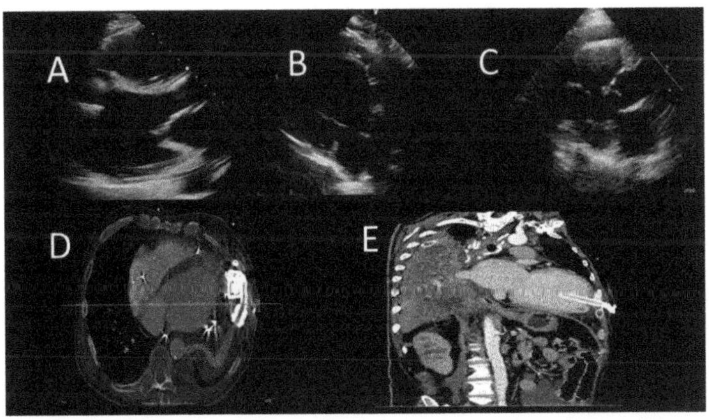

Figure 5. Evaluation after left ventricle assist device (LVAD) (**A**) Transthoracic echocardiography (TTE) evaluation parasternal long axis (PLAX) shows normal position of interventricular septum (IVS) and the inflow cannula; (**B**) TTEPLAX view of LVAD patient, showing incorrect right-convex position of the interventricular septum; (**C**) TTE evaluation (PLAX) of LVAD patient, showing incorrect left-convex position of the IVS; (**D**) Cardiac computed tomography (CCT) showing hematoma around LV cannula; (**E**) CCT showing small left ventricular apical thrombus.

2.3.3. Advanced Echocardiography in LVAD Patients

Some patients with LVADs have very difficult acoustic access in the traditional transthoracic view. Several factors influence poor image quality in LVAD patients. First, LVAD inflow and outflow cannula limit the acoustic window. Furthermore, the device may cause artifacts, and due to the device, the probe positioning during the examination may not be optimal. In such cases, ultrasound-enhancing agents (UEAs) are a good alternative—they are feasible, safe, and reproducible [75]. UEAs allow for a better definition of endocardial borders; this is useful for better quantification of the LV end-diastolic diameter and residual function. It also increases the possibility of detecting intracavitary thrombi. Moreover, it permits better visualization of the RV and helps to identify RV dysfunction and recognize patients at higher risk of RV failure. Finally, during the follow-up, UEAs can reveal the presence of pseudoaneurysms demonstrating a bidirectional flow between the pseudoaneurysm and the LV [73].

TEE is utilized to exclude right-to-left shunting and to monitor air trapping caused by the LVAD coring of the LV apex during implantation and to direct subsequent de-airing movements. TEE is also recommended in the setting of a bloodstream infection to assess vegetations and abnormal flow across the LVAD [76].

2.3.4. Role of Cardiac Computed Tomography and Nuclear Imaging in LVAD Patients

CMR is contraindicated in patients with LVADs; therefore, a CCT scan represents an opportunity for a noninvasive evaluation of the function of the device and its complications [76–78]. A limitation of echocardiography in patients with LVADs is the incomplete visualization of the outflow cannula; the latter is well seen with the help of the CCT scan. During the follow-up, CCT can reveal complications such as compression of the right ventricle (due to pericardial clots), thrombosis, malposition, and kinking of the outflow cannula. Indications for CCT in LVAD patients include suspicion of:

(1) inflow-cannula malposition (i.e., in case of unexplained frequent LVAD suction events, recurring ventricular dysrhythmias, or residual HF due to only partial LV unloading).

(2) Pump thrombosis involving the inflow cannula or outflow tract with evidence of hemolysis.

(3) LVAD malfunction due to outflow-graft kinking, excluding an intracardiac and/or aortic root clot in patients with an unexplained transient ischemic attack or stroke.

Pre-implantation cannula placement can be optimized using CT-derived anatomy, 3D printing, and virtual modeling; nonetheless, this method needs further research [77]. Finally, whenever poor acoustic windows prevent appropriate assessment of ventricular size and function, it is possible to use either multiple-gated acquisition equilibrium radionuclide angiography or electrocardiographically gated CCT as a second-line alternative test [76].

One-fifth of LVAD recipients experience driveline infections, which can cause sepsis and/or death [78]. It has been suggested to use CT and ultrasound to detect infections in the driveline, pump, and cannula; however, due to general discoveries of metal artifacts, the usefulness of these modalities has been severely constrained. Recently, it has been shown that 18F-fluorodeoxyglucose (18F-FDG) PET/CT may be used to diagnose driveline infections in LVAD patients. Moreover, SPECT imaging has been validated to assess myocardial viability, the extension of fibrosis, and the recovery of LV function [76]. Table 6 provides the timing and role of different imaging modalities in LVAD patients.

Table 6. Timing and role of transthoracic echocardiography (TTE), advanced echocardiography, and cardiac computed tomography (CCT) and nuclear imaging in left ventricle assist device (LVAD) patients.

	TTE	TTE with Echocontrast	CT	Nuclear Imaging
Role	• LV volume and function. • Position of interventricular septum and cannula. • RV size and function. • Assessment of AV and MV	• Better definition of endocardial border for quantification of LV volume and residual function. • Identification of patients at higher risk of RV dysfunction.	• Identification of specific complications.	• Identification of specific complications.
Identification of complications	• Evidence of the intracardiac thrombi.	• Increases the possibility to detect intracavitary thrombi.	• Compression of RV. • Thrombosis. • Malposition and kinking of outflow cannula.	• Driveline, pump and cannula infection (PET). • Assessment of myocardial viability (SPECT).

PET = Positron Emission Tomography, SPECT = Single-Photon Emission Computed Tomography.

2.4. *Imaging in Orthotopic Cardiac Transplant (OTC)*

TTE is essential in the follow-up of OTC patients. It has a role both in the immediate post-operative period and in the surveillance of short- and long-term complications [79].

Over the initial three-month period, there is an elevation in ventricular thicknesses and mass, attributed to the infiltration of inflammatory cells and graft-related edema. Prolonged persistence of ventricular hypertrophy beyond this phase could be associated with either immunosuppressive treatment or recurrent instances of acute rejection. Generally, within the first decade, LV function and regional wall motion remain intact [77]. Indeed, according to data provided by the 2019 report from the International Society for Heart and Lung Transplantation (ISHLT) registry, the occurrence of CAV after OTC was recorded at 8% after

1 year, 29% after 5 years, and 47% after 10 years [80]. An early decline in LV EF might signal either the rejection of the transplanted organ or the development of vasculopathy [79].

Diastolic function can be difficult to evaluate since cardiac denervation and the subsequent high heart rate can cause E and A wave fusion. E′ and a′ waves are of smaller amplitudes than in the normal population. A restrictive filling pattern may be present in the early post-transplant stages. Its persistence can be linked to inflammation, fibrosis and the vasculopathy of the allograft [28]. Elevated pulmonary capillary wedge pressure (PCWP) can be accurately predicted by echocardiographic signs of increased right atrial pressure (RAP) or with three out of five specific parameter values (E/A, DT, IVRT, E/E′ lateral, and Doppler PASP) exceeding cut-off values, with positive likelihood ratios between 9 and 15.3, while normal RAP or parameters below cut-off values effectively rule out elevated PCWP, supported by negative likelihood ratios ranging from 0.07 to 0.19 [81].

After cardiac surgery, the longitudinal parameters are abnormal; therefore, they are not considered sensitive parameters (including TAPSE and RV TVI). As for the atrial morphology, in the historical bi-atrial technique, an atrial enlargement and the presence of a ridge at the anastomosis are visualized. In the more recent technique, bi-caval atrial reservoir function is significantly diminished in OCT recipients, primarily associated with increased PCWP and LA enlargement, while in the RA, it is correlated with impaired longitudinal RV function [28].

Normally, valve morphology and the function of transplanted hearts are normal. There may be mild tricuspid and mitral regurgitation. Mitral regurgitation can be linked to papillary muscle edema and tends to decrease over time [63]. Tricuspid regurgitation can be detected during the first phase due to the increased pulmonary pressures, while in more advanced stages it can be linked to valve damage due to frequent biopsies or the dilatation of right chambers [79].

The presence of severe pericardial effusion leading to cardiac tamponade is rare and may be related to the presence of hearts that are smaller compared to the body surface. When a pericardial effusion is found, it is important to perform serial echocardiographic examinations (every 1–3 months) to evaluate the size, extent, and hemodynamic impact of the effusion [82].

2.4.1. Advanced Echocardiography

STE may help in identifying acute cell rejection (ACR) [83]. Several studies have explored the potential of STE in detecting acute cell rejection (ACR) grade ≥2R in heart transplant recipients [84]. Promising findings include the identification of specific strain measurements, such as LV GLS and RV FWLS, as well as LV radial strain, which have shown high negative predictive values for ACR grade ≥2R [85]. Further validation in prospective trials could potentially reduce the need for frequent biopsies, especially for patients with ACR grade 2R or greater. Moreover, it has been shown that the reduction of LV torsion by at least 25% predicts, with high specificity and a high negative predictive value, ACR of at least a second degree [86].

Stress echocardiography (SE), mainly with dobutamine, is recommended in patients with a prohibitive risk for invasive coronary angiography, according to the ISHLTV guidelines. Commonly, it is acknowledged that dobutamine SE (DSE) offers initial evaluations that can help determine whether further invasive follow-up procedures are necessary [84]. A recent meta-analysis demonstrated that SE has a very low sensitivity (about 60%) in the detection of CAV and mostly cannot detect mild and moderated CAV degrees [87]). The Post-Systolic Strain Index (PSI) has been also used to evaluate CAV through DSE. To calculate PSI using specialized software, it is essential to calculate end-systolic (e-sys) and peak strain (peak-s). The PSI is calculated by finding the ratio of [peak-s–e-sys] to peak-s. If this ratio is greater than 34%, it suggests a potential presence of CAV in the patient's heart. A study by Eroglu et al. found that this threshold has a high sensitivity of 88% in identifying patients with CAV [88].

Doppler echocardiography can be employed to gauge the velocity of blood flow within the coronary arteries and evaluate CAV, as outlined in a study by Tona et al. [89]. Coronary flow reserve (CFR) is a useful parameter, representing the maximum increase in blood flow observed between periods of rest and stress. A CFR value below 2.9, as determined by research [87], is indicative of CAV with a notably high sensitivity.

2.4.2. Cardiac Magnetic Resonance

CMR enables the early identification of rejection and CAV in patients who have undergone OCT. Emerging mapping techniques might play a role in OCT rejection diagnosis [89–91]. A recent study [74] showed that combining GLS > −16% and T1 time ≥ 1060 ms defined grade 1 rejection with 91% sensitivity and 92% negative predictive value, providing a potential noninvasive alternative to guide endomyocardial biopsies. Moreover, T1-mapping has demonstrated a reduction after successful treatment, serving as an excellent indicator with a negative predictive value for noninvasive rejection detection [90]. Indeed, research has demonstrated that a combined CMR strategy, incorporating both T2 mapping and extracellular volume fraction (ECV) quantification, shows a strong ability to accurately diagnose acute rejection, potentially leading to a reduction in the necessity for routine endomyocardial biopsies in these patients [91]. This multiparametric approach serves to enhance the diagnostic precision of CMR in identifying ACR [92], as shown in Figure 6. These findings were confirmed by Dolan et al. [93], who found that a combination of CMR-derived myocardial T2 and ECV holds potential as a noninvasive tissue biomarker for detecting ACR, suggesting its promise as an alternative to endomyocardial biopsy. Nevertheless, the advancement of multiparametric CMR for surveillance in transplant recipients requires additional extensive studies, particularly during instances of ACR.

Finally, stress perfusion CMR offers promise in the assessment of microvascular disease through the estimation of myocardial perfusion reserve (MPR). This CMR-based approach addresses microvasculopathy and explores its connection with myocardial perfusion reserve (MPRI) and diastolic strain rate [92]. This interesting study's outcomes underscore the potential of CMR as a noninvasive tool for the early detection of transplant-related microvasculopathy, preceding the onset of epicardial CAV, which could potentially enhance surveillance strategies and ultimately contribute to improved patient outcomes [92].

2.4.3. Cardiac Computed Tomography Angiography and Nuclear Imaging

CCT has increasingly been used to detect CAV in OTC patients [94–96]. Wever-Pinzon et al. in a meta-analysis of 13 studies evaluated 615 HTx patients, demonstrating a high diagnostic specificity, sensitivity, and accuracy of CCT in comparison with invasive coronary angiography (ICA) for the detection of any CAV and significant CAV using 16- and 64-slice CCT [95]. In addition, CAC > 0 was associated with an increased risk of MACE, death, and graft loss. Moreover, the absence of CAC predicted a low prevalence of International Society for Heart and Lung Transplantation (ISHLT) CAV 2–3 grade [96].

Newer CCT technologies, such as dual-source CT and multidetector CT, increasing temporal and spatial resolution, allow for a better acquisition even at higher rate—as in the denervated transplanted heart [94–96]. More recently, Nous et al. [97] in a prospective observational study on 129 OTC patients demonstrated that CCT (using 2° and 3° generation dual-source CT) could be a safe and accurate alternative to ICA in CAV evaluation (Figure 7).

SPECT is a nuclear imaging method utilizing gamma-ray emissions. Several research studies have provided a range of sensitivity values (from 21% to 92%) and specificity values (from 55% to 100%) for CAV diagnosis [98]. Recent studies have generally shown improved diagnostic accuracy [99,100].

Moreover, a recent study aimed [101] to assess the effectiveness of using cadmium-zinc-telluride (CZT) SPECT with 99mTc and 201Tl tracers to measure myocardial blood flow (MBF) and myocardial flow reserve (MFR) for diagnosing CAV. The results were further compared and validated against 13 N-NH3 PET. Key findings included a strong correlation between CZT SPECT-derived stress MBF and MFR values, obtained with both 201Tl and 99mTc tracers, and those from 13 N-NH3 PET. CZT SPECT was effective in detecting low MFR (<2.0) and moderate-to-severe CAV, with results comparable to 13 N-NH3 PET.

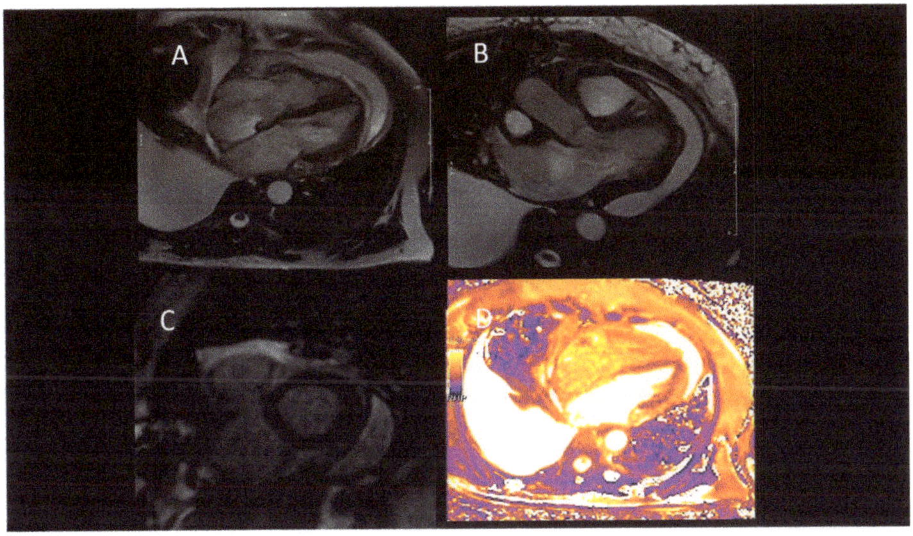

Figure 6. Representative case of use of CMR (cardiac magnetic resonance) in OTC (orthotopic cardiac transplantation) patients. (**A**,**B**) Immuno-mediated rejection with pericardial and pleural effusion (diastolic frame on A and B, respectively, four and three long-axis views); (**C**) Post contrast sequences (short-axis view) demonstrated the absence of late gadolinium enhancement (LGE) and the T2-mapping was negative for inflammation (**D**). The absence of late gadolinium enhancement (LGE) and normal mapping confirmed their prognostic role since the patient demonstrated a full recovery after modification of immunosuppressive therapy.

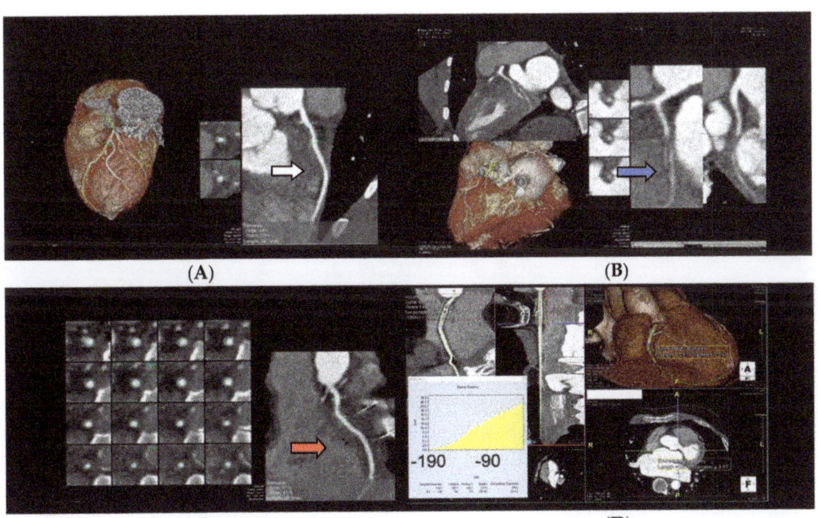

Figure 7. Evaluation of cardiac plaques in OTC (orthotopic cardiac transplantation) patients by CCT (cardiac computed tomography). The squares represent details of the extent of coronary stenosis. (**A**) Mild LAD (left anterior descending artery) circumferential soft plaque (white arrow); (**B**) Occlusion of LCx (left circumflex) artery (blue arrow); (**C**) Mild RCA (right coronary artery soft plaque (red arrow); (**D**) Increased pericoronary fat attenuation index values suggestive of coronary artery inflammation. Pictures from our archive.

Additionally, it is important to note that the use of PET has been investigated for CAV diagnosis, and these studies have yielded positive results [102,103]. A study by Wu et al. focused on evaluating the effectiveness of PET as a noninvasive method for detecting early stages of CAV [103]. MBF was assessed using dynamic PET, both at rest and during adenosine-induced hyperemia [103]. The researchers calculated myocardial perfusion reserve (MPR) by comparing hyperemic MBF to resting MBF. They also used a scoring system for regional PET assessments. Key findings from the study included strong correlations between MBF and MPR in different coronary artery territories. The summed stress score and summed difference score showed a moderate inverse correlation with MPR but not with intravascular ultrasound (IVUS) measurements. MPR was inversely related to plaque volume but not to maximal luminal stenosis, as determined by IVUS.

Another study [104] aimed to ascertain the simultaneous involvement of both the epicardial and intramyocardial arteries during the initial stages of CAV, highlighting that CAV is a progressive condition affecting both the epicardial and microvascular coronary systems.

One of the most clinically robust modalities used in the OTC population to screen for CAV is nuclear imaging with Rubidium-PET (Rb-PET). A recent study [105] revealed that in patients who have OTC for an extended period, there is an elevated level of resting MBF), coupled with a diminished coronary flow reserve (CFR), indicating a reduced ability to respond to stress, likely due to impaired vasodilation. This impairment is further exacerbated by the presence of CAV. Rb-PET was also shown to have prognostic significance, as serial evaluation of CFR independently predicted late mortality in OTC patients [106].

Interestingly, in a small retrospective study, quantitative coronary wall assessment and plaque analysis allowed for the early detection of CAV not detected by ICA [107]. Finally, Budde et al. demonstrated that 25% of OTC patients with focal stenosis >30% showed a low value of FFR-CT. Even without a focal stenosis, FFR-CT values were often found to be abnormal in Htx patients [108]. Table 7 describes the timing and role of different imaging modalities in OCT.

Table 7. Timing and role of TTE (transthoracic echocardiography), advanced echocardiography, and CCT (cardiac computed tomography) in HT (heart transplant) patients.

	TTE	Advanced Echo	CMR	CT	Nuclear Imaging
Role	LV wall thickness and mass. LV volume and function. Diastolic function. Valve morphology and function. Pericardium.	LV torsion (speckle tracking). Cardiac ischemia (stress echocardiography).	LV wall thickness and mass. LV volume and function. Myocardial perfusion reserve (stress).	Coronary stenosis. Coronary plaque.	Myocardial blood flow Myocardial blood flow reserve
Timing	Immediate post-operative. Short-term period. Long-term period.	Short-term period. Long-term period.	Short-term period. Long-term period	Short-term period. Long-term period.	Short-term period. Long-term period.
Identification of complications	Allograft rejection. Primary or secondary valvopathies. Pericardial effusion.	Acute cell rejection. Cardiac allograft vasculopathy.	Acute cell rejection. Cardiac allograft vasculopathy.	Cardiac allograft vasculopathy.	Cardiac allograft vasculopathy. Microvascular vasculopathy

TTE = transthoracic echocardiography, TEE = transesophageal echocardiography, CCT = cardiac computed tomography, LV = left ventricular.

3. Conclusions (Take Home Messages) and Future Perspectives

This paper aims to highlight the steady advances in multimodality imaging techniques in AHF, which offer a unique opportunity for a comprehensive evaluation of such complex scenarios. In this literature review, we aim to suggest a practical, stepwise algorithm with an integrative multimodality imaging approach for the better assessment of underlying mechanisms, patterns of progression and possible complications in patients with end-stage HF and supported with short- or long-term MSD. Finally, we did not include in the present review BiVAD and TAH, aiming to provide some reflections on this future direction. Device-based therapies for HF with preserved or mildly reduced EF, encompassing atrial shunts, LV expanders, electrical and neurostimulators, and MCS devices, are still under development or used in clinical trials. These innovative approaches show promise in potentially revolutionizing HF management, offering hope for enhanced patient survival and improved quality of life. Moreover, the role of new imaging markers such as the pericoronary fat attenuation index (pFAI) in predicting cardiovascular outcomes and CAV in TCO patients should be investigated in prospective studies.

Author Contributions: Conceptualization, V.P. and G.P.; methodology, V.P., M.P.M. and G.M.; validation, S.I. and P.P.F.; writing—original draft preparation, F.A., C.M.D., M.C.P. and G.M.; writing—review and editing, S.M., M.C., A.I.G. and R.M.; visualization, S.N.; supervision, S.D., A.D. and R.P. All authors have read and agreed to the published version of the manuscript.

Funding: This research received no external funding.

Data Availability Statement: Not applicable.

Acknowledgments: We thank Laura Evangelista for her support.

Conflicts of Interest: The authors declare no conflict of interest.

References

1. McDonagh, T.A.; Metra, M.; Adamo, M.; Gardner, R.S.; Baumbach, A.; Böhm, M.; Burri, H.; Butler, J.; Čelutkienė, J.; Chioncel, O.; et al. 2021 ESC Guidelines for the diagnosis and treatment of acute and chronic heart failure. *Eur. Heart J.* **2021**, *42*, 3599–3726, Erratum in *Eur. Heart J.* **2021**, *42*, 4901. [CrossRef] [PubMed]
2. Heidenreich, P.A.; Bozkurt, B.; Aguilar, D.; Allen, L.A.; Byun, J.J.; Colvin, M.M.; Deswal, A.; Drazner, M.H.; Dunlay, S.M.; Evers, L.R.; et al. 2022 AHA/ACC/HFSA Guideline for the Management of Heart Failure: A Report of the American College of Cardiology/American Heart Association Joint Committee on Clinical Practice Guidelines. *Circulation* **2022**, *145*, E895–E1032, Erratum in *Circulation* **2022**, *145*, e1033; Erratum in *Circulation* **2022**, *146*, e185; Erratum in *Circulation* **2023**, *147*, e674. [CrossRef]
3. Savarese, G.; Lund, L.H. Global Public Health Burden of Heart Failure. *Card. Fail. Rev.* **2017**, *3*, 7–11. [CrossRef] [PubMed]
4. Xanthakis, V.; Enserro, D.M.; Larson, M.G.; Wollert, K.C.; Januzzi, J.L.; Levy, D.; Aragam, J.; Benjamin, E.J.; Cheng, S.; Wang, T.J.; et al. Prevalence, Neurohormonal Correlates, and Prognosis of Heart Failure Stages in the Community. *JACC Heart Fail.* **2016**, *4*, 808–815. [CrossRef] [PubMed]
5. Giannitsi, S.; Bougiakli, M.; Bechlioulis, A.; Kotsia, A.; Michalis, L.K.; Naka, K.K. 6-minute walking test: A useful tool in the management of heart failure patients. *Ther. Adv. Cardiovasc. Dis.* **2019**, *13*, 1753944719870084. [CrossRef] [PubMed]
6. Dunlay, S.M.; Roger, V.L.; Killian, J.M.; Weston, S.A.; Schulte, P.J.; Subramaniam, A.V.; Blecker, S.B.; Redfield, M.M. Advanced Heart Failure Epidemiology and Outcomes: A Population-Based Study. *JACC Heart Fail.* **2021**, *9*, 722–732. [CrossRef]
7. Subramaniam, A.V.; Weston, S.A.; Killian, J.M.; Schulte, P.J.; Roger, V.L.; Redfield, M.M.; Blecker, S.B.; Dunlay, S.M. Development of Advanced Heart Failure: A Population-Based Study. *Circ. Heart Fail.* **2022**, *15*, e009218. [CrossRef]
8. Francis, G.S.; Bartos, J.A.; Adatya, S. Inotropes. *J. Am. Coll. Cardiol.* **2014**, *63*, 2069–2078. [CrossRef]
9. Kittleson, M.M.; Shah, P.; Lala, A.; McLean, R.C.; Pamboukian, S.; Horstmanshof, D.A.; Thibodeau, J.; Shah, K.; Teuteberg, J.; Gilotra, N.A.; et al. INTERMACS profiles and outcomes of ambulatory advanced heart failure patients: A report from the REVIVAL Registry. *J. Heart Lung Transplant.* **2019**, *39*, 16–26. [CrossRef]
10. Barge-Caballero, E.; Almenar-Bonet, L.; Gonzalez-Vilchez, F.; Lambert-Rodríguez, J.L.; González-Costello, J.; Segovia-Cubero, J.; Castel-Lavilla, M.A.; Delgado-Jiménez, J.; Garrido-Bravo, I.P.; Rangel-Sousa, D.; et al. Clinical outcomes of temporary mechanical circulatory support as a direct bridge to heart transplantation: A nationwide Spanish registry. *Eur. J. Heart Fail.* **2017**, *20*, 178–186. [CrossRef]
11. Mehra, M.M.R.; Cleveland, J.C., Jr.; Uriel, N.; Cowger, J.A.; Hall, S.; Horstmanshof, D.; Naka, Y.; Salerno, C.T.; Chuang, J.; Msc, C.W.; et al. Primary results of long-term outcomes in the MOMENTUM 3 pivotal trial and continued access protocol study phase: A study of 2200 HeartMate 3 left ventricular assist device implants. *Eur. J. Heart Fail.* **2021**, *23*, 1392–1400. [CrossRef]
12. Cameli, M.; Pastore, M.C.; Campora, A.; Lisi, M.; Mandoli, G.E. Donor shortage in heart transplantation: How can we overcome this challenge? *Front. Cardiovasc. Med.* **2022**, *9*, 1001002. [CrossRef]
13. Dandel, M.; Javier, M.F.d.M.; Delmo, E.M.d.J.; Hetzer, R. Accurate assessment of right heart function before and after long-term left ventricular assist device implantation. *Expert Rev. Cardiovasc. Ther.* **2020**, *18*, 289–308. [CrossRef] [PubMed]
14. Kapur, N.K.; Esposito, M.L.; Bader, Y.; Morine, K.J.; Kiernan, M.S.; Pham, D.T.; Burkhoff, D. Mechanical Circulatory Support Devices for Acute Right Ventricular Failure. *Circulation* **2017**, *136*, 314–326. [CrossRef] [PubMed]
15. Shehab, S.; Hayward, C.S. Choosing Between Left Ventricular Assist Devices and Biventricular Assist Devices. *Card. Fail. Rev.* **2019**, *5*, 19–23. [CrossRef]
16. Mehra, M.R.; Canter, C.E.; Hannan, M.M.; Semigran, M.J.; Uber, P.A.; Baran, D.A.; Danziger-Isakov, L.; Kirklin, J.K.; Kirk, R.; Kushwaha, S.S.; et al. The 2016 International Society for Heart Lung Transplantation listing criteria for heart transplantation: A 10-year update. *J. Heart Lung Transplant.* **2016**, *35*, 1–23. [CrossRef] [PubMed]
17. Oras, J.; Doueh, R.; Norberg, E.; Redfors, B.; Omerovic, E.; Dellgren, G. Left ventricular dysfunction in potential heart donors and its influence on recipient outcomes. *J. Thorac. Cardiovasc. Surg.* **2020**, *159*, 1333–1341.e6. [CrossRef] [PubMed]
18. Hassan, O.K.A.; Higgins, A.R. The role of multimodality imaging in patients with heart failure with reduced and preserved ejection fraction. *Curr. Opin. Cardiol.* **2022**, *37*, 285–293. [CrossRef] [PubMed]

19. Porter, T.R.; Xie, F. Contrast Echocardiography: Latest Developments and Clinical Utility. *Curr. Cardiol. Rep.* **2015**, *17*, 569. [CrossRef]
20. Lang, R.M.; Badano, L.P.; Mor-Avi, V.; Afilalo, J.; Armstrong, A.; Ernande, L.; Flachskampf, F.A.; Foster, E.; Goldstein, S.A.; Kuznetsova, T.; et al. Recommendations for Cardiac Chamber Quantification by Echocardiography in Adults: An Update from the American Society of Echocardiography and the European Association of Cardiovascular Imaging. *Eur. Heart J. Cardiovasc. Imaging* **2015**, *16*, 233–270, Erratum in *Eur. Heart J. Cardiovasc.* **2016**, *17*, 412. Erratum in *Eur. Heart J. Cardiovasc.* **2016**, *17*, 969. [CrossRef]
21. Takada, T.; Nakata, Y.; Matsuura, K.; Minami, Y.; Kishihara, M.; Watanabe, S.; Shirotani, S.; Abe, T.; Yoshida, A.; Hasegawa, S.; et al. Left Ventricular End-Systolic Diameter May Predict Persistent Heart Failure with Reduced Ejection Fraction. *Int. Heart J.* **2023**, *64*, 1095–1104. [CrossRef] [PubMed]
22. Mandoli, G.E.; Benfari, G.; Baggiano, A.; Florea, R.; Cameli, M. Editorial: Advances in cardiac imaging and heart failure management. *Front. Cardiovasc. Med.* **2023**, *9*, 1095829. [CrossRef]
23. Sugimoto, T.; Dulgheru, R.; Bernard, A.; Ilardi, F.; Contu, L.; Addetia, K.; Caballero, L.; Akhaladze, N.; Athanassopoulos, G.D.; Barone, D.; et al. Echocardiographic reference ranges for normal left ventricular 2D strain: Results from the EACVI NORRE study. *Eur. Heart J. Cardiovasc. Imaging* **2017**, *18*, 833–840. [CrossRef]
24. Karlsen, S.; Dahlslett, T.; Grenne, B.; Sjøli, B.; Smiseth, O.; Edvardsen, T.; Brunvand, H. Global longitudinal strain is a more reproducible measure of left ventricular function than ejection fraction regardless of echocardiographic training. *Cardiovasc. Ultrasound* **2019**, *17*, 18. [CrossRef] [PubMed]
25. Galderisi, M.; Cosyns, B.; Edvardsen, T.; Cardim, N.; Delgado, V.; Di Salvo, G.; Donal, E.; Sade, L.E.; Ernande, L.; Garbi, M.; et al. Standardization of adult transthoracic echocardiography reporting in agreement with recent chamber quantification, diastolic function, and heart valve disease recommendations: An expert consensus document of the European association of cardiovascular imaging. *Eur. Heart J. Cardiovasc. Imaging* **2017**, *18*, 1301–1310. [CrossRef] [PubMed]
26. Pastore, M.C.; Mandoli, G.E.; Aboumarie, H.S.; Santoro, C.; Bandera, F.; D'andrea, A.; Benfari, G.; Esposito, R.; Evola, V.; Sorrentino, R.; et al. Basic and advanced echocardiography in advanced heart failure: An overview. *Heart Fail. Rev.* **2020**, *25*, 937–948. [CrossRef]
27. Nagueh, S.F.; Smiseth, O.A.; Appleton, C.P.; Byrd, B.F., 3rd; Dokainish, H.; Edvardsen, T.; Flachskampf, F.A.; Gillebert, T.C.; Klein, A.L.; Lancellotti, P.; et al. Recommendations for the Evaluation of Left Ventricular Diastolic Function by Echocardiography: An Update from the American Society of Echocardiography and the European Association of Cardiovascular Imaging. *J. Am. Soc. Echocardiogr.* **2016**, *29*, 277–314. [CrossRef] [PubMed]
28. Bech-Hanssen, O.; Pergola, V.; Al-Admawi, M.; Fadel, B.M.; Di Salvo, G. Atrial function in heart transplant recipients operated with the bicaval technique. *Scand. Cardiovasc. J.* **2016**, *50*, 42–51. [CrossRef]
29. Carluccio, E.; Biagioli, P.; Lauciello, R.; Zuchi, C.; Mengoni, A.; Bardelli, G.; Alunni, G.; Gronda, E.G.; Ambrosio, G. Superior Prognostic Value of Right Ventricular Free Wall Compared to Global Longitudinal Strain in Patients with Heart Failure. *J. Am. Soc. Echocardiogr.* **2019**, *32*, 836–844.e1. [CrossRef]
30. Mauro, C.; Chianese, S.; Cocchia, R.; Arcopinto, M.; Auciello, S.; Capone, V.; Carafa, M.; Carbone, A.; Caruso, G.; Castaldo, R.; et al. Acute Heart Failure: Diagnostic–Therapeutic Pathways and Preventive Strategies—A Real-World Clinician's Guide. *J. Clin. Med.* **2023**, *12*, 846. [CrossRef]
31. Via, G.; Hussain, A.; Wells, M.; Reardon, R.; ElBarbary, M.; Noble, V.E.; Tsung, J.W.; Neskovic, A.N.; Price, S.; Oren-Grinberg, A.; et al. International Evidence-Based Recommendations for Focused Cardiac Ultrasound. *J. Am. Soc. Echocardiogr.* **2014**, *27*, 683.e1–683.e33. [CrossRef]
32. Gargani, L. Ultrasound of the Lungs. *Heart Fail. Clin.* **2019**, *15*, 297–303. [CrossRef] [PubMed]
33. Pellicori, P.; Platz, E.; Dauw, J.; ter Maaten, J.M.; Martens, P.; Pivetta, E.; Cleland, J.G.; McMurray, J.J.; Mullens, W.; Solomon, S.D.; et al. Ultrasound imaging of congestion in heart failure: Examinations beyond the heart. *Eur. J. Heart Fail.* **2021**, *23*, 703–712. [CrossRef]
34. Coiro, S.; Rossignol, P.; Ambrosio, G.; Carluccio, E.; Alunni, G.; Murrone, A.; Tritto, I.; Zannad, F.; Girerd, N. Prognostic value of residual pulmonary congestion at discharge assessed by lung ultrasound imaging in heart failure. *Eur. J. Heart Fail.* **2015**, *17*, 1172–1181. [CrossRef]
35. Contaldi, C.; Dellegrottaglie, S.; Mauro, C.; Ferrara, F.; Romano, L.; Marra, A.M.; Ranieri, B.; Salzano, A.; Rega, S.; Scatteia, A.; et al. Role of Cardiac Magnetic Resonance Imaging in Heart Failure. *Heart Fail. Clin.* **2021**, *17*, 207–221. [CrossRef] [PubMed]
36. Vöhringer, M.; Mahrholdt, H.; Yilmaz, A.; Sechtem, U. Significance of Late Gadolinium Enhancement in Cardiovascular Magnetic Resonance Imaging (CMR). *Herz* **2007**, *32*, 129–137. [CrossRef] [PubMed]
37. Memon, S.; Ganga, H.V.; Kluger, J. Late Gadolinium Enhancement in Patients with Nonischemic Dilated Cardiomyopathy. *Pacing Clin. Electrophysiol.* **2016**, *39*, 731–747. [CrossRef]
38. Aquaro, G.D.; De Gori, C.; Faggioni, L.; Parisella, M.L.; Cioni, D.; Lencioni, R.; Neri, E. Diagnostic and prognostic role of late gadolinium enhancement in cardiomyopathies. *Eur. Heart J. Suppl.* **2023**, *25*, C130–C136. [CrossRef]
39. Nagueh, S.F.; Nabi, F.; Chang, S.M.; Al-Mallah, M.; Shah, D.J.; Bhimaraj, A. Imaging for implementation of heart failure guidelines. *Eur. Heart J. Cardiovasc. Imaging* **2023**, *24*, 1283–1292. [CrossRef] [PubMed]

40. Karamitsos, T.D.; Piechnik, S.K.; Banypersad, S.M.; Fontana, M.; Ntusi, N.B.; Ferreira, V.M.; Whelan, C.J.; Myerson, S.G.; Robson, M.D.; Hawkins, P.N.; et al. Noncontrast T1 Mapping for the Diagnosis of Cardiac Amyloidosis. *JACC Cardiovasc. Imaging* **2013**, *6*, 488–497. [CrossRef]
41. Markatis, E.; Afthinos, A.; Antonakis, E.; Papanikolaou, I.C. Cardiac sarcoidosis: Diagnosis and management. *Rev. Cardiovasc. Med.* **2020**, *21*, 321–338. [CrossRef] [PubMed]
42. Child, N.M.; Das, R. Is cardiac magnetic resonance imaging assessment of myocardial viability useful for predicting which patients with impaired ventricles might benefit from revascularization? *Interact. Cardiovasc. Thorac. Surg.* **2012**, *14*, 395–398. [CrossRef] [PubMed]
43. Katikireddy, C.K.; Samim, A. Myocardial viability assessment and utility in contemporary management of ischemic cardiomyopathy. *Clin. Cardiol.* **2022**, *45*, 152–161. [CrossRef] [PubMed]
44. Aziz, W.; Claridge, S.; Ntalas, I.; Gould, J.; de Vecchi, A.; Razeghi, O.; Toth, D.; Mountney, P.; Preston, R.; Rinaldi, C.A.; et al. Emerging role of cardiac computed tomography in heart failure. *ESC Heart Fail.* **2019**, *6*, 909–920. [CrossRef]
45. Ramanathan, R.; Anumandla, A.K.; Haramati, L.B.; Spevack, D.M.; Godelman, A.; Jain, V.R.; Kazam, J.; Burton, W.B.; Levsky, J.M. Evaluation of the Cardiac Chambers on Axial CT. *J. Comput. Assist. Tomogr.* **2014**, *38*, 53–60. [CrossRef] [PubMed]
46. Taylor, A.J.; Cerqueira, M.; Hodgson, J.M.; Mark, D.; Min, J.; O'Gara, P.; Rubin, G.D.; Kramer, C.M.; Berman, D.; Brown, A.; et al. ACCF/SCCT/ACR/AHA/ASE/ASNC/NASCI/SCAI/SCMR 2010 Appropriate Use Criteria for Cardiac Computed Tomography. *J. Cardiovasc. Comput. Tomogr.* **2010**, *4*, 407.e1–407.e33. [CrossRef]
47. Penso, M.; Babbaro, M.; Moccia, S.; Baggiano, A.; Carerj, M.L.; Guglielmo, M.; Fusini, L.; Mushtaq, S.; Andreini, D.; Pepi, M.; et al. A deep-learning approach for myocardial fibrosis detection in early contrast-enhanced cardiac CT images. *Front. Cardiovasc. Med.* **2023**, *10*, 1151705. [CrossRef] [PubMed]
48. Treibel, T.A.; Bandula, S.; Fontana, M.; White, S.K.; Gilbertson, J.A.; Herrey, A.S.; Gillmore, J.D.; Punwani, S.; Hawkins, P.N.; Taylor, S.A.; et al. Extracellular volume quantification by dynamic equilibrium cardiac computed tomography in cardiac amyloidosis. *J. Cardiovasc. Comput. Tomogr.* **2015**, *9*, 585–592. [CrossRef]
49. Baggiano, A.; Conte, E.; Spiritigliozzi, L.; Mushtaq, S.; Annoni, A.; Carerj, M.L.; Cilia, F.; Fazzari, F.; Formenti, A.; Frappampina, A.; et al. Quantification of extracellular volume with cardiac computed tomography in patients with dilated cardiomyopathy. *J. Cardiovasc. Comput. Tomogr.* **2023**, *17*, 261–268. [CrossRef]
50. Selvakumar, D.; Brown, P.; Geenty, P.; Barnett, R.; AB Saunders, C.; Altman, M.; Thomas, L. Comparative Assessments of Left and Right Ventricular Function by Two-Dimensional, Contrast Enhanced and Three-Dimensional Echocardiography with Gated Heart Pool Scans in Patients Following Myocardial Infarction. *Am. J. Cardiol.* **2020**, *134*, 14–23. [CrossRef]
51. Printezi, M.I.; Yousif, L.I.E.; Kamphuis, J.A.M.; van Laake, L.W.; Cramer, M.J.; Hobbelink, M.G.G.; Asselbergs, F.W.; Teske, A.J. LVEF by Multigated Acquisition Scan Compared to Other Imaging Modalities in Cardio-Oncology: A Systematic Review. *Curr. Heart Fail. Rep.* **2022**, *19*, 136–145. [CrossRef] [PubMed]
52. Mittal, B.R.; Santhosh, S.; Kashyap, R.; Bhattacharya, A.; Singh, B.; Bahl, A. Ventricular ejection fraction in patients with dilated cardiomyopathy calculated by gated blood pool SPET processing software: Correlation with multigated acquisition and first pass radionuclide ventriculography. *Hell. J. Nucl. Med.* **2011**, *14*, 234–238. [PubMed]
53. Xie, B.-Q.; Tian, Y.-Q.; Zhang, J.; Zhao, S.-H.; Yang, M.-F.; Guo, F.; Wang, D.-Y.; Wei, H.-X.; Chu, K.-W.; He, Z.-X. Evaluation of Left and Right Ventricular Ejection Fraction and Volumes from Gated Blood-Pool SPECT in Patients with Dilated Cardiomyopathy: Comparison with Cardiac MRI. *J. Nucl. Med.* **2012**, *53*, 584–591. [CrossRef] [PubMed]
54. Odak, M.; Kayani, W.T. MUGA Scan. In *StatPearls*; StatPearls Publishing: Treasure Island, FL, USA, 2023.
55. Mangla, A.; Oliveros, E.; Williams, K.A.; Kalra, D.K. Cardiac Imaging in the Diagnosis of Coronary Artery Disease. *Curr. Probl. Cardiol.* **2017**, *42*, 316–366. [CrossRef] [PubMed]
56. Miller, T.D.; Askew, J.W.; Anavekar, N.S. Noninvasive Stress Testing for Coronary Artery Disease. *Heart Fail. Clin.* **2016**, *12*, 65–82. [CrossRef]
57. Agdamag, A.C.; Riad, S.; Maharaj, V.; Jackson, S.; Fraser, M.D.; Charpentier, V.B.; Nzemenoh, B.; Martin, C.M.; Alexy, T. Temporary Mechanical Circulatory Support Use and Clinical Outcomes of Simultaneous Heart/Kidney Transplant Recipients in the Pre- and Post-Heart Allocation Policy Change Eras. *Transplantation* **2023**, *107*, 1605–1614. [CrossRef]
58. Randhawa, V.K.; Al-Fares, A.; Tong, M.Z.; Soltesz, E.G.; Hernandez-Montfort, J.; Taimeh, Z.; Weiss, A.J.; Menon, V.; Campbell, J.; Cremer, P.; et al. A Pragmatic Approach to Weaning Temporary Mechanical Circulatory Support. *JACC Heart Fail.* **2021**, *9*, 664–673. [CrossRef]
59. Zein, R.; Patel, C.; Mercado-Alamo, A.; Schreiber, T.; Kaki, A. A Review of the Impella Devices. *Interv. Cardiol.* **2022**, *17*, e05. [CrossRef]
60. Sef, D.; Kabir, T.; Lees, N.J.; Stock, U. Valvular complications following the Impella device implantation. *J. Card. Surg.* **2021**, *36*, 1062–1066. [CrossRef]
61. Anand, S.; Barry, T.; Arsanjani, R.; LeMond, L. Echocardiography in Cardiac Assist Devices. *Rev. Cardiovasc. Med.* **2022**, *23*, 253. [CrossRef]
62. Crowley, J.; Cronin, B.; Essandoh, M.; D'Alessandro, D.; Shelton, K.; Dalia, A.A. Transesophageal Echocardiography for Impella Placement and Management. *J. Cardiothorac. Vasc. Anesthesia* **2019**, *33*, 2663–2668. [CrossRef] [PubMed]
63. Pieri, M.; Pappalardo, F. Bedside insertion of impella percutaneous ventricular assist device in patients with cardiogenic shock. *Int. J. Cardiol.* **2020**, *316*, 26–30. [CrossRef]

64. Yastrebov, K.; Brunel, L.; Paterson, H.S.; Williams, Z.A.; Wise, I.K.; Burrows, C.S.; Bannon, P.G. Implantation of Impella CP left ventricular assist device under the guidance of three-dimensional intracardiac echocardiography. *Sci. Rep.* **2020**, *10*, 17485, Erratum in *Sci. Rep.* **2021**, *11*, 5091. [CrossRef]
65. Nakao, Y.; Aono, J.; Namiguchi, K.; Nishimura, T.; Izutani, H.; Higashi, H.; Inaba, S.; Nishimura, K.; Inoue, K.; Ikeda, S.; et al. Usefulness of contrast computed tomography for diagnosing left ventricular thrombus before impella insertion. *J. Cardiol. Cases* **2020**, *22*, 291–293. [CrossRef] [PubMed]
66. Swedzky, F.; Barbagelata, A.; Perrone, S.; Kaplinsky, E.; Ducharme, A. Emerging concepts in heart failure management and treatment: Circulatory support with extracorporeal membrane oxygenation (ECMO). *Drugs Context* **2023**, *12*, 2022-7-7. [CrossRef] [PubMed]
67. Hockstein, M.A.; Singam, N.S.; Papolos, A.I.; Kenigsberg, B.B. The Role of Echocardiography in Extracorporeal Membrane Oxygenation. *Curr. Cardiol. Rep.* **2023**, *25*, 9–16. [CrossRef]
68. Tian, L.; Zhang, S.; Xu, J.; Han, X. Extracorporeal Membrane Oxygenation as a Bridge between Transfer and Perioperative Periods in Refractory Cardiogenic Shock Secondary to a Large Left Atrial Myxoma. *Heart Surg. Forum* **2021**, *24*, E215–E216. [CrossRef]
69. Ostadal, P.; Vondrakova, D.; Popkova, M.; Hrachovina, M.; Kruger, A.; Janotka, M.; Naar, J.; Kittnar, O.; Neuzil, P.; Mlcek, M. Aortic stenosis and mitral regurgitation modify the effect of venoarterial extracorporeal membrane oxygenation on left ventricular function in cardiogenic shock. *Sci. Rep.* **2022**, *12*, 17076. [CrossRef]
70. Platts, D.G.; Sedgwick, J.F.; Burstow, D.J.; Mullany, D.V.; Fraser, J.F. The Role of Echocardiography in the Management of Patients Supported by Extracorporeal Membrane Oxygenation. *J. Am. Soc. Echocardiogr.* **2012**, *25*, 131–141, Erratum in *J. Am. Soc. Echocardiogr.* **2012**, *25*, 427. [CrossRef]
71. Kim, D.; Jang, W.J.; Park, T.K.; Cho, Y.H.; Choi, J.-O.; Jeon, E.-S.; Yang, J.H. Echocardiographic Predictors of Successful Extracorporeal Membrane Oxygenation Weaning After Refractory Cardiogenic Shock. *J. Am. Soc. Echocardiogr.* **2021**, *34*, 414–422.e4. [CrossRef]
72. Lee, S.; Chaturvedi, A. Imaging adults on extracorporeal membrane oxygenation (ECMO). *Insights Imaging* **2014**, *5*, 731–742. [CrossRef] [PubMed]
73. Stainback, R.F.; Estep, J.D.; Agler, D.A.; Birks, E.J.; Bremer, M.; Hung, J.; Kirkpatrick, J.N.; Rogers, J.G.; Shah, N.R. Echocardiography in the Management of Patients with Left Ventricular Assist Devices: Recommendations from the American Society of Echocardiography. *J. Am. Soc. Echocardiogr.* **2015**, *28*, 853–909. [CrossRef] [PubMed]
74. Vriz, O.; Mushtaq, A.; Shaik, A.; El-Shaer, A.; Feras, K.; Eltayeb, A.; Alsergnai, H.; Kholaif, N.; Al Hussein, M.; Albert-Brotons, D.; et al. Reciprocal interferences of the left ventricular assist device and the aortic valve competence. *Front. Cardiovasc. Med.* **2023**, *9*, 1094796. [CrossRef] [PubMed]
75. Pergola, V.; Tarzia, V.; Baroni, G.; Iliceto, S.; Gerosa, G.; Mele, D. Utilization of an Ultrasound-Enhancing Agent Improves the Evaluation of the Right Ventricle in Patients with Left Ventricular Assist Device. *J. Am. Soc. Echocardiogr.* **2022**, *36*, 337–339. [CrossRef] [PubMed]
76. Almarzooq, Z.I.; Varshney, A.S.; Vaduganathan, M.; Pareek, M.; Stewart, G.C.; Estep, J.D.; Mehra, M.R. Expanding the Scope of Multimodality Imaging in Durable Mechanical Circulatory Support. *JACC Cardiovasc. Imaging* **2020**, *13*, 1069–1081. [CrossRef] [PubMed]
77. Pontone, G.; Rossi, A.; Guglielmo, M.; Dweck, M.R.; Gaemperli, O.; Nieman, K.; Pugliese, F.; Maurovich-Horvat, P.; Gimelli, A.; Cosyns, B.; et al. Clinical applications of cardiac computed tomography: A consensus paper of the European Association of Cardiovascular Imaging—Part I. *Eur. Heart J. Cardiovasc. Imaging* **2022**, *23*, 299–314, Erratum in *Eur. Heart J. Cardiovasc. Imaging* **2022**, *23*, e274. [CrossRef] [PubMed]
78. Shroff, G.S.; Ocazionez, D.; Akkanti, B.; Vargas, D.; Garza, A.; Gupta, P.; Patel, J.A.; Patel, M.K.; Gregoric, I.D. CT Imaging of Complications Associated with Continuous-Flow Left Ventricular Assist Devices (LVADs). In *Seminars in Ultrasound, CT and MRI*; WB Saunders: Philadelphia, PA, USA, 2017; Volume 38, pp. 616–628. [CrossRef]
79. Masarone, D.; Kittleson, M.; Gravino, R.; Valente, F.; Petraio, A.; Pacileo, G. The Role of Echocardiography in the Management of Heart Transplant Recipients. *Diagnostics* **2021**, *11*, 2338. [CrossRef]
80. Khush, K.K.; Cherikh, W.S.; Chambers, D.C.; Harhay, M.O.; Hayes, D.; Hsich, E.; Meiser, B.; Potena, L.; Robinson, A.; Rossano, J.W.; et al. The International Thoracic Organ Transplant Registry of the International Society for Heart and Lung Transplantation: Thirty-sixth adult heart transplantation report—2019; focus theme: Donor and recipient size match. *J. Heart Lung Transplant.* **2019**, *38*, 1056–1066, Erratum in *J. Heart Lung Transplant.* **2020**, *39*, 91. [CrossRef]
81. Bech-Hanssen, O.; Al-Habeeb, W.; Ahmed, W.; Di Salvo, G.; Pergola, V.; Al-Admawi, M.; Al-Amri, M.; Al-Shahid, M.; Al-Buraiki, J.; Fadel, B.M. Echocardiography Detects Elevated Left Ventricular Filling Pressures in Heart Transplant Recipients. *Echocardiography* **2015**, *32*, 411–419. [CrossRef]
82. Badano, L.P.; Miglioranza, M.H.; Edvardsen, T.; Colafranceschi, A.S.; Muraru, D.; Bacal, F.; Nieman, K.; Zoppellaro, G.; Braga, F.G.M.; Binder, T.; et al. European Association of Cardiovascular Imaging/Cardiovascular Imaging Department of the Brazilian Society of Cardiology recommendations for the use of cardiac imaging to assess and follow patients after heart transplantation. *Eur. Heart J. Cardiovasc. Imaging* **2015**, *16*, 919–948. [CrossRef]
83. Narang, A.; Blair, J.E.; Patel, M.B.; Mor-Avi, V.; Fedson, S.E.; Uriel, N.; Lang, R.M.; Patel, A.R. Myocardial perfusion reserve and global longitudinal strain as potential markers of coronary allograft vasculopathy in late-stage orthotopic heart transplantation. *Int. J. Cardiovasc. Imaging* **2018**, *34*, 1607–1617. [CrossRef]

84. Mingo-Santos, S.; Moñivas-Palomero, V.; Garcia-Lunar, I.; Mitroi, C.D.; Goirigolzarri-Artaza, J.; Rivero, B.; Oteo, J.F.; Castedo, E.; González-Mirelis, J.; Cavero, M.A.; et al. Usefulness of Two-Dimensional Strain Parameters to Diagnose Acute Rejection after Heart Transplantation. *J. Am. Soc. Echocardiogr.* **2015**, *28*, 1149–1156. [CrossRef] [PubMed]
85. Ruiz Ortiz, M.; Peña, M.L.; Mesa, D.; Delgado, M.; Romo, E.; Santisteban, M.; Puentes, M.; López Granados, A.; Castillo, J.C.; Arizón, J.M.; et al. Impact of asymptomatic acute cellular rejection on left ventricle myocardial function evaluated by means of two-dimensional speckle tracking echocardiography in heart transplant recipients. *Echocardiography* **2015**, *32*, 229. [CrossRef] [PubMed]
86. Sato, T.; Kato, T.S.; Kamamura, K.; Hashimoto, S.; Shishido, T.; Mano, A.; Oda, N.; Takahashi, A.; Ishibashi-Ueda, H.; Nakatani, T.; et al. Utility of left ventricular systolic torsion derived from 2-dimensional speckle-tracking echocardiography in monitoring acute cellular rejection in heart transplant recipients. *J. Heart Lung Transplant.* **2011**, *30*, 536. [CrossRef] [PubMed]
87. Elkaryoni, A.; Abu-Sheasha, G.; Altibi, A.M.; Hassan, A.; Ellakany, K.; Nanda, N.C. Diagnostic accuracy of dobutamine stress echocardiography in the detection of cardiac allograft vasculopathy in heart transplant recipients: A systematic review and meta-analysis study. *Echocardiography* **2019**, *36*, 528–536. [CrossRef] [PubMed]
88. Eroglu, E.; D'Hooge, J.; Sutherland, G.R.; Marciniak, A.; Thijs, D.; Droogne, W.; Herbots, L.; Van Cleemput, J.; Claus, P.; Bijnens, B.; et al. Quantitative dobutamine stress echocardiography for the early detection of cardiac allograft vasculopathy in heart transplant recipients. *Heart* **2008**, *94*, e3. [CrossRef]
89. Tona, F.; Osto, E.; Tarantini, G.; Gambino, A.; Cavallin, F.; Feltrin, G.; Montisci, R.; Caforio, A.L.P.; Gerosa, G.; Iliceto, S. Coronary Flow Reserve by Transthoracic Echocardiography Predicts Epicardial Intimal Thickening in Cardiac Allograft Vasculopathy. *Am. J. Transplant.* **2010**, *10*, 1677–1685. [CrossRef]
90. Sade, L.E.; Hazirolan, T.; Kozan, H.; Ozdemir, H.; Hayran, M.; Eroglu, S.; Pirat, B.; Sezgin, A.; Muderrisoglu, H. T1 mapping by cardiac magnetic resonance and multidimensional speckle-tracking strain by echocardiography for the detection of acute cellular rejection in cardiac allograft recipients. *JACC Cardiovasc. Imaging* **2019**, *12 Pt 2*, 1601–1614. [CrossRef]
91. Vermes, E.; Pantaléon, C.; Auvet, A.; Cazeneuve, N.; Machet, M.C.; Delhommais, A.; Bourguignon, T.; Aupart, M.; Brunereau, L. Cardiovascular magnetic resonance in heart transplant patients: Diagnostic value of quantitative tissue markers: T2 mapping and extracellular volume fraction, for acute rejection diagnosis. *J. Cardiovasc. Magn. Reson.* **2018**, *20*, 59. [CrossRef] [PubMed]
92. Erbel, C.; Mukhammadaminova, N.; Gleissner, C.A.; Osman, N.F.; Hofmann, N.P.; Steuer, C.; Akhavanpoor, M.; Wangler, S.; Celik, S.; Doesch, A.O.; et al. Myocardial Perfusion Reserve and Strain-Encoded CMR for Evaluation of Cardiac Allograft Microvasculopathy. *JACC Cardiovasc. Imaging* **2016**, *9*, 255–266. [CrossRef]
93. Dolan, R.S.; Rahsepar, A.A.; Blaisdell, J.; Suwa, K.; Ghafourian, K.; Wilcox, J.E.; Khan, S.S.; Vorovich, E.E.; Rich, J.D.; Anderson, A.S.; et al. Multiparametric Cardiac Magnetic Resonance Imaging Can Detect Acute Cardiac Allograft Rejection After Heart Transplantation. *JACC Cardiovasc. Imaging* **2019**, *12*, 1632–1641. [CrossRef]
94. Shah, N.R.; Blankstein, R.; Villines, T.; Imran, H.; Morrison, A.R.; Cheezum, M.K. Coronary CTA for Surveillance of Cardiac Allograft Vasculopathy. *Curr. Cardiovasc. Imaging Rep.* **2018**, *11*, 26, Erratum in *Curr. Cardiovasc. Imaging Rep.* **2019**, *12*, 1. [CrossRef] [PubMed]
95. Wever-Pinzon, O.; Romero, J.; Kelesidis, I.; Wever-Pinzon, J.; Manrique, C.; Budge, D.; Drakos, S.G.; Piña, I.L.; Kfoury, A.G.; Garcia, M.J.; et al. Coronary Computed Tomography Angiography for the Detection of Cardiac Allograft Vasculopathy. *J. Am. Coll. Cardiol.* **2014**, *63*, 1992–2004. [CrossRef]
96. Günther, A.; Andersen, R.; Gude, E.; Jakobsen, J.; Edvardsen, T.; Sandvik, L.; Abildgaard, A.; Aaberge, L.; Gullestad, L. The predictive value of coronary artery calcium detected by computed tomography in a prospective study on cardiac allograft vasculopathy in heart transplant patients. *Transpl. Int.* **2018**, *31*, 82–91. [CrossRef] [PubMed]
97. Nous, F.M.A.; Roest, S.; Dijkman, E.D.; Attrach, M.; Caliskan, K.; Brugts, J.J.; Nieman, K.; Hirsch, A.; Constantinescu, A.A.; Manintveld, O.C.; et al. Clinical implementation of coronary computed tomography angiography for routine detection of cardiac allograft vasculopathy in heart transplant patients. *Transpl. Int.* **2021**, *34*, 1886–1894. [CrossRef] [PubMed]
98. Labarrere, C.A.; Patel, B.; Ahuja, A.; Kassab, G.S.; Labarrere, C.A. Diagnosis of cardiac allograft vasculopathy Challenges and opportunities. *Front. Biosci.* **2017**, *9*, 141–161. [CrossRef] [PubMed]
99. Wu, Y.-W.; Yen, R.-F.; Lee, C.-M.; Ho, Y.-L.; Chou, N.-K.; Wang, S.-S.; Huang, P.-J. Diagnostic and Prognostic Value of Dobutamine Thallium-201 Single-Photon Emission Computed Tomography After Heart Transplantation. *J. Heart Lung Transplant.* **2005**, *24*, 544–550. [CrossRef] [PubMed]
100. Veenis, J.F.; Boiten, H.J.; Berge, J.C.v.D.; Caliskan, K.; Maat, A.P.W.M.; Valkema, R.; Constantinescu, A.A.; Manintveld, O.C.; Zijlstra, F.; van Domburg, R.T.; et al. Prediction of long-term (>10 year) cardiovascular outcomes in heart transplant recipients: Value of stress technetium-99m tetrofosmin myocardial perfusion imaging. *J. Nucl. Cardiol.* **2019**, *26*, 845–852. [CrossRef]
101. Ko, K.-Y.; Ko, C.-L.; Lee, C.-M.; Cheng, J.-S.; Wu, Y.-W.; Hsu, R.-B.; Chen, Y.-S.; Wang, S.-S.; Yen, R.-F.; Cheng, M.-F. Myocardial Flow Assessment after Heart Transplantation Using Dynamic Cadmium-Zinc-Telluride Single-Photon Emission Computed Tomography with ^{201}Tl and ^{99m}Tc Tracers and Validated by ^{13}N-NH$_3$ Positron Emission Tomography. *Circ. Cardiovasc. Imaging* **2023**, *16*, e015034. [CrossRef]
102. Wu, Y.-W.; Chen, Y.-H.; Wang, S.-S.; Jui, H.-Y.; Yen, R.-F.; Tzen, K.-Y.; Chen, M.-F.; Lee, C.-M. PET Assessment of Myocardial Perfusion Reserve Inversely Correlates with Intravascular Ultrasound Findings in Angiographically Normal Cardiac Transplant Recipients. *J. Nucl. Med.* **2010**, *51*, 906–912. [CrossRef]

103. Lee, C.-M.; Wu, Y.-W.; Jui, H.-Y.; Yen, R.-F.; Tzen, K.-Y.; Chou, N.-K.; Wang, S.-S. Intravascular Ultrasound Correlates with Coronary Flow Reserve and Predicts the Survival in Angiographically Normal Cardiac Transplant Recipients. *Cardiology* **2008**, *109*, 93–98. [CrossRef]
104. Chih, S.; Chong, A.Y.; Erthal, F.; Dekemp, R.A.; Davies, R.A.; Stadnick, E.; So, D.Y.; Overgaard, C.; Wells, G.; Mielniczuk, L.M.; et al. PET Assessment of Epicardial Intimal Disease and Microvascular Dysfunction in Cardiac Allograft Vasculopathy. *J. Am. Coll. Cardiol.* **2018**, *71*, 1444–1456. [CrossRef] [PubMed]
105. Shrestha, U.M.; Sciammarella, M.; Pampaloni, M.H.; Botvinick, E.H.; Gullberg, G.T.; DeMarco, T.; Seo, Y. Assessment of late-term progression of cardiac allograft vasculopathy in patients with orthotopic heart transplantation using quantitative cardiac 82Rb PET. *Int. J. Cardiovasc. Imaging* **2021**, *37*, 1461–1472. [CrossRef] [PubMed]
106. Nelson, L.M.; Christensen, T.E.; Rossing, K.; Hasbak, P.; Gustafsson, F. Prognostic value of myocardial flow reserve obtained by 82-rubidium positron emission tomography in long-term follow-up after heart transplantation. *J. Nucl. Cardiol.* **2022**, *29*, 2555–2567. [CrossRef]
107. Miller, R.J.; Kwiecinski, J.; Shah, K.S.; Eisenberg, E.; Patel, J.; Kobashigawa, J.A.; Azarbal, B.; Tamarappoo, B.; Berman, D.S.; Slomka, P.J.; et al. Coronary computed tomography–angiography quantitative plaque analysis improves detection of early cardiac allograft vasculopathy: A pilot study. *Am. J. Transplant.* **2020**, *20*, 1375–1383. [CrossRef] [PubMed]
108. Budde, R.P.J.; Nous, F.M.A.; Roest, S.; Constantinescu, A.A.; Nieman, K.; Brugts, J.J.; Koweek, L.M.; Hirsch, A.; Leipsic, J.; Manintveld, O.C. CT-derived fractional flow reserve (FFRct) for functional coronary artery evaluation in the follow-up of patients after heart transplantation. *Eur. Radiol.* **2022**, *32*, 1843–1852. [CrossRef]

Journal of
Clinical Medicine

MDPI

Review

The Ross Procedure: Imaging, Outcomes and Future Directions in Aortic Valve Replacement

Domenico Galzerano [1,2,†], Naji Kholaif [1,2,*,†], Bandar Al Amro [1,2], Mohammed Al Admawi [1], Abdalla Eltayeb [1], Amal Alshammari [1], Giovanni Di Salvo [3] and Zohair Y. Al-Halees [1]

1 Heart Center Department, King Faisal Specialist Hospital and Research Center, Riyadh 11564, Saudi Arabia; domenicogalzerano@libero.it (D.G.); b.alamro@hotmail.com (B.A.A.); al-admawi@hotmail.com (M.A.A.); abdullaheltayeb2002@gmail.com (A.E.); amalmubarak888@gmail.com (A.A.); alhalees@kfshrc.edu.sa (Z.Y.A.-H.)
2 College of Medicine, Alfaisal University, Riyadh 11533, Saudi Arabia
3 Department of Cardiac, Thoracic, Vascular Sciences and Public Health, Medical School, University of Padua, 35122 Padua, Italy; giodisal@yahoo.it
* Correspondence: dr.kholaif@gmail.com
† These authors contributed equally to this work both are considered first authors.

Abstract: The Ross procedure is gaining recognition as a significant option for aortic valve replacement (AVR), and is particularly beneficial in specific patient groups. Although categorized as a class IIb recommendation in the 2020 American College of Cardiology (ACC)/American Heart Association (AHA), and the European Society of Cardiology (ESC) management guidelines on valvular heart disease, recent studies bolster its credibility. Research, including a propensity-matched study, underlines the Ross procedure's association with enhanced long-term survival and reduced adverse valve-related events compared to other AVR types. This positions the Ross procedure as a primary option for AVR in young and middle-aged adults within specialized centers, and potentially the only choice for children and infants requiring AVR. This review meticulously examines the Ross procedure, covering historical perspectives, surgical techniques, imaging, and outcomes, including hemodynamic performance and quality of life, especially focusing on pediatric and young adult patients. It explores contemporary techniques and innovations like minimally invasive approaches and tissue engineering, underscoring ongoing research and future directions. A summarization of comparative studies and meta-analyses reiterates the Ross procedure's superior long-term outcomes, valve durability, and preservation of the left ventricular function, accentuating the crucial role of patient selection and risk stratification, and pinpointing areas for future research.

Keywords: Ross procedure; prosthetic aortic valve; aortic valve replacement; valvular heart disease; adverse valve-related events; surgical techniques; valve imaging; valve hemodynamics; contemporary surgical techniques and innovations; tissue engineering

1. Introduction

The Ross procedure, also known as pulmonary autograft replacement of the aortic valve, is a surgical technique by which the patient's diseased valve is replaced by their own pulmonary valve (autograft). The used pulmonary valve is replaced by a pulmonary allograft or other suitable valve prosthesis. The rationale behind this procedure stems from the many advantages it offers. These include superior durability, better hemodynamics than any other aortic valve substitute, the potential for growth in younger patients and not requiring anticoagalation therapy with its well-known limitations. This translates into improved long-term outcomes and better quality of life [1,2].

The Ross procedure has gained significant attention as an alternative to other aortic value substitutes, particularly in young and active patients. The growth potential of the autograft valve makes it an attractive option for pediatric patents including infants and neonates requiring aortic valve replacement, potentially avoiding the need for repeat surgeries [3,4]. However, the Ross procedure is not without limitations. It is technically a demanding surgery that requires a skilled surgical team. It is associated with longer aortic cross-clamp and operative times compared to other aortic valve replacement procedures. Additionally, there is the risk of a replaced pulmonary valve dysfunction long-term, potentially necessitating a reoperation or percutaneous reintervention in some patients [5]. As a result of these concerns and despite the growing body of evidence showing the excellent long-term outcomes, the Ross procedure remains a class IIb recommendation in the most recent 2020 ACC/AHA and 2021 ESC guidelines on valvular heart disease [6,7].

The Ross procedure's usefulness has gained renewed interest after the publication of many studies including a propensity-matched study showing that it is associated with better long-term survival and freedom from adverse valve-related events compated to bioprosthetic or mechanical AVR. Therefore, in specialized cardiac centers with expertise, the Ross procedure can be considered the optimal option for adult and middle-aged adults undergoing AVR [8,9]. Needless to say, it may be the only option for infants and neonates requiring AVR for non-repairable aortic valve disease [4].

By examining the existing literature and synthesizing the available evidence, this review aims to shed light on the benefits, limitations, and appropriate patient selection for the Ross procedure. We hope that this will ultimately assist clinicians in making informed decisions regarding the utilization of the procedure in their clinical practice.

2. Historical Perspective

2.1. *Overview of the Development and Evolution of the Ross Procedure*

The Ross procedure, named after its pioneering surgeon Donald Ross, has undergone significant development and evolution since its inception. It was first introduced in the 1960s as a novel technique for aortic valve replacement using the patient's own pulmonary valve. In his original paper describing the technique, Ross also suggested that the pulmonary autograft can be used to replace the mitral valve as well (later referred to as the Ross II procedure) [10,11]. Over the years, advancements in surgical techniques, perioperative management, and excellent long-term outcomes have led to considerable interest in the procedure. Initially, it was primarily offered to adults and older patients with various aortic valve pathologies, including patients with rheumatic aortic valve disease manifesting as aortic valve regurgitation/stenosis or both [12]. Its application was expanded to include younger patients with congenital aortic valve disease and metabolic diseases such as familial hypercholesterolemia [13].

2.2. *Milestones and Key Contributors in Advancing the Technique*

Several milestones and key contributors have played a significant role in advancing the Ross procedure. Donald Ross first described the technique and performed the initial series of surgeries [10]. His pioneering work laid the foundation for the procedure and demonstrated the potential benefits of using the patient's own pulmonary valve to replace the aortic or mitral valve. Subsequently, other cardiac surgeons worldwide further refined the surgical technique, expanding its indications and improving outcomes. The emphasis was on AVR. Mitral valve replacement using the pulmonary valve (Ross II) did not gain as much attention [14].

Notable contributors include Dr. Magdi Yacoub, who contributed to the advancements in the Ross procedure and its widespread adoption. His work included the only randomized controlled trial comparing Ross with a homograft aortic root replacement in adults with aortic valve disease, demonstrating the superiority of the Ross procedure [15]. It took about 20 years for the Ross procedure to catch on in the United States and Canada. But then, North American surgeons including Ronald Elkins, Paul Stelzer, Tirone David, John Oswalt, and many others made significant contributions to the understanding and refinement of the Ross procedure [16,17]. Zohair Al Halees, who performed one of the largest series worldwide, highlighted the importance of candidate selection in the long-term results of the Ross procedure, emphasizing the need for careful patient selection to achieve optimal outcomes [18].

3. Surgical Technique

The Ross procedure involves several key steps. First, the patient is placed on the cardiopulmonary bypass and the aorta is cross-clamped and cardioplegia is given. The aortic valve is then carefully examined and if not repairable is excised and the aortic annulus is sized. There should not be much discrepancy in size between the aortic and the pulmonary annuli. Not more than a 2–3 mm discrepancy should be accepted. Very little RV muscle is kept below the pulmonary valve and only a few mms of the pulmonary artery are kept above pulmonary valve commissures. The pulmonary valve is then sutured to the aortic annulus, creating a new normally functioning neoaortic valve. There are several techniques to implant the autograft However, the technique of a freestanding aortic root with a coronary transfer is the most commonly used today. Subsequently, a pulmonary allograft or a prosthetic valve is implanted in the pulmonary position. Finally, the aorta is unclamped, and the patient is weaned off a cardiopulmonary bypass [19].

Surgeon's Expertise

The Ross procedure necessitates a high level of surgical expertise due to its complexity and technical demands. Surgeons must possess specialized experience in aortic root surgery, as the techniques required for the Ross procedure are similar to those used in complex root surgeries, such as familiarity with root anatomy and replacement as well as homograft root replacement. In centers with experience of and a high volume in performing the Ross procedure, long-term survival and freedom from valve-related complications are better than alternative procedures in young and middle-aged patients [20].

4. Patient Selection Criteria

Patient selection for the Ross procedure requires careful consideration. The procedure is most suitable for younger patients with aortic valve disease, in whom stenosis is the predominant hemodynamic manifestation, particularly those who desire freedom from lifelong anticoagulation therapy or who are engaged in high-impact physical activities [21]. Patients with a rheumatic aortic valve disease should be carefully assessed as it has been demonstrated that the pulmonary autograft becomes susceptible to rheumatic fever [22]. In general, patients with severe aortic valve regurgitation and with a dilated aortic root of more than 27–28 mm may not be as good candidates as those with aortic stenosis and normal aortic roots [23]. Additional measures to stabilize the aortic root and prevent progressive dilatation need to be undertaken. Patients with connective tissue disorders such as Marfan and Loeys–Dietz syndrome are not good candidates for the procedures [24].

Candidates should have a normally functioning pulmonary valve without a significant pathology. It is not advisable to use a bicuspid or a quadricuspid pulmonary valve or a pulmonary valve with too many large fenestrations [19].

The Ross procedure may not be suitable for older patients and those with significant comorbidities, as they may have a higher risk of complications. The procedure may still be an option in patients with combined mitral and aortic valve disease if a good mitral valve repair can be accomplished [25].

Therefore, careful patient selection and consideration of the procedure's technical challenges and potential drawbacks are crucial factors in achieving optimal outcomes.

5. Outcomes and Complications

5.1. Analysis of Short-Term and Long-Term Survival Rates

The Ross procedure has demonstrated favorable short-term and long-term survival rates in various studies. Regarding short-term outcomes, several studies have reported low operative mortality rates ranging from 0% to 4% [25]. Long-term survival rates after the Ross procedure have also been encouraging. Long-term outcomes showed 10-year survival rates ranging from 81% to 94%, while 20-year survival rates ranged from 65% to 92% [26]. These results suggest that the Ross procedure can provide durable survival benefits for appropriately selected patients. In a propensity-matched study, the Ross procedure demonstrated conferring a survival advantage when compared with mechanical valve replacement [27]. In a more recent study, the procedure was associated with better long-term survival when compared to patients with mechanical or bioprosthetic AVR. Therefore, in cardiac centers with expertise, the Ross procedure is considered the primary option for young and middle-aged adults undergoing AVR [28]. Table 1 summarizes the short- and long-term outcomes of the Ross procedure.

Table 1. Short- and long-term outcomes of the Ross procedure in different studies. N denote number of patients, date denote date of study publication.

Relevant Study	Ross Procedure Outcomes
El-Hamamsy et al., RCT n(228) 2010 [9]	10 Year Survival 97%
Ryan et al., 2021 n(225) [26]	20 Year Survival 81.3% (74.8–88.3%)
	Mortality (In-hospital) 0.9% (30 day) 2.2%
Pergola et al., n(536) 2020 [18]	15 Year Freedom from all Re-operation 83%
	Freedom from Autograft reoperation 81%
David et al., n(212) 2019 [23]	20 Year Mortality 10.8%
Stelzer et al., n(702) 2021 [25]	Perioperative Mortality 1%
Aboud et al., n(2444) 2021 [28]	25 Year Survival 75.8%
	Early mortality 1%

5.2. Evaluation of Postoperative Complications and Their Management

Early complications include technical issues causing autograft malfunction, bleeding, infection, arrhythmias, and coronary artery problems leading to left ventricular dysfunction. Later complications include valve-related issues, such as autograft dysfunction and/or pulmonary valve substitute dysfunction. Autograft dysfunction can occur due to valve regurgitation, stenosis or both or due to annular or aortic root dilatation. Progressive aortic root dilatation was observed frequently in the early series, particularly in young adults (Figures 1 and 2). This actually at one stage dampened the enthusiasm for the procedure [29]. Strict blood pressure control to avoid hypertension particularly early is very important in avoiding this complication. Techniques to prevent this were introduced, including aortic root reinforcement ± sino-tubular junction reinforcement or placing the autograft inside a cylinder Dacron vascular graft with or without sinuses of Valsalva (Figure 3) [30,31].

Recently, a personalized external aortic root support (PEARS), a custom-made macroporous mesh, was used to stabilize a dilated aortic root (Exstent limited®). This approach was adapted to the Ross procedure (ROSS-PEARS) (Figure 4) [32]. However, the long-term outcome of such modifications is yet to be validated. [33]. Pulmonary valve substitute dysfunction can be stenosis, regurgitation, or both. This remains the weak link in the procedure to the extent that some call it "turning a single-valve disease into a double-valve disease". The management of this complication may require surgical or percutaneous intervention. The increased interventional cardiologists' experience and the availability of many percutaneous pulmonary valve substitutes reduced apprehension about this potential problem.

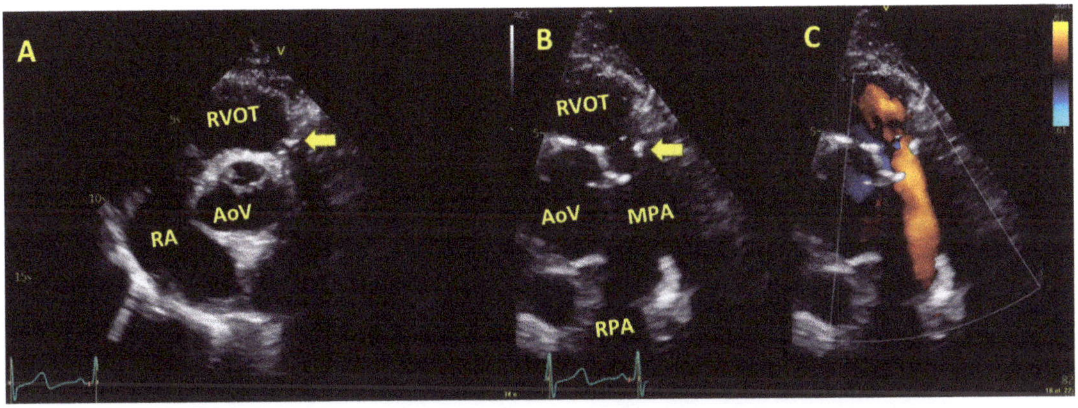

Figure 1. Transthoracic echocardiography Parasternal short axis view; Panel (**A**): Degenerative homograft cusps (yellow arrow, diastolic phase); Panel (**B**): Degenerative homograft cusps (yellow arrow, systolic phase); Panel (**C**): color Doppler showing the regurgitation originating from the right pulmonary artery suggestive of severe regurgitation; Abbreviations: RVOT: Right ventricular outflow track, RA: Right atrium, AoV: Aortic valve, MPA: Main trunk of pulmonary artery, RPA: Right main branch of pulmonary artery.

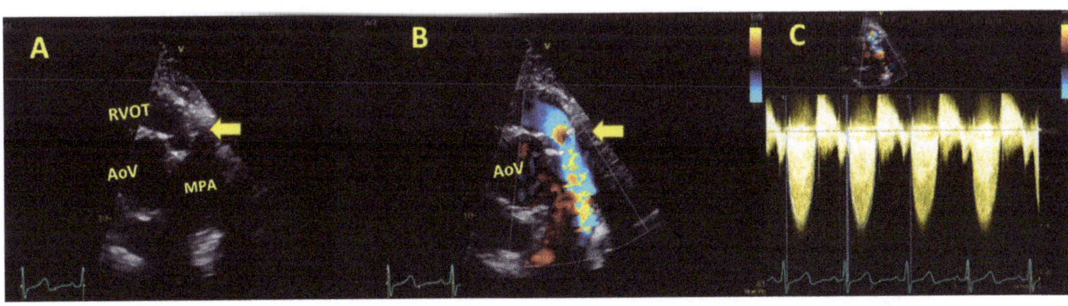

Figure 2. Panel (**A**) Parasternal short-axis (PSAX) view at aortic valve level short-axis (PSAX) view showing severe homograft stenosis with degenerative homograft cusps (yellow arrow) RVOT and MPA. Panel (**B**); color Doppler demonstrating systolic flow acceleration starting at the level of pulmonic homograft (yellow arrow) indicating pulmonic valve stenosis (PS). Panel (**C**); Continuous-flow (CW) Doppler across the pulmonic valve showing severe PS with peak and mean gradients of 69 and 42 mmHg, respectively; Abbreviations: AoV: aortic valve, RVOT: right ventricle out-flow tract, MPA: main pulmonary artery.

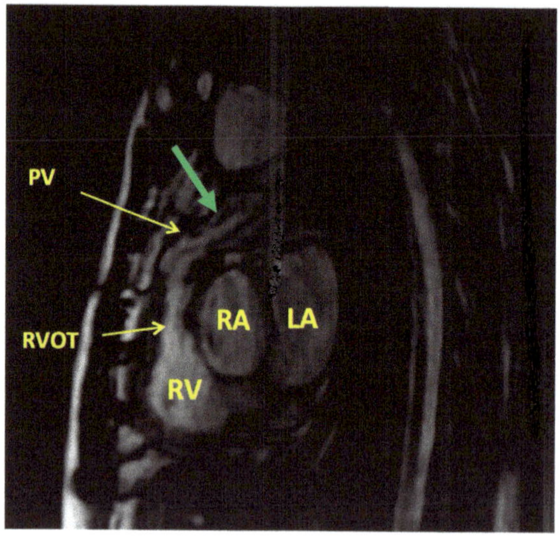

Figure 3. Cardiac magnetic resonance (CMR) with oblique sagittal stack cine cuts at different level showing pulmonic homograft stenosis. Green arrow showing defacing (showing significant stenosis); Abbreviations: PV: pulmonary valve, RVOT: right ventricular outflow track, RA: right atrium. RV: right ventricle, LA: left atrium.

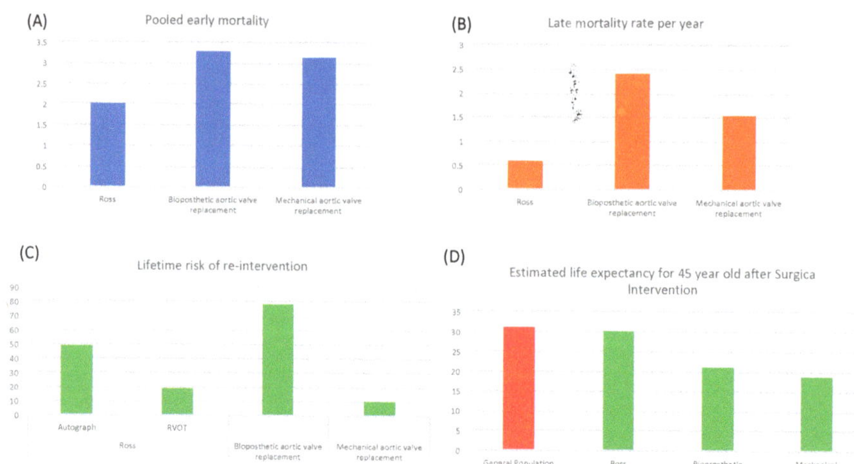

Figure 4. This figure presents a systematic review encompassing three distinct patient populations from studies reporting outcomes in adult patients aged between 18 and 55 years who have undergone the Ross procedure [34], bioprosthetic aortic valve replacement [35], and mechanical aortic valve replacement [36]. Panel (**A**) illustrates the aggregated early mortality rates, represented on the Y-axis, across different cohorts subjected to the three aforementioned surgical procedures. Panel (**B**) displays the aggregated annual late mortality rates as percentages. Panel (**C**) delineates the lifetime risk percentages for re-intervention in the Ross procedure, with separate data for the autograft in the aortic position and right ventricular outflow tract (RVOT) surgical interventions, as well as for bioprosthetic and mechanical aortic valve replacements. Panel (**D**) involves pooled data input into a microsimulation model, estimating the life expectancy, in years, of a 45-year-old patient following different aortic valve replacement surgeries. These estimates are compared (highlighted in red) with the projected life expectancy, post-45 years, of the general population that has not undergone any surgical interventions.

The autograft must function perfectly or "unfortunately the patient will end up with a different valve in the aortic position and lose the original pulmonary valve to a substitute requiring life-long surveillance" [37]. Valve sparing reoperations are possible for failed pulmonary autografts. Although this depends on the mechanism of autograft failure, still up to 50% salvage rates can be achieved in experienced hands [38].

5.3. Comparison of Outcomes with Alternative Procedures

When comparing the outcomes of the Ross procedure with alternative procedures, such as a mechanical valve, bioprosthetic or homograft aortic root replacement, several factors need to be considered. A mechanical valve replacement provides excellent durability but requires lifelong anticoagulation therapy, which may increase the risk of bleeding complications. A bioprosthetic AVR or homograft aortic root replacement avoids the need for anticoagulation therapy but has limited durability due to degeneration. The younger the patient is, the faster will be the degeneration and need for re-intervention.

Comparative studies have shown similar or improved survival rates and lower rates of valve-related complications with the Ross procedure compared to other aortic valve replacement options. One study comparing the Ross procedure to a mechanical valve replacement in young patients demonstrated similar long-term survival rates but significantly lower rates of reoperation in the Ross group [39]. Another study comparing the Ross procedure to a homograft aortic root replacement found comparable long-term survival rates but a higher incidence of valve-related complications in the homograft group [15].

In propensity-matched studies, the Ross procedure was associated with better long-term survival and freedom from adverse valve-related events compared with mechanical or bioprosthesis AVR [9].

Today, dealing with the durability, when comparing the Ross procedure with the bioprosthetic valve replacement, we have to take in consideration the possibility of treating the bioprosthetic valve dysfunction by a transcatheter valve in the procedure. It is true that this is not a surgical reintervention but nevertheless another procedure with an incurred cost. At present, a valve in valve therapy is not an option for a failed autograft.

In terms of quality of life, the Ross procedure has been shown to provide better functional outcomes and higher patient satisfaction compared to a mechanical valve replacement, likely due to the avoidance of anticoagulation therapy and an optimal autograft function. Additionally, the Ross procedure has been associated with lower rates of thromboembolic events compared to a mechanical valve replacement. This translates to a better survival [40].

It is important to note that the choice of procedure should be individualized based on patient characteristics, including age, comorbidities, lifestyle, and surgeon expertise. Long-term follow-up and further research are necessary to continue evaluating and comparing the outcomes of the Ross procedure with alternative procedures in different patient populations. It is therefore imperative to consider the creation of Ross centers of excellence for achieving the best results.

5.4. Comparison of Outcomes with Alternative Procedures Entered in Microsimulation

Etnel and colleagues performed an extensive meta-analysis and systematic review focusing on patients younger than 55 years who underwent the Ross procedure (Figure 4) [34], bioprosthetic aortic valve replacement [35], and mechanical aortic valve replacement [36]. The rates of various events were compiled and fed into a microsimulation model, which was utilized to calculate both the life expectancy and the aggregate rate of events over a lifetime. Observations indicated that patients undergoing the Ross procedure exhibited a reduced incidence of perioperative mortality. Comparative analysis suggested more favorable long-term outcomes for the Ross procedure compared to a bioprosthetic or mechanical aortic valve replacement. When incorporated into the microsimulation, the probability of requiring re-operation over a lifetime was found to be low, and the projected life expectancy aligned closely with that of the general population.

6. Imaging in Ross Procedure

The Ross procedure imaging scenario necessitates a dedicated professional figure with specific expertise in this procedure. Multimodality imaging is paramount in the Ross procedure. As its clinical application grows, knowledge of the various imaging modalities used is required for the imager and beneficial for the interventional and surgical teams. The purpose of this review is to describe the key steps of the procedural imaging pathway.

6.1. Pre-Procedural Imaging

Pre-procedure cardiac multimodality imaging in the candidate selection, screening and planning for the Ross procedure is the guidelines recommended pathway in valvular and congenital heart disease. It includes a multimodality comprehensive assessment of cardiac pathologies and functions and associated great vessels anomalies like patent ductus arteriosus and coarctation of the aorta, which are sometimes challenging in the clinical arena [18,41,42]. It can determine patient eligibility based on anatomic features and measurements, provide measurements for appropriate homograft sizing, predict the risks of potential procedural complications and their likelihood of success. In this phase, the whole imaging armamentarium plays a role. In sizing, the AV and PV annulus, echocardiography represents the technique of choice even though cardiac CT allows a more precise sizing.

6.2. Intraoperative Imaging

Intraoperative imaging includes the use of transesophageal echocardiography able to confirm the preprocedural features and postoperatively detect the normal functioning of both the autograft and homograft as well as the ventricular function.

Multimodality imaging follow-up evaluations, including echocardiography and magnetic resonance imaging (MRI), allow early detection of any potential issues, optimizing reintervention decision-making and improving long-term outcomes.

6.3. Post-Operative and Long-Term Follow-Up Imaging

In the follow-up imaging pathway, echocardiography represents the first step. It is able to diagnose and follow over time the autograph and homograft behavior as well as the cardiac function. However, MRI and cardiac computed tomography are paramount tools in the imaging pathway in order to better assess the right ventricular function, the degree of the regurgitation as well as assessing both the coronary arteries and the great vessels (Figures 1–3).

7. Hemodynamic Performance

Hemodynamic performance is a crucial aspect of evaluating the success of the Ross procedure. Studies have shown favorable hemodynamic outcomes in patients who have undergone the procedure. The pulmonary autograft, when used as an aortic valve replacement, has demonstrated excellent hemodynamic properties, including low transvalvular gradients, larger effective orifice areas, and improved left ventricular function [1,3]. These findings indicate that the Ross procedure provides favorable hemodynamic outcomes and contributes to optimal cardiac function.

8. Quality of Life and Functional Outcomes

8.1. Postoperative Quality of Life Measures

Several studies have investigated the impact of the Ross procedure on postoperative quality of life. These studies have utilized various validated instruments, such as the SF-36 Health Survey and the EuroQol-5D, to assess physical, emotional, and social well-being. Overall, these studies have consistently reported favorable postoperative quality of life outcomes in patients who have undergone the Ross procedure. Patients often experience improvements in symptoms, functional capacity, and overall satisfaction with their cardiac health [43,44].

8.2. Assessment of Functional Outcomes and Exercise Capacity

Functional outcomes and exercise capacity are important indicators of the success of the Ross procedure. Studies evaluating these aspects have shown that patients who undergo the Ross procedure often exhibit excellent functional outcomes and have the ability to engage in regular physical activities. Exercise stress testing, including peak oxygen consumption (VO_2 max) measurements, has demonstrated good exercise capacity in these patients, comparable to or even superior to other valve replacement options [44]. While most valve prostheses will have an increase in AV gradient during exercise, the autograft exhibits hemodynamic characteristics similar to normal human AV even under conditions of enhanced cardiac output [45].

8.3. Comparison of Quality of Life and Functional Outcomes with Alternative Procedures

When comparing the quality of life and functional outcomes of the Ross procedure with alternative procedures, such as mechanical valve replacement and bioprosthetic valve replacement, several factors need to be considered. Mechanical valve replacement, while durable, may impact the quality of life and restrict certain activities. Bioprosthetic valve replacement avoids the need for anticoagulation but has limitations in terms of durability and hence the need for future re-intervention. Comparative studies have shown that the Ross procedure can provide similar or superior quality of life and functional outcomes compared to alternative procedures.

9. Patient Selection and Risk Stratification

Optimal patient selection is crucial for achieving successful outcomes with the Ross procedure. Several patient characteristics have been identified as favorable for considering the Ross procedure. These include a younger age, an absence of significant coronary artery disease, an absence of aortic root dilatation with aortic stenosis, and an absence of significant left ventricular dysfunction. Patients with these characteristics are more likely to benefit from the Ross procedure due to their potential for long-term durability and improved quality of life [18,46]. Table 2 summarizes candidates that do better and do worse.

Table 2. Summarizing patient who will do better or worse after the Ross procedure.

Candidate Selection	
Better	**Worse**
Congenital etiology	Rheumatic
Aortic stenosis	Pure Aortic regurgitation
Aortic root diameter < 15 mm/m^2	Older age (homograft re-intervention)

Studies evaluating the outcomes and long-term follow-up of the Ross procedure in pediatric and young adult patients have reported promising results. These studies have demonstrated excellent survival rates, favorable hemodynamic performance, and low rates of reoperation. Additionally, long-term follow-up studies have shown low incidences of valve-related complications such as neoaortic regurgitation and neoaortic root dilatation [47,48].

Performing the Ross procedure in pediatric patients including infants and neonates presents unique challenges and considerations. The smaller size of pediatric hearts requires the adaptation of surgical techniques and the use of appropriately sized homografts to replace the used pulmonary valve. Careful assessment of the aortic annulus and root dimensions is crucial to ensure proper matching of the autograft and the aortic root. Usually, under such circumstances, the autograft is larger than the aortic root as the most common lesion in this age group is aortic stenosis with a generally smaller aortic annulus. Enlarging the aortic annulus should be done just enough to match the size of the autograft. The autograft will grow with the child's growth and most of the time match the somatic growth [49]. Ongoing growth and development necessitate long-term follow-up as reoperation to change the pulmonary valve substitute is inevitable.

The management of pediatric patients also requires multidisciplinary collaboration involving pediatric cardiac surgeons, pediatric cardiologists, and other specialists experienced in treating congenital heart diseases. Preoperative evaluation and risk stratification, as well as postoperative care and follow-up, should be tailored to the unique needs of pediatric patients.

While the Ross procedure has demonstrated favorable outcomes in the pediatric and young adult population, further studies with larger cohorts and longer follow-up are needed to assess the durability and long-term benefits in this specific patient group.

Aortic valve pathology and hemodynamic manifestations are important in selecting patients for the Ross procedure. Patients with dilated aortic roots and pure aortic valve regurgitation do not do as well, particularly if this is related to rheumatic heart disease and associated with mitral valve involvement. Patients with aortic valve disease related to connective tissue disorders are generally not good candidates for the procedure [50].

The Ross Procedure for the Treatment of Infective Endocarditis

Traditionally, management of infective endocarditis (IE) has involved the utilization of biologic homografts or mechanical valves. However, the Ross procedure emerges as a viable alternative for young adults. It offers a reduced reoperation incidence compared to biologic homografts and eliminates the need for anticoagulation required by mechanical valves—a significant consideration for younger patients, who may exhibit lower compliance. In the absence of randomized controlled trials, small clinical series provide the most reliable evidence. An early series of 28 patients [51], where 14 of the cases were emergency surgeries, reported an in-hospital mortality of 10.7%. The 10-year survival stood at 47%, with three cases of recurrent IE documented. Another cohort of 20 patients [52], including 10 with bicuspid aortic valves, showed only one early mortality and no IE recurrence over a 47-month follow-up, with stable postoperative hemodynamics. A more recent series by Loobuyck et al. [53] encompassed 38 patients with a mean age of 33.9 years, yielding an in-hospital mortality of 5.3% and an overall survival of 82%. Recurrent IE was observed in two patients, and six required reinterventions due to autograft or homograft failure. Despite the limited evidence from small clinical series, the procedure's favorable outcomes are underscored by relatively low in-hospital mortality and a decent long-term survival rate. Nevertheless, there remains the need for larger, randomized studies to further validate these findings and establish more definitive treatment guidelines for this population.

10. Contemporary Techniques and Innovations

In recent years, there have been significant advances in cardiac surgical techniques, including the development of minimally invasive, endoscopic and robotic approaches. Such techniques aim to reduce surgical trauma, shorten the hospital stay and enhance postoperative recovery. These approaches may be utilized in performing the Ross procedure, though this is a complex surgical procedure requiring special expertise. Nevertheless, potential benefits for patients undergoing the Ross procedure are there [54].

Tissue engineering is another area of innovation in cardiac surgery. Researchers are exploring strategies to develop bioengineered grafts and valves using a combination of synthetic materials and patient-specific cells. These bioengineered constructs have the potential to improve the durability and functionality of the pulmonary valve substitutes after the Ross procedure, reducing the need for reoperations and long-term complications [55,56]. Additionally, development of durable patch material may result in improvements in aortic valve repair and reconstruction techniques including the neo-cuspidization (Ozaki) procedure reducing the need for aortic valve replacement in general [57].

Future directions in valve surgery include the exploration of tissue-engineered scaffolds and valve substitutes and the integration of regenerative medicine approaches, aiming to further enhance the outcomes and long-term success and ultimately improving the quality of life of patients requiring a valve replacement.

Ongoing research in the field of the Ross procedure focuses on several areas. Researchers are investigating novel imaging techniques, such as 3D echocardiography and cardiac magnetic resonance imaging, to improve preoperative planning, intraoperative guidance, and postoperative follow-up [58]. Additionally, long-term studies are being conducted to evaluate the durability and outcomes of contemporary Ross procedures, particularly in high-risk patient populations [25,59].

11. Conclusions

In conclusion, the Ross procedure, one of the most scrutinized surgical procedures in literature, has emerged as a viable excellent option for aortic valve replacement offering unique advantages in certain patient populations. The pulmonary autograft as an aortic valve substitute is probably currently the closest to an ideal valve substitute. It provides excellent long-term survival matching the normal population, favorable and durable hemodynamic performance and proven potential for growth in the pediatric age group, including neonates and infants (Table 3).

Table 3. Table demonstrating the characteristics of the autograft as an ideal valve. the number of +++ denotes more benefits relative other procedures.

Features	Benefit
Silent	++++
Non-thrombogenic	++++
Normal Hemodynamic	++++
Readily Available–Low cost	++++
Has Potential for growth	+++
Infection Resistant	+++
Easy to Implant	++
Durable-Non-Rheumatics -Rheumatics	++++ ++

The strength of evidence supporting the benefits of the Ross procedure comes from a combination of retrospective observational studies, prospective registries, and meta-analysis. While the level of evidence varies between studies, there is a consistent trend showing favorable outcomes. Nevertheless, direct head-to-head randomized controlled trials comparing the Ross procedure to alternative aortic valve replacement options are limited. It is important, however, to acknowledge that the procedure does have some limitations. Further research, including well-designed prospective studies, is needed to validate and strengthen the current evidence base.

The Ross procedure should be considered a valuable option in the armamentarium of adult and congenital cardiac surgeons. Careful selection is of utmost importance for a successful long-lasting outcome and should be individualized based on the patient's characteristics and preferences.

In that regard, we support "a hard look at current practices and a call for re-evaluation of the current guidelines" [60,61].

Funding: This research received no external funding.

Institutional Review Board Statement: Not applicable.

Informed Consent Statement: Not applicable.

Data Availability Statement: Not applicable.

Conflicts of Interest: The authors declare no conflict of interest.

References

1. Takkenberg, J.J.; Klieverik, L.M.; Schoof, P.H.; van Suylen, R.J.; van Herwerden, L.A.; Zondervan, P.E.; Roos-Hesselink, J.W.; Eijkemans, M.J.; Yacoub, M.H.; Bogers, A.J. The Ross procedure: A systematic review and meta-analysis. *Circulation* **2009**, *119*, 222–228. [CrossRef] [PubMed]
2. Ercan, S.; Koçak, I.; Özkan, F. Valve performance classification in 630 subcoronary Ross patients over 22 years. *J. Thorac. Cardiovasc. Surg.* **2012**, *144*, 413–420. [CrossRef]
3. Sharabiani, M.T.; Dorobantu, D.M.; Mahani, A.S.; Turner, M.; Tometzki, A.J.P.; Angelini, G.D.; Parry, A.J.; Caputo, M.; Stoica, S.C. Aortic Valve Replacement and the Ross Operation in Children and Young Adults. *J. Am. Coll. Cardiol.* **2016**, *67*, 2858–2870. [CrossRef] [PubMed]
4. Mookhoek, A.; Charitos, E.I.; Hazekamp, M.G.; Bogers, A.J.; Hörer, J.; Lange, R.; Hetzer, R.; Sachweh, J.S.; Riso, A.; Stierle, U.; et al. Ross Procedure in Neonates and Infants: A European Multicenter Experience. *Ann. Thorac. Surg.* **2015**, *100*, 2278–2284. [CrossRef] [PubMed]
5. Stulak, J.M.; Burkhart, H.M.; Sundt, T.M.; Connolly, H.M.; Suri, R.M.; Schaff, H.V.; Dearani, J.A. Spectrum and Outcome of Reoperations after the Ross Procedure. *Circulation* **2010**, *122*, 1153–1158. [CrossRef] [PubMed]
6. Otto, C.M.; Nishimura, R.A.; Bonow, R.O.; Carabello, B.A.; Gentile, F.; Jneid, H.; Krieger, E.V.; Mack, M.; McLeod, C.; O'Gara, P.T.; et al. 2020 ACC/AHA Guideline for the Management of Patients with Valvular Heart Disease: Executive Summary: A Report of the American College of Cardiology/American Heart Association Joint Committee on Clinical Practice Guidelines. *Circulation* **2021**, *143*, e35–e71. [CrossRef] [PubMed]
7. Vahanian, A.; Beyersdorf, F.; Praz, F.; Milojevic, M.; Baldus, S.; Bauersachs, J.; Capodanno, D.; Conradi, L.; De Bonis, M.; De Paulis, R.; et al. ESC/EACTS Scientific Document Group. 2021 ESC/EACTS Guidelines for the management of valvular heart disease. *Eur. Heart J.* **2022**, *43*, 561–632. [CrossRef] [PubMed]
8. Mazine, A.; Rocha, R.V.; El-Hamamsy, I.; Ouzounian, M.; Yanagawa, B.; Bhatt, D.L.; Verma, S.; Friedrich, J.O. Ross Procedure vs Mechanical Aortic Valve Replacement in Adults: A Systematic Review and Me-ta-analysis. *JAMA Cardiol.* **2018**, *3*, 978–987. [CrossRef]
9. El-Hamamsy, I.; Toyoda, N.; Itagaki, S.; Stelzer, P.; Varghese, R.; Williams, E.E.; Erogova, N.; Adams, D.H. Propensity-Matched Comparison of the Ross Procedure and Prosthetic Aortic Valve Re-placement in Adults. *J. Am. Coll. Cardiol.* **2022**, *79*, 805–815. [CrossRef]
10. Ross, D. Replacement of aortic and mitral valves with a pulmonary autograft. *Lancet* **1967**, *2*, 956–958. [CrossRef]
11. Al Halees, Z.; Awad, M.M.; Pieters, F.; Shahid, M.S.; Al Amri, M.A. Six-year follow-up of a pulmonary autograft in the mitral position: The Ross II procedure. *J. Thorac. Cardiovasc. Surg.* **1999**, *117*, 614–616. [CrossRef] [PubMed]
12. Kumar, N.; Gallo, R.; Gometza, B.; Al-Halees, Z.; Duran, C.M. Pulmonary autograft for aortic valve replacement in rheumatic disease—An ideal solution? *J. Heart Valve Dis.* **1994**, *3*, 384–387. [PubMed]
13. Kholaif, N.; Mohamed, T.I.; Alharbi, I.S.; Aljenedil, S.A.; AlHumaidan, H.; Al-Ashwal, A.; Almahfouz, A.; Algorashi, S.; Almasood, A.; Baqal, O.J. Management and clinical outcomes of patients with homozygous familial hypercholesteremia in Saudi Arabia. *Monaldi Arch Chest Dis.* **2023**, *93*. [CrossRef] [PubMed]
14. Kabbani, S.; Jamil, H.; Nabhani, F.; Hamoud, A.; Katan, K.; Sabbagh, N.; Koudsi, A.; Kabbani, L.; Hamed, G. Analysis of 92 mitral pulmonary autograft replacement (Ross II) operations. *J. Thorac. Cardiovasc. Surg.* **2007**, *134*, 902–908.e7. [CrossRef] [PubMed]
15. El-Hamamsy, I.; Eryigit, Z.; Stevens, L.-M.; Sarang, Z.; George, R.; Clark, L.; Melina, G.; Takkenberg, J.J.; Yacoub, M.H. Long-term outcomes after autograft versus homograft aortic root replacement in adults with aortic valve disease: A randomised controlled trial. *Lancet* **2010**, *376*, 524–531. [CrossRef] [PubMed]
16. Elkins, R.C.; Thompson, D.M.; Lane, M.M.; Elkins, C.C.; Peyton, M.D. Ross operation: 16-year experience. *J. Thorac. Cardiovasc. Surg.* **2008**, *136*, 623–630.e5. [CrossRef] [PubMed]
17. Stelzer, P. The Ross Procedure: State of the Art 2011. *Semin. Thorac. Cardiovasc. Surg.* **2011**, *23*, 115–123. [CrossRef] [PubMed]
18. Pergola, V.; Di Salvo, G.; Fadel, B.; Galzerano, D.; Al-Shaid, M.; Al-Admawi, M.; Al Amri, M.; Al-Ahmadi, M.; Al-Halees, Z. The long term results of the Ross procedure: The importance of candidate selection. *Int. J. Cardiol.* **2020**, *320*, 35–41. [CrossRef]
19. AlHalees, Z. Chapter 20-The Pulmonary Autograft for Aortic Valve Replacement. In *Operative Cardiac Surgery*, 6th ed.; Spray, T.L., Acker, M.A., Eds.; CRC Press: Boca Raton, FL, USA, 2019; pp. 227–230.
20. Mazine, A.; David, T.E.; Stoklosa, K.; Chung, J.; Lafreniere-Roula, M.; Ouzounian, M. Improved Outcomes Following the Ross Procedure Compared with Bioprosthetic Aortic Valve Replacement. *J. Am. Coll. Cardiol.* **2022**, *79*, 993–1005. [CrossRef]
21. Ouzounian, M.; Mazine, A.; David, T.E. The Ross procedure is the best operation to treat aortic stenosis in young and middle-aged adults. *J. Thorac. Cardiovasc. Surg.* **2017**, *154*, 778–782. [CrossRef]
22. Al-Halees, Z.; Kumar, N.; Gallo, R.; Gometza, B.; Duran, C.M. Pulmonary autograft for aortic valve replacement in rheumatic disease: A caveat. *Ann. Thorac. Surg.* **1995**, *60* (Suppl. 2), S172–S176, discussion S176. [CrossRef] [PubMed]
23. David, T.E.; Ouzounian, M.; David, C.M.; Lafreniere-Roula, M.; Manlhiot, C. Late results of the Ross procedure. *J. Thorac. Cardiovasc. Surg.* **2019**, *157*, 201–208. [CrossRef] [PubMed]

24. Chauvette, V.; Lefebvre, L.; Chamberland, M.; Williams, E.E.; El-Hamamsy, I. Contemporary Review of the Ross Procedure. *Struct. Heart* **2021**, *5*, 11–23. [CrossRef]
25. Stelzer, P.; Mejia, J.; Varghese, R. Operative risks of the Ross procedure. *J. Thorac. Cardiovasc. Surg.* **2021**, *161*, 905–915.e3. [CrossRef] [PubMed]
26. Ryan, W.H.; Squiers, J.J.; Harrington, K.B.; Goodenow, T.; Rawitscher, C.; Schaffer, J.M.; DiMaio, J.M.; Brinkman, W.T. Long-term outcomes of the Ross procedure in adults. *Ann. Cardiothorac. Surg.* **2021**, *10*, 499–508. [CrossRef] [PubMed]
27. Alsoufi, B.; Al-Halees, Z.; Manlhiot, C.; McCrindle, B.W.; Al-Ahmadi, M.; Sallehuddin, A.; Canver, C.C.; Bulbul, Z.; Joufan, M.; Fadel, B. Mechanical valves versus the Ross procedure for aortic valve replacement in children: Propensity-adjusted comparison of long-term outcomes. *J. Thorac. Cardiovasc. Surg.* **2009**, *137*, 362–370.e9. [CrossRef] [PubMed]
28. Aboud, A.; Charitos, E.I.; Fujita, B.; Stierle, U.; Reil, J.-C.; Voth, V.; Liebrich, M.; Andreas, M.; Holubec, T.; Bening, C.; et al. Long-Term Outcomes of Patients Undergoing the Ross Procedure. *J. Am. Coll. Cardiol.* **2021**, *77*, 1412–1422. [CrossRef]
29. Laudito, A.; Brook, M.M.; Suleman, S.; Bleiweis, M.S.; Thompson, L.D.; Hanley, F.L.; Reddy, V. The Ross procedure in children and young adults: A word of caution. *J. Thorac. Cardiovasc. Surg.* **2001**, *122*, 147–153. [CrossRef]
30. Gebauer, R.; Cerny, S. A modification of the Ross procedure to prevent pulmonary autograft dilatation. *Eur. J. Cardio-Thoracic Surg.* **2009**, *36*, 195–197. [CrossRef]
31. Starnes, V.A.; Bowdish, M.E.; Cohen, R.G.; Baker, C.J.; Elsayed, R.S. The Ross procedure utilizing the pulmonary autograft inclusion technique in adults. *JTCVS Tech.* **2021**, *10*, 372–376. [CrossRef]
32. Kenny, L.A.; Austin, C.; Golesworthy, T.; Venugopal, P.; Alphonso, N. Personalized External Aortic Root Support (PEARS) for Aortic Root Aneurysm. *Oper. Tech. Thorac. Cardiovasc. Surg.* **2021**, *26*, 290–305. [CrossRef]
33. Williams, E.; El-Hamamsy, I. Commentary: The Ross procedure in a graft: A word of caution. *JTCVS Tech.* **2021**, *10*, 377–378. [CrossRef] [PubMed]
34. Etnel, J.R.; Grashuis, P.; Huygens, S.A.; Pekbay, B.; Papageorgiou, G.; Helbing, W.A.; Roos-Hesselink, J.W.; Bogers, A.J.; Mokhles, M.M.; Takkenberg, J.J. The Ross Procedure: A Systematic Review, Meta-Analysis, and Microsimulation. *Circ. Cardiovasc. Qual. Outcomes* **2018**, *11*, e004748. [CrossRef] [PubMed]
35. Etnel, J.R.; Huygens, S.A.; Grashuis, P.; Pekbay, B.; Papageorgiou, G.; Hesselink, J.W.R.; Bogers, A.J.; Takkenberg, J.J. Bioprosthetic Aortic Valve Replacement in Nonelderly Adults: A Systematic Review, Meta-Analysis, Microsimulation. *Circ. Cardiovasc. Qual. Outcomes* **2019**, *12*, e005481. [CrossRef]
36. Korteland, N.M.; Etnel, J.R.G.; Arabkhani, B.; Mokhles, M.M.; Mohamad, A.; Roos-Hesselink, J.W.; Bogers, A.J.J.C.; Takkenberg, J.J.M. Mechanical aortic valve replacement in non-elderly adults: Meta-analysis and microsimulation. *Eur. Hear. J.* **2017**, *38*, 3370–3377. [CrossRef] [PubMed]
37. Al Halees, Z. Commentary: The pulmonary autograft, too valuable to repeal. *JTCVS Tech.* **2021**, *10*, 415–416. [CrossRef] [PubMed]
38. Goldstone, A.B.; Woo, Y.J. Valve-sparing reoperations for failed pulmonary autografts. *JTCVS Tech.* **2021**, *10*, 408–412. [CrossRef]
39. Yokoyama, Y.; Kuno, T.; Toyoda, N.; Fujisaki, T.; Takagi, H.; Itagaki, S.; Ibrahim, M.; Ouzounian, M.; El-Hamamsy, I. Ross Procedure Versus Mechanical Versus Bioprosthetic Aortic Valve Replacement: A Network Meta-Analysis. *J. Am. Heart Assoc.* **2023**, *12*, e8066. [CrossRef]
40. Aicher, D.; Holz, A.; Feldner, S.; Köllner, V.; Schäfers, H.-J. Quality of life after aortic valve surgery: Replacement versus reconstruction. *J. Thorac. Cardiovasc. Surg.* **2011**, *142*, e19–e24. [CrossRef]
41. Fadel, B.M.; Mohty, D.; Husain, A.; Dahdouh, Z.; Al-Admawi, M.; Pergola, V.; Di Salvo, G. The Various Hemodynamic Profiles of the Patent Ductus Arteriosus in Adults. *Echocardiography* **2015**, *32*, 1172–1178. [CrossRef]
42. Baumgartner, H.; De Backer, J.; Babu-Narayan, S.V.; Budts, W.; Chessa, M.; Diller, G.-P.; lung, B.; Kluin, J.; Lang, I.M.; Meijboom, F.; et al. 2020 ESC Guidelines for the management of adult congenital heart disease. *Eur. Heart J.* **2021**, *42*, 563–645. [CrossRef] [PubMed]
43. Mueller, G.C.; Becker, O.; Mir, T.; Arndt, F.; Kozlik-Feldmann, R.; Dodge-Khatami, A. Functional Outcomes after the Ross Procedure. *Thorac. Cardiovasc. Surg.* **2015**, *63*. [CrossRef]
44. Marino, B.S.; Pasquali, S.K.; Wernovsky, G.; Bockoven, J.R.; McBride, M.; Cho, C.J.; Spray, T.L.; Paridon, S.M. Exercise performance in children and adolescents after the Ross procedure. *Cardiol. Young* **2006**, *16*, 40–47. [CrossRef] [PubMed]
45. Doty, D.B.; Flores, J.H.; Yanowitz, F.G.; Oury, J.H. Maximum Exercise after Aortic Valve Replacement with Pulmonary Autograft. *Asian Cardiovasc. Thorac. Ann.* **1999**, *7*, 37–39. [CrossRef]
46. Alsoufi, B.; Manlhiot, C.; Fadel, B.; Al-Ahmadi, M.; Tamim, M.; McCrindle, B.W.; Canver, C.C.; Al-Halees, Z. The Ross procedure in children: Preoperative haemodynamic manifestation has significant effect on late autograft re-operation. *Eur. J. Cardio-Thorac. Surg.* **2010**, *38*, 547–555. [CrossRef] [PubMed]
47. Al-Halees, Z.; Pieters, F.; Qadoura, F.; Shahid, M.; Al-Amri, M.; Al-Fadley, F. The Ross procedure is the procedure of choice for congenital aortic valve disease. *J. Thorac. Cardiovasc. Surg.* **2002**, *123*, 437–442. [CrossRef] [PubMed]
48. Fadel, B.M.; Manlhiot, C.; Al-Halees, Z.; Di Salvo, G.; Al-Ahmadi, M.; McCrindle, B.; Alsoufi, B. The fate of the neoaortic valve and root after the modified Ross–Konno procedure. *J. Thorac. Cardiovasc. Surg.* **2013**, *145*, 430–437.e1. [CrossRef] [PubMed]
49. Al Halees, Z. The Mini-Ross–Konno procedure. *Eur. J. Cardio-Thorac. Surg.* **2011**, *39*, 1067–1069. [CrossRef]
50. Alsoufi, B.; Manlhiot, C.; Fadel, B.; Al-Fayyadh, M.; McCrindle, B.W.; Alwadai, A.; Al-Halees, Z. Is the ross procedure a suitable choice for aortic valve replacement in children with rheumatic aortic valve disease? *World J. Pediatr. Congenit. Heart Surg.* **2012**, *3*, 8–15. [CrossRef]

51. Le Guillou, V.; Bouchart, F.; Gay, A.; Nafeh-Bizet, C.; Hubscher, C.; Tabley, A.; Bessou, J.P.; Doguet, F. The Ross procedure in endocarditis: A report of 28 cases. *Eur. J. Cardio-Thoracic Surg.* **2014**, *45*, 153–158. [CrossRef]
52. Ratschiller, T.; Sames-Dolzer, E.; Paulus, P.; Schimetta, W.; Müller, H.; Zierer, A.F.; Mair, R. Long-term Evaluation of the Ross Procedure in Acute Infective Endocarditis. In *Seminars in Thoracic and Cardiovascular Surgery*; WB Saunders: Philadelphia, PA USA, 2017. [CrossRef]
53. Loobuyck, V.; Soquet, J.; Moussa, M.D.; Coisne, A.; Pinçon, C.; Richardson, M.; Rousse, N.; Mugnier, A.; Juthier, F.; Marechaux S.; et al. Active Aortic Endocarditis in Young Adults: Long-term Results of the Ross Procedure. *Ann. Thorac. Surg.* **2020**, *110* 856–861. [CrossRef] [PubMed]
54. Lamelas, J. Minimally invasive aortic valve replacement: The "Miami Method". *Ann. Cardiothorac. Surg.* **2015**, *4*, 71–77. [PubMed]
55. Huygens, S.A.; Rutten-van Mölken, M.P.M.H.; Noruzi, A.; Etnel, J.R.G.; Corro Ramos, I.; Bouten, C.V.C.; Kluin, J.; Takkenberg J.J.M. What Is the Potential of Tissue-Engineered Pulmonary Valves in Children? *Ann. Thorac. Surg.* **2019**, *107*, 1845–1853 [CrossRef] [PubMed]
56. Dohmen, P.M.; Lembcke, A.; Holinski, S.; Kivelitz, D.; Braun, J.P.; Pruss, A.; Konertz, W. Mid-Term Clinical Results Using a Tissue-Engineered Pulmonary Valve to Re-construct the Right Ventricular Outflow Tract During the Ross Procedure. *Ann. Thorac. Surg.* **2007**, *84*, 729–736. [CrossRef] [PubMed]
57. Karamlou, T.; Pettersson, G.; Nigro, J.J. Commentary: A pediatric perspective on the Ozaki procedure. *J. Thorac. Cardiovasc. Surg.* **2021**, *161*, 1582–1583. [CrossRef] [PubMed]
58. Drullinsky, D.; Mehta, C.K.; Scott, M.B.; Crawford, E.; Markl, M.; Bonow, R.O.; Mendelson, M.A.; El-Hamamsy, I.; Malaisrie, S.C. Four-Dimensional Magnetic Resonance after Ross Procedure for Unicuspid Aortic Valve. *Circ. Cardiovasc. Imaging* **2021**, *14*, e011500. [CrossRef] [PubMed]
59. Knott-Craig, C.J.; Goldberg, S.P.; Pastuszko, P.; Peyton, M.D.; Kirklin, J.K. The Ross operation for aortic valve disease: Previous sternotomy results in improved long-term outcome. *J. Heart Valve Dis.* **2007**, *16*, 394–397.
60. El-Hamamsy, I.; Bouhout, I. The Ross procedure: Time for a hard look at current practices and a reexamination of the guidelines. *Ann. Transl. Med.* **2017**, *5*, 142. [CrossRef]
61. Misfeld, M.; Borger, M.A. The Ross procedure: Time to reevaluate the guidelines. *J. Thorac. Cardiovasc. Surg.* **2019**, *157*, 211–212. [CrossRef]

Journal of
Clinical Medicine

MDPI

Review

The Postoperative Paradoxical Septum (POPS): A Comprehensive Review on Physio-Pathological Mechanisms

Emanuele Di Virgilio [1], Paolo Basile [2], Maria Cristina Carella [2], Francesco Monitillo [2], Daniela Santoro [2], Michele Davide Latorre [2], Silvia D'Alessandro [3], Laura Fusini [4], Fabio Fazzari [4], Gianluca Pontone [4,5] and Andrea Igoren Guaricci [2,*]

1 Cardiology Unit, Hospital of Corato, ASL Bari, 70033 Corato, Italy; emanueledrit@gmail.com
2 University Cardiology Unit, Interdisciplinary Department of Medicine, "Aldo Moro" University School of Medicine, AOUC Polyclinic, 70121 Bari, Italy; paolo.basile@uniba.it (P.B.); m.c.carella92@gmail.com (M.C.C.); dr.francescomonitillo@gmail.com (F.M.); danina2012@gmail.com (D.S.); latorre.michele.d@gmail.com (M.D.L.)
3 Neurology Unit, Hospital of Altamura, 70022 Altamura, Italy
4 Department of Perioperative Cardiology and Cardiovascular Imaging, Centro Cardiologico Monzino IRCCS, 20138 Milan, Italy; laura.fusini@cardiologicomonzino.it (L.F.); fabio.fazzari@cardiologicomonzino.it (F.F.); gianluca.pontone@cardiologicomonzino.it (G.P.)
5 Department of Biomedical, Surgical and Dental Sciences, University of Milan, 20122 Milan, Italy
* Correspondence: andreaigoren.guaricci@uniba.it; Tel.: +39-080-559-2740

Abstract: The interventricular septum (IVS) is a core myocardial structure involved in biventricular coupling and performance. Physiologically, during systole, it moves symmetrically toward the center of the left ventricle (LV) and opposite during diastole. Several pathological conditions produce a reversal or paradoxical septal motion, such as after uncomplicated cardiac surgery (CS). The postoperative paradoxical septum (POPS) was observed in a high rate of cases, representing a *unicum* in the panorama of paradoxical septa as it does not induce significant ventricular morpho-functional alterations nor negative clinical impact. Although it was previously considered a postoperative event, evidence suggests that it might also appear during surgery and gradually resolve over time. The mechanism behind this phenomenon is still debated. In this article, we will provide a comprehensive review of the various theories generated over the past fifty years to explain its pathological basis. Finally, we will attempt to give a heuristic interpretation of the biventricular postoperative motion pattern based on the switch of the ventricular anchor points.

Keywords: postoperative paradoxical septum; abnormal septal motion; cardiac imaging

1. Introduction

Following cardiac surgery (CS), patients often exhibit a new abnormal motion of the interventricular septum (IVS) during echocardiographic follow-up. This issue has been reported since the early 1970s [1–5]. Although other imaging techniques can detect it, echocardiography remains the most common method [6–11]. This abnormal septal motion is known by different names, such as reversed septal movement, pseudo-paradoxical septum, or simply abnormal septal motion (ASM). In this review, we will use "ASM" to indicate generic alteration of septal movement and "postoperative paradoxical septum" (POPS) for specific postoperative septal kinetic alterations. The definition of POPS has evolved with technology advancements and imaging techniques. It can be comprehensively defined as a new-onset postoperative non-respirophasic flat or centrifugal systolic motion of the IVS with normal septal wall thickening, preserved left ventricular geometry, unchanged global systolic function, and normal septal perfusion and metabolism. POPS represents a *unicum* in the panorama of paradoxical septa as it does not induce significant ventricular morpho-functional alterations nor negative clinical impact. However, a dyskinetic IVS can be observed in various pathological conditions, such as myocardial ischemia or necrosis, intraventricular conduction delays, pre-excitation, constriction physiology, pericardial effusion, right heart overload, or congenital absence of the pericardium (CAP) [12–16]. Some of these conditions can complicate the postoperative period [10,17–19]. Furthermore, changes in the lateral wall can also occur, complicating the overall assessment of the postoperative systolic function of the left ventricle (LV) [20–23].

The pathophysiological basis of postoperative septal behavior is still debated, and several theories have been proposed over the years, including intraoperative myocardial damage and altered wall synchrony. However, current theories focus on extrinsic factors related to increased heart mobility and new anatomical relationships with the thoracic walls during the cardiac cycle [3,20,21,24]. Postoperative changes in the morphological and systolic function patterns of the right ventricle (RV) are also believed to play a pathogenetic role [25–28]. In this article, we provide a comprehensive review of the current state-of-the-art knowledge about POPS, tracing its essential stages from the initial observations to the most recent developments.

2. Epidemiology

A paradoxical septal bouncing is observed in a relatively large number of cases during the postoperative period. The reported incidence ranges from 29% to 100% in the early perioperative follow-up. Most studies have primarily focused on male adult or elderly patients undergoing various types of CS. Notably, a significant number of studies have specifically investigated coronary artery bypass graft surgery (CABG) [29], while there is limited data available on other types of cardiac interventions (Table 1).

In the largest population examined, consisting of 3292 cases, an overall POPS incidence of 39% was reported. Valvular heart surgery (VHS), particularly mitral valve surgery (MVS), showed the highest rate of POPS (60% of cases). Multivariate analysis indicated that the development of POPS was independently associated with the type of surgical approach, patient's age, and cross-clamp time ($p < 0.001$), while gender had no significant impact [9]. A cohort of 256 subjects undergoing VHS had a similar overall incidence, although aortic valve surgery (AVS) had a significantly higher POPS incidence than MVS (64% vs. 36%, $p < 0.01$) [30]. Other authors also reported no statistically significant differences in the POPS incidence between CABG and VHS. They also reported a notable improvement in septal dyskinesia after a 12-month follow-up [31]. In a prospective study of 165 patients, the type of surgery and approach did not influence the development of POPS, with a decrease in prevalence from 73% to 25% during the late follow-up [24]. Similarly, previous studies based on small cohorts in the 70s and 80s consistently described a progressive POPS resolution during follow-up [3,20,32].

In contrast, Okada et al. reported the presence of POPS in all subjects during perioperative control and in the late follow-up using gated blood-pool scans with technetium-99m-pyrophosphate (Tc-99m-PYP-GBPS) [33]. Moreover, using rest-gated single photon emission computed tomography (SPECT), POPS was observed in over two-thirds of the subjects during routine 2-year imaging follow-up after CABG [22]. Patients undergoing AVS showed similar findings after 19 months of follow-up using radionuclide angiocardiography (RNA) [34]. Therefore, the choice of imaging tool may affect the assessment of septal kinesis. However, there is a lack of comparative data between echocardiography and other imaging techniques. For example, in a qualitative assessment using Nuclear Magnetic Resonance (NMR), the presence of POPS was observed after 3 months from CABG, with different results reported between the echocardiographic evaluation and NMR [26]. De Nardo et al. found consistent results evaluating 34 patients after 10 days of uncomplicated CABG, with both echocardiography and RNA showing POPS, although RNA detected a higher prevalence. They also highlighted a high rate of postoperative increase in segmental ejection fraction in the posterolateral wall using RNA, without significant differences in the systolic thickening fraction of the posterior wall (PW) examined by echo-Motion-Mode (M-mode) [35]. It seems that techniques other than ultrasound tend to overestimate wall displacement when compared to echocardiography. This difference could be due to the varying definitions of POPS used. Ultrasound techniques often use quantitative assessment, while other methods rely on a qualitative approach. However, recent echocardiographic studies have reported a high prevalence of POPS using both qualitative and quantitative approaches during late follow-up [36].

It is worth noting that the method of approach can impact the diagnosis of POPS, even when using the same imaging tool. Lehman et al. discovered that the incidence of POPS was 100% and 76% when using qualitative and quantitative approaches, respectively [21]. Additionally, the visibility of POPS can be affected by the choice of tomographic cut. Recent echocardiography evaluations have identified POPS in approximately 43% and 50% of patients using apical and parasternal windows, respectively [37]. However, ultrasound-based studies in this area used different cut plans for wall motion assessment and definitions of POPS, leading to variability in the results.

In summary, POPS can be predicted in about half of the patients, regardless of gender and type of CS. The prevalence of POPS is significantly influenced by various factors, including the timing of surgery and examination, the imaging technique used, and the definition applied.

Table 1. Characteristics of patients in previous studies. AVR: Aortic Valve Replacement; IVS: Interventricular Septum; CABG: Coronary Artery Bypass Graft; CPB: Cardiopulmonary Bypass; GBPS: Gated Blood Pool Scintigraphy; MVR/Rep: Mitral Valve Replacement/Repair; M-Mode: Motion-mode imaging; NMR: Nuclear Magnetic Resonance; POPS: Post-operative Paradoxical Septum; PTV: Parasternal Views; PW: Posterior Wall; RV: Right Ventricle; SPECT: Single Photon Emission Computed Tomography; TEE: Transoesophageal Echocardiogram; VHS: Valve Heart Surgery; VVI: Velocity Vector Imaging; 4CHV: Four-chamber Apical View.

Author/Year	N. TOT	Male (%)	Mean Age of Patient	Type of Surgery	% POPS *		Imaging other than TTE M-Mode and 2d	Explanation Theories
					<3 Months **	Follow-Up		
Burggraf, 1975 [2]	50	50	38	19 AVR 17 MVR 14 Other VHS	51 §	15	-	Related to CPB
Righetti, 1977 [3]	40	77	57	40 CABG	57	20	Radionuclide angiography	Transient ischemic injury and exaggerated cardiac mobility due to pericardiotomy
Vignola, 1979 [4]	45	-	51	7 CABG 14 AVR 14 MVR 10 Others	53	-	GBPS	Related to CPB
Matsumoto, 1980 [5]	24	67	58	12 CABG 7 AVR 5 MVR	10	-	Intraoperative TEE	Exaggerated cardiac mobility due to pericardiotomy
Waggoner, 1982 [38]	17	56	56 ± 13	12 CABG 3 AVR 2 Others	60	-	Intraoperative direct-M-Mode post-operative 2D TTE	Exaggerated cardiac mobility due to pericardiotomy
Rubenson, 1982 [23]	20	90	62 ± 15	20 CABG	58	-	TTE 2D	-
Kerber, 1982 [32]	25	-	-	4 AVR 14 MVR 6 Others	56	28	TEE 2D	Exaggerated cardiac mobility due to limited RV free wall mobility
Gourdier, 1982 [30]	256	/	/	256 VHS	44	-	-	Exaggerated cardiac mobility
Force, 1983 [39]	20	20	59	17 CABG 2 AVR + CABG 1 AVR	68	-	TTE 2D (floating axis) radionuclide ventriculography	Exaggerated cardiac mobility
Akins, 1984 [40]	22	68	52	22 CABG	50	-	Resting GBPS or ventricular angiography	Related to CPB and/or myocardial preservation techniques.

Table 1. *Cont.*

Author/Year	N. TOT	Male (%)	Mean Age of Patient	Type of Surgery	% POPS *		Imaging other than TTE M-Mode and 2d	Explanation Theories
					<3 Months **	Follow-Up		
Schroeder, 1985 [31]	324	/	/	110 CABG 214 HVS	69	14	-	Exaggerated cardiac mobility due to pericardiotomy
Schnittger, 1985 [41]	21	-	-	14 CABG 6 HSV 1 Other	76	-	Intraoperative direct M-Mode	Exaggerated cardiac mobility due to pericardiotomy
Feneley, 1987 [20]	16	87	52	15 CABG 1 Other	56	0	Intraoperative direct M-Mode post-operative TEE	Exaggerated cardiac mobility
De Nardo, 1989 [35]	34	88	55.2 ± 7.0	34 CABG	41 (Radionuclide angiocardiography) 29 (echocardiography)	-	Radionuclide angiocardiography	Exaggerated cardiac mobility due to pericardiotomy
van der Wall, 1990 [34]	12	75	41	12 AVR	-	92	Radionuclide angiography	Rigid ring of prosthesis limiting septal excursion
Lehmann, 1990 [21]	21	76	59.6 ± 9.6	18 CABG 2 HVS 1 Other	100 qualitatively 76 quantitatively	-	Intraoperative TEE	Related to CPB
Okada, 1992 [33]	16	100	59	16 CABG	100	100	Thallium-201 Scintigraphy Gated blood pool scan Tc 99m	Excluded ischemic injury
Wranne, 1993 [25]	19	52	54	4 CABG 4 CABG + HVS 6 MVR/Rep 3 AVR 2 Others	29 (before chest closure) 84 (after chest closure)	-	Intraoperative TEE	Recruitments of IVS to maintain RV global performance
Gigli, 1995 [42]	10	80	60 ± 9	10 CABG	50	-	TEE cyclic gray-level variation study	Excluded ischemic injury
Giubbini, 2004 [22]	82	86	67.8 ± 9.6	82 CABG	-	93	SPECT Tc 99	Excluded ischemic injury
Hedman, 2004 [43]	99	86	65 ± 9	99 CABG	-	96	-	Recruitments of IVS to maintain RV global performance
Toyoda, 2004 [44]	12	83	62 ± 11	12 CABG	75 (not specified the interval time from the intervention)		TDI	Exaggerated cardiac mobility
Reynolds, 2007 [9]	2979	-	-	1808 CABG 687 AVR 759 MVR/Rep 45 Others	40 (not specified the interval time from the intervention)		None	Related to the type of surgery and surgical approach
Joshi, 2008 [26]	23	73	64	23 CABG	-	100	NMR	Recruitments of IVS to maintain RV global performance
Roshanali, 2008 [36]	240	79	58.3 ± 11.3	240 CABG	-	97	TDI	Recruitments of IVS to maintain RV global performance
Choi, 2010 [45]	18	56	58 ± 12	18 CABG	-	56	NMR rest/stress	Exaggerated cardiac mobility due to pericardiotomy
Codreanu, 2011 [46]	18	100	67 ± 7	18 CABG	-	100	NMR high temporal resolution tissue phase mapping	Adhesion limiting the rotational motion of LV pushing IVS anteriorly during systole
Michaux, 2011 [47]	50		65 ± 8 cohort A 61 ± 9 cohort B	50 CABG	32	-	TDI	No correlation with CPB
Kang, 2014 [24]	165	56	60 ± 13	59 CABG 99 VHS 7 Other	73	25	TOE-VVI	Related to subtle conduction disturbance
Moya Mur, 2018 [37]	30	60	69.9 ± 13.3	7 CABG 11 AVR 2 MVR 10 Other	50 in PTV 43 in 4CHV	-	TTE-STI	Exaggerated cardiac mobility due to limited RV free wall mobility

* The percentage refers to the actual cases studied that do not always correspond to the starting number of subjects, mainly during the follow-up. ** The early evaluation varies a lot among studies. Some studies performed early and late follow-ups within three months after the intervention. In this case, we reported the higher incidence observed in the period. § They performed the early follow-up within two months and the late beyond.

3. Normal and Paradoxical Interventricular Septum

The IVS represents the keystone for interventricular coupling and the biventricular performance [27,48]. Unlike the other ventricular walls, IVS is directly exposed to both intraventricular pressures and influenced by the systolic and diastolic trans-ventricular gradients. Under normal conditions, it thickens during systole, increases its curvature, moves towards the LV center, and returns to its original position during diastole [49]. Breathing patterns can influence IVS motion during diastole, with inspiration displacing it posteriorly and expiration moving it in the opposite direction. This breathing-related effect on IVS motion is minimal under normal circumstances but can be more significant in pathological conditions [8,19]. When the IVS moves in the opposite direction to the physiological motion, it is called a "paradoxical" septum (Figure 1). A differential diagnosis is important for interpreting other paradoxical septa (Table 2) [50], but a comprehensive discussion of them is beyond the scope of this review.

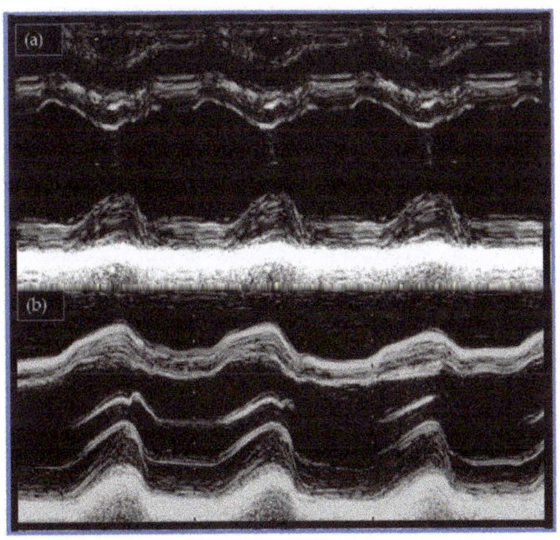

Figure 1. (**a**) Normal septal motion pattern (**b**) Postoperative paradoxical septal motion (Motion-mode imaging).

Table 2. Characteristics and types of abnormal septal motion. IV: Intraventricular; IVS: Interventricular Septum; LBBB: Left Bundle Branch Block; LV: Left Ventricle; POPS: post-operative paradoxical septum; RV: Right Ventricle; (*) could also be diastolic (**) could be systolic and/or diastolic.

Characteristics of Abnormal Septal Motion	Common Causes of Abnormal Septal Motion						
	POPS	LBBB/RV Pacing Rhythm	Ischemia	Rv Pressure/ Volume Overload	Constrictive Pericarditis	Pericardial Tamponade	Obstructive Pulmonary Diseases/Mechanical Ventilation
Systolic	+	+	+ (*)	+ (**)	–	–	–
Normal Iv Conduction	+	–	+	+	+	+	+
Preserved Ivs Perfusion	+	+	–	+	+	+	+
Normal Ivs Metabolism	+	+	–	+	+	+	+
Normal Lv Geometry	+	–	–	–	–	–	–
Normal Lv Global Systolic Function	+	+	+/–	+/–	+/–	+/–	+/–
Respirophasic Motion	–	–	–	–	+	+	+
Stress Related	–	+/–	+/–	–	–	–	–

4. The Septal Injury Theory

During the perioperative period, patients may experience complications such as type 5 acute myocardial infarction (MI) and procedure-related myocardial injury, particularly during cardiopulmonary bypass (CPB) [51–53]. Burggraf and Craige, in 1975, were the first to suggest that CPB-related myocardial injury may contribute to the development of POPS [2]. Studies conducted in the 70s and 80s confirmed a higher incidence of POPS when CPB was performed, with different possible explanations being speculated, such as transient CPB-related damage and graft-related coronary steal phenomenon [3,4,30,54]. It is important to note that in these studies, evidence of ischemia was primarily based on a reduction in wall thickening as observed in M-Mode. In many cases, there was no other evidence of myocardial injury.

However, recent literature has criticized the ischemic hypothesis, as there is no electrocardiographic or laboratory evidence supporting the myocardial damage required to cause such acute and localized kinetic alterations [21,25,30,32]. Moreover, the presence of POPS in patients undergoing uncomplicated CS with patent coronary arteries in the pre-surgical angiographic control makes the ischemic hypothesis unlikely [32,34]. Additionally, studies using 2D imaging found no significant reduction in septal systolic wall thickening (SSWT) in the POPS subgroup [24,35,37,41,45]. However, a stunning localized effect with minimal release of myocardial enzymes, such as in Takotsubo syndrome, should be considered [51]. Anyway, no differences in ventricular deformation pattern, perfusion, and late gadolinium enhancement (LGE) in the POPS group were reported [24,26,45,46].

There is also conflicting evidence on the role of CPB in causing damage during CS. A prospective study on 22 patients found that POPS incidence was significantly higher after uncomplicated on-pump CABG compared to off-pump CABG ($p < 0.0005$) [40]. Other studies also reported a higher incidence of POPS in on-pump CABG and found that POPS was independently associated with the CPB time and preoperative septal perfusion on multivariate analysis [9,55,56]. However, some studies have found no differences in postoperative septal motion patterns between the two cohorts [24]. In a recent study, Michaux et al. randomized 50 patients for on-pump vs. off-pump CABG and found no differences in POPS incidence after 3 months [47].

To summarize, myocardial ischemia is considered an unlikely cause of septal dyskinesia after uncomplicated CS and POPS seem to involve a dissociation between wall thickening and displacement.

5. The Timing

The temporal aspect of POPS is significant, as it occurs after CS. Typically, it is observed on transthoracic echocardiography (TTE) performed within a week after the procedure.

Intraoperative imaging studies helped to define the timing and shed light on the underlying pathophysiological mechanism. Early studies using intraoperative M-Mode echocardiography from an anterior approach yielded intriguing results. In a 1982 study, 17 patients undergoing CS were examined before and after pericardiotomy and just before chest closure. Surprisingly, no patients exhibited ASM at the end of the operation, including those with preoperative paradoxical IVS on TTE. However, after a week, approximately 60% of patients showed POPS, with no significant changes in LV dimensions or function [38]. Similar findings were observed in a subsequent study involving a comparable population [41]. Feneley et al. reported normal IVS motion during all intraoperative stages in 16 patients undergoing uncomplicated CS. However, about 50% of a subgroup of patients exhibited POPS when assessed by transoesophageal echocardiography (TEE) within two hours after surgery [20]. These findings indicated that POPS developed early after chest closure, but the precise moment remained to be determined.

In a shift of perspective, Lehmann et al. employed intraoperative TEE in a cohort of 21 patients undergoing their first CS. They quantitatively assessed LV motion during various intraoperative steps, comparing them with the baseline. Interestingly, they observed a sudden onset of ASM and compensatory lateral hyperkinesis immediately after discontinuation of CPB in 76% of subjects. No significant changes were noted in regional or global ventricular kinetics during previous steps. This discovery demonstrated the intraoperative detectability of POPS, reinforcing the association with CPB while dismissing myocardial injury as a probable cause [21]. Similar partially overlapping observations were made by Wranne et al. using a similar intraoperative approach, where ASM appeared either after CPB discontinuation or soon after chest closure [25]. Other authors confirmed the intraoperative development of ASM [42].

In summary, the timing of POPS is crucial, occurring after CS and typically detectable on TTE within a week post-surgery. Intraoperative imaging studies have provided valuable insights, revealing the early development of POPS after chest closure or CPB discontinuation.

6. The Reference System

The choice of observation system significantly affects the assessment of postoperative septal motion. Contact-based imaging methods remove the relative motion between the heart and the probe, which could affect the detection of POPS. In line with this observation, a study by Waggoner et al. revealed that intraoperative evaluation did not show any alterations in patients with preoperative ASM, which was due to previous CS. In contrast, patients who had right-side overload showed paradoxical IVS until the atrial defect was corrected [38]. Reoperated patients with POPS have been less studied, but the presence of a true paradoxical IVS should be evident regardless of the imaging technique used or external factors [25]. In 1973, Miller et al. first described POPS in patients after uncomplicated MVR. Moreover, they found unexpectedly that patients with significant residual mitral or aortic regurgitation had normal septal motion. After correcting the LV volume overload, those patients paradoxically developed an ASM [1]. It seemed that after CS, the normal IVS motion could be reversed. Consequently, some authors have suggested excluding the IVS from postoperative LV kinetic evaluations.

The "floating system method" overcomes the limitations of M-mode imaging by superimposing traced endocardial end-diastolic and end-systolic 2D images using a defined intraventricular point of reference known as the "centroid".

Various approaches have been employed (Figure 2). In their study, Waggoner et al. used the centroid (Figure 2a) to show a significant anteriorization of the LV after CS compared to unoperated healthy subjects. However, their method, which was similar to M-Mode imaging, did not provide information on the LV geometry [38]. To address this limitation, a more advanced approach was introduced, which defined both a center and an axis of reference (Figure 2b). Patients with POPS exhibited a notable anterior shift in the centroid, coupled with decreased septal kinesis and augmented kinesis of the lateral wall using an external reference. On the contrary, there were no noticeable differences in the kinetics of the LV walls when utilizing the floating system method [39].

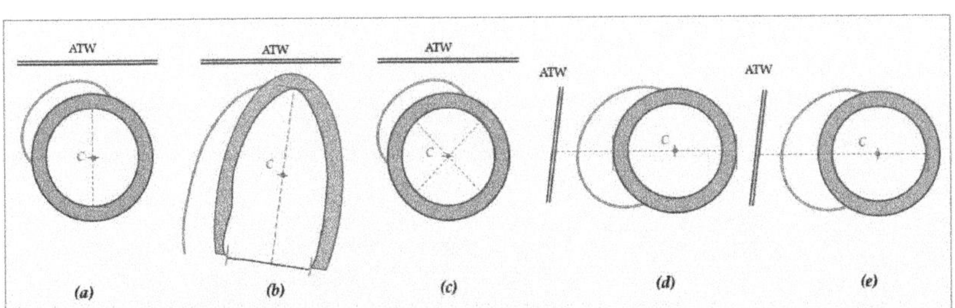

Figure 2. Schematic representation of left ventricular centroids used in the literature for post-operative septal motion assessment: (**a**) intermediate point between the IVS and the PW endocardium from short-axis view. (**b**) intermediate point between the apex and the mitral valve plane midpoint from the apical four-chamber view. (**c**) center of two perpendicular lines bisecting the cross-sectional area from a parasternal short-axis view. (**d**) the intermediate point between the IVS and the PW epicardium from a short-axis view. (**e**) intermediate point between the IVS and the PW endocardium from a short-axis view. ATW: Anterior Thoracic Wall; C: Centroid.

Subsequent studies using TEE and NMR further supported the use of mobile reference systems. Intraoperative studies described the simultaneous appearance of wall kinetics anomalies and the significant increase in anteromedial translation of the centroid (Figure 2c) [21]. This finding was also corroborated by NMR in a subsequent study using a similar Waggoner's approach after uncomplicated CABG (Figure 2d). They measured a significant increase in the postoperative systolic anterior displacement of the IVS, LV lateral wall, and LV centroid after intervention ($p = 0.001$) [26]. Other studies corroborated this evidence, showing decreased postoperative septal displacement in the ASM group, while SSWT remained unchanged (Figure 2e) [45].

In cases of uncomplicated CS, these findings suggest that LV experiences an increased postoperative anteromedial translational motion. The translation motion and wall thickening in the same range of values support the development of an appreciable optical effect explained by the composition of motions (Figure 3).

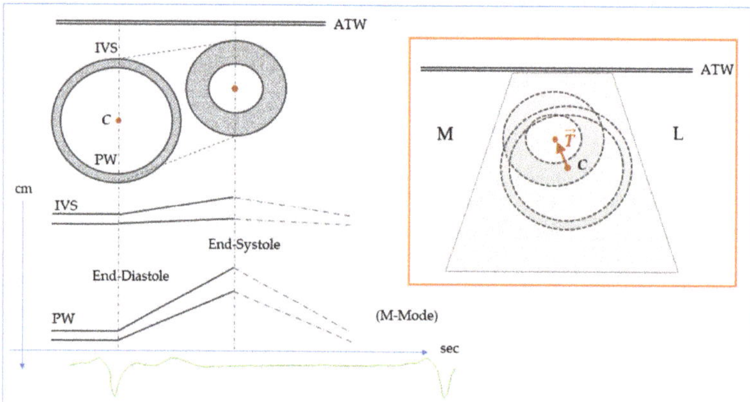

Figure 3. Schematic representation of the systolic left ventricular anterior translation movement (**above**) and corresponding mono-dimensional echocardiography pattern (**below**). In the orange box: schematic representation of the anterior-medial translation of the left ventricle from a parasternal-short axis view. The combined ventricular movement of anteromedial translation and radial contraction produces a hypokinetic septum and hyperkinetic posterior wall in the Motion-Mode scan. ATW: Anterior Thoracic Wall; C: Centroid; IVS: interventricular septum; L: Lateral side; M: Medial side; M-Mode: Motion-mode Imaging; PW: posterior wall; T: centroid translational vector.

7. Curvature and Deformation

In addition to the floating system method, 2D imaging offers another way to evaluate kinetic independent of any translational motions. The LV has an approximately conical shape and physiologically maintains a concave shape throughout the cardiac cycle. When dealing with paradoxical IVS, such as in pulmonary hypertension, the curvature radius of the IVS increases [57]. However, studies have shown that the curvature of the LV and the LV's eccentricity index remain unchanged after uncomplicated CS [20,21,32,58].

To obtain objective results and address the challenges posed by translation and traction motions when evaluating the postoperative LV regional kinetics, the study of LV curvature and a floating system have been used.

Additionally, tissue characterization and deformation evaluation techniques have emerged as valuable tools to differentiate between IVS function and mere displacement [15,22,59–62]. In this regard, Giubbini et al. retrospectively compared subjects with previous anterior MI (all with pre-operative hypokinetic IVS) and others with stable angina (with pre-operative normokinetic LV) after CABG. After the intervention, both cohorts expressed a similarly high incidence of ASM. However, only patients with previous MI showed a significant reduction in normalized septal thickening and perfusion

($p < 0.0001$) [22]. Similarly, one study found that patients with previous anterior MI had a reduction in strain parameters compared to those with stable angina after CABG, despite both groups having a similar rate of ASM. The CABG group also demonstrated significant anteromedial displacement of the LV, resulting in reduced tissue Doppler septal velocity when sampled from an apical approach or inverted when sampled from a parasternal approach [44]. Moreover, others have shown intact septal thickening and similar deformation parameters between cohorts with and without POPS, supporting the idea of a preserved septal function in both cases [37,46]. In a prospective study of 165 patients, LV global and regional peak circumferential strain and strain rate remained similar pre- and post-operatively. However, the POPS cohort showed significantly reduced radial systolic velocities of IVS. The authors ruled out the possibility of IVS injury based on intact septal thickening and similar deformation parameters between the groups [24]. While some authors suggested that the differences in segmental rotation velocities were due to friction to the anterior thoracic wall [46], others proposed that minor postoperative conduction disorders could be the reason for POPS [63]. However, the absence of intraventricular conduction delays on postoperative electrocardiograms casts doubt on this explanation [24]. Moreover, no correlation between LV dyssynchrony and previous CABG was observed in a large, heterogeneous cohort using SPECT or positron emission tomography (PET) [64].

The lack of alterations in LV geometry and function reported in various studies has shifted attention toward extrinsic factors as potential contributors to POPS. The exaggerated anterior motion of the LV during systole has been suggested as a possible mechanism, although the underlying cause of this translation motion is still subject to debate after many years of research.

8. The Role of the Pericardium

The pericardium plays a crucial role in stabilizing the heart and facilitating its physiological movements without friction. After CS, it was often left open, leading some researchers to suggest that the lack of pericardial integrity may contribute to postoperative exaggerated heart mobility [5,25,31,35,41,45]. In agreement with this assumption, patients who have had CS or those with CAP exhibit similar echocardiographic features, including ASM, excessive heart mobility, and increased PW displacement [17,65]. Consistently, the development of post-pericardiectomy ASM was described in [66]. However, the absence of intraoperative changes in septal kinetics after pericardiotomy has led to reevaluating the pericardium's role [21,25,58]. Additionally, closure of the pericardium after CS does not appear to affect the development of ASM, as evidenced by a study by Lindqvist et al., which found no significant differences in bi-ventricular function and morphology during follow-up after pericardial repair at the end of AVS [67].

Other factors, such as the removal of the anterior mediastinal tissue, have been proposed as potential contributors to the development of exaggerated heart motion [39].

Over time, researchers have moved from thinking that excessive cardiac mobility was due to the pericardiotomy to believing that friction between the heart and surrounding tissues can lead to POPS.

9. The Right Ventricle: The Other Side of The Coin

It has been observed that RV longitudinal function (RVLF) tends to decrease after surgical procedures. There is an intriguing relationship between postoperative RV function adaptation, excessive heart motion, and POPS.

Kerber et al. first speculated on the role of RV in the POPS genesis. In their hypothesis, the RV attached to the anterior thoracic wall drags the entire heart anteriorly, contracting [32]. Friction between the heart and anterior mediastinum may explain the reduction of rotational and radial septal velocities described after uncomplicated CS [24,46]. Consistently, post-interventional systolic anteriorization of the heart has been observed using NMR [26]. Moreover, STI studies have demonstrated a postoperative shift of the ventricular longitudinal static reference point from the LV apex to the RV-free wall [37].

This resulted in a postoperative reduction of RV basal longitudinal velocity, strain, and displacement while bi-ventricular global systolic function remained stable [37].

The return to normal values of tricuspid annular plane systolic excursion (TAPSE) after adhesiolysis in patients who underwent a second cardiac intervention supports these findings [25].

However, the traction of the heart due to adhesions and containment of the anterior thoracic wall fails to explain the intraoperative ASM development [21].

In 1993, Wranne et al. demonstrated that RVLF impairment and POPS occurred during the same intraoperative phases [25]. Several subsequent studies reported similar findings, leading to the hypothesis that postoperative reduced RVLF may lead to compensatory movement of the IVS to maintain stable ventricular function [25,28,58]. This is supported by studies that show a significant correlation between septal systolic anterior motion and reduced TAPSE ($r = 0.60$; $p < 0.001$) [67], as well as between septal systolic anterior motion and RV ejection fraction ($r = 0.47$; $p = 0.023$) [26]. Moreover, patients with normokinetic IVS showed preserved RVLF [36]. Some experimental models with a dysfunctional RV-free wall showed that IVS compensates for RV-impaired systolic function [68].

The RV contraction comprises three mechanisms: the base-apical displacement (the most important in the normal setting, contributing to up to two-thirds of the output), the radial contraction, and the traction of the free wall by the twisting-LV [48,69]. Postoperatively, the RV shows a peculiar functional adaptation consisting of reduced longitudinal displacement with increased radial wall displacement and unaltered global function [28,37,45,58,70]. Some authors have also reported a relative RV distension [4,71]. Postoperative changes in RV morphology and function occur rapidly but may persist for a prolonged period [36,43].

While there are commonalities between excessive heart motion, POPS, and RVLF impairment, they are not always interconnected, and the degree of RV dysfunction required for POPS development remains unclear. The hypothesis of adaptive IVS compensation for RV function aligns with the intraoperative development of POPS and excessive heart motion and the maintenance of RV global function [72].

10. A New Heuristic Hypothesis for POPS

The postoperative kinetic pattern of the LV characterized by anteroseptal hypo- and posterolateral hyperkinesis can be interpreted in different ways. One possibility is that it represents septal dysfunction compensated by PW hyperkinesis, resulting in an unchanged LVEF. However, this pattern is not consistent with the nature of injury-related postoperative complications, as there is a lack of significant markers of injury and normal ventricular perfusion and wall thickening [22,24,35,37,46]. Another interpretation is that the combined systolic displacement of the entire heart and LV walls produces the observed motion pattern when viewed from a fixed observational system like TTE. This scheme may account for the apparent discrepancy between LV function and motion. The anterior displacement of the centroid and PW associated with an unchanged SSWT supported this view [20,21,38,39]. The septal kinetics abnormalities observed in patients with POPS may be reversible during a second CS and tend to resolve over time [25]. Moreover, the return to a normal centroid displacement range during follow-up also reinforces this idea [38,39]. However, despite knowing when it manifests during surgery, when and how it resolves remains debated. In an uncomplicated setting, POPS does not seem to have significant clinical consequences, and changes in pharmacological management are not currently recommended since data on the negative clinical impact of POPS are lacking [36,43,73].

Impaired RVLF after CS has been proposed as a possible cause of POPS. Both POPS and RVLF impairment develop intraoperatively and can normalize over time [25,26,28,36]. Postoperatively, the RV motion's pattern and geometry change, while LV morphology does not, leading to speculation that the RV plays a central role in the biventricular motion pattern changes. The POPS may represent a compensative mechanism for the impaired RVLF [25,26,58,67]. The exact trigger for RVLF impairment and its transmission to the LV is not fully understood, but it appears to be linked to the surgery itself, independent of other variables [74]. Biventricular motion patterns change rapidly after CS without significant ventricular dysfunction. The possibility of an acute postoperative myopathic state of the endocardial fibers has been considered. However, several studies have demonstrated the preservation of ventricular contractility using strain parameters [28,37,46,67]. Moreover, most reports indicate that global ventricular function and clinical status remain unchanged or improve after CS despite the impaired RVLF [26,28,36,43,58,67]. These findings challenge the idea of compensatory mechanisms due to abrupt functional asymmetry between the ventricles.

A heuristic geometric explanation for the biventricular kinetic pattern changes is proposed. The contraction of the LV involves twisting, shortening, and thickening motion, with myocardial fibers arranged in a specific pattern moving from one to another coplanar point on the cardiac fibrous skeleton [27,48,49]. During contraction, they move centripetally towards the base and the central axis. Yet, there is a prevailing movement of the base towards the apex due to the relative fixation of the phrenic cardiac surface and the apex cordis. We wonder how the kinetics of a normal heart hanging on its hilum vary. It could be different than a heart in situ, despite maintaining normal function. In the described condition, the medial ventricular segments remain longitudinally static, and the contraction of the RV-free wall drags the LV anteriorly, eliminating the need for any friction mechanism (Figure 4). The postoperative increase in anteromedial LV rotation supports our conjecture [20,39]. This mechanism may explain the intraoperative development and its correlation with the CPB of both the POPS and the RVLF impairment. Additionally, it does not indicate any functional asymmetry between the ventricles.

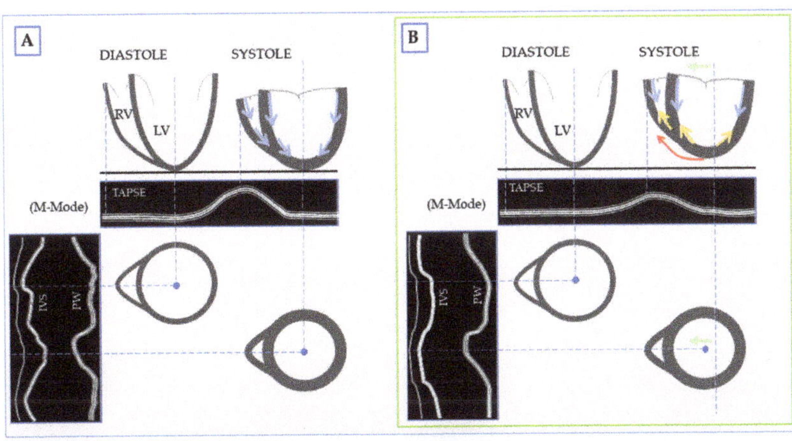

Figure 4. The connection between postoperative paradoxical septum (POPS) and right ventricular longitudinal function (RVLF). (**A**) Schematic representation of normal bi-ventricular motion. (**B**) Post-operative bi-ventricular motion according to our hypothesis. After surgery, the reduced relative apical fixation produces an anterior heart displacement (green arrow) accounting for POPS and a reduced basal-apical tricuspid annular displacement. An accentuated rotation (red arrow) could contribute to the post-operative reduction of TAPSE and septal MAPSE. The blue and yellow arrows indicate the prevailing longitudinal direction displacement of the left ventricle during systole. IVS: interventricular septum; M-Mode: Motion-mode Imaging; LV: Left Ventricle; MAPSE: mitral annular plane systolic excursion; PW: posterior wall; RV: Right Ventricle; TAPSE: tricuspid annular plane systolic excursion.

Removal of anterior mediastinal tissue and the CBP-related impairment of the right atrium may also contribute to this mechanism [38,39,67].

After chest closure, friction and adhesions between the heart and thoracic tissues could further enhance this pattern by fixing the mid-basal sternal cardiac surface [32,37,46].

11. Conclusions

In conclusion, after uncomplicated CS, there are changes in the bi-ventricular kinetic pattern without negative clinical impact, maintaining preserved systolic function. Various theories intended to explain this phenomenon. Selective IVS damage and significant conduction disturbances are considered unlikely causes of POPS. Currently, the most widely accepted hypothesis is that a combination of left ventricular contraction and anterior translation is responsible for increased cardiac motility. Although it was initially believed that the absence of pericardial constrictions was the primary cause, recent evidence suggests that it may increase friction with the surrounding mediastinum. Early studies focused primarily on the LV and interpreted its motion as that of the entire heart. However, the RV appears more static postoperatively with impaired longitudinal performance. Some researchers have suggested that POPS compensates for impaired RVLF, but the idea of significant functional asymmetry between the ventricles is criticized. We conjecture that postoperative bi-ventricular kinetic changes could be related to a shift in anchor ventricular points from the apex toward the anteromedial basal portion. Intraoperatively, anterior mediastinal tissue removal and CPB may contribute, while adhesions with the anterior thorax appear to be the main determinant after chest closure. According to this perspective, the paradoxical motion pattern may express normal biventricular kinetics in the postoperative period.

Author Contributions: Conceptualization, A.I.G. and E.D.V.; methodology, M.C.C.; investigation, F.M. and D.S.; data curation, M.D.L.; writing—original draft preparation, E.D.V. and P.B.; writing—review and editing, G.P., F.F. and L.F.; visualization, S.D.; supervision, A.I.G. All authors have read and agreed to the published version of the manuscript.

Funding: This research received no external funding.

Institutional Review Board Statement: Not applicable.

Informed Consent Statement: Not applicable.

Data Availability Statement: Not applicable.

Conflicts of Interest: The authors declare no conflicts of interest.

References

1. Miller, H.C.; Gibson, D.G.; Stephens, J.D. Role of echocardiography and phonocardiography in diagnosis of mitral paraprosthetic regurgitation with Starr-Edwards prostheses. *Br. Heart J.* **1973**, *35*, 1217–1225. [CrossRef]
2. Burggraf, G.W.; Craige, E. Echocardiographic studies of left ventricular wall motion and dimensions after valvular heart surgery. *Am. J. Cardiol.* **1975**, *35*, 473–480. [CrossRef] [PubMed]
3. Righetti, A.; Crawford, M.H.; O'Rourke, R.A.; Schelbert, H.; Daily, P.O.; Ross, J., Jr. Interventricular septal motion and left ventricular function after coronary bypass surgery: Evaluation with echocardiography and radionuclide angiography. *Am. J. Cardiol.* **1977**, *39*, 372–377. [CrossRef]
4. Vignola, P.A.; Boucher, C.A.; Curfman, G.D.; Walker, H.J.; Shea, W.H.; Dinsmore, R.E.; Pohost, G.M. Abnormal interventricular septal motion following cardiac surgery: Clinical, surgical, echocardiographic and radionuclide correlates. *Am. Heart J.* **1979**, *97*, 27–34. [CrossRef]
5. Matsumoto, M.; Oka, Y.; Strom, J.; Frishman, W.; Kadish, A.; Becker, R.M.; Frater, R.W.; Sonnenblick, E.H. Application of transesophageal echocardiography to continuous intraoperative monitoring of left ventricular performance. *Am. J. Cardiol.* **1980**, *46*, 95–105. [CrossRef]
6. Guaricci, A.I.; Bulzis, G.; Pontone, G.; Scicchitano, P.; Carbonara, R.; Rabbat, M.; De Santis, D.; Ciccone, M.M. Current interpretation of myocardial stunning. *Trends Cardiovasc. Med.* **2018**, *28*, 263–271. [CrossRef] [PubMed]
7. Todiere, G.; Barison, A.; Baritussio, A.; Cipriani, A.; Guaricci, A.I.; Pica, S.; Indolfi, C.; Pontone, G.; Dellegrottaglie, S. Acute clinical presentation of nonischemic cardiomyopathies: Early detection by cardiovascular magnetic resonance. *J. Cardiovasc. Med.* **2023**, *24*, e36–e46. [CrossRef]
8. Guaricci, A.I.; Basso, C.; Tarantini, G. Recurrent syncope on effort due to concealed constrictive pericarditis. *Eur. Heart J.* **2013**, *34*, 1817. [CrossRef] [PubMed]
9. Reynolds, H.R.; Tunick, P.A.; Grossi, E.A.; Dilmanian, H.; Colvin, S.B.; Kronzon, I. Paradoxical septal motion after cardiac surgery: A review of 3,292 cases. *Clin. Cardiol.* **2007**, *30*, 621–623. [CrossRef]

10. Mori, S.; Nakatani, S.; Kanzaki, H.; Yamagata, K.; Take, Y.; Matsuura, Y.; Kyotani, S.; Nakanishi, N.; Kitakaze, M. Patterns of the interventricular septal motion can predict conditions of patients with pulmonary hypertension. *J. Am. Soc. Echocardiogr.* **2008**, *21*, 386–393. [CrossRef]
11. Perone, F.; Bernardi, M.; Redheuil, A.; Mafrica, D.; Conte, E.; Spadafora, L.; Ecarnot, F.; Tokgozoglu, L.; Santos-Gallego, C.G.; Kaiser, S.E.; et al. Role of Cardiovascular Imaging in Risk Assessment: Recent Advances, Gaps in Evidence, and Future Directions. *J. Clin. Med.* **2023**, *12*, 5563. [CrossRef] [PubMed]
12. Ghio, S.; Acquaro, M.; Agostoni, P.; Ambrosio, G.; Carluccio, E.; Castiglione, V.; Colombo, D.; D'Alto, M.; Delle Grottaglie, S.; Dini, F.L.; et al. Right heart failure in left heart disease: Imaging, functional, and biochemical aspects of right ventricular dysfunction. *Heart Fail. Rev.* **2023**, *28*, 1009–1022. [CrossRef] [PubMed]
13. Gaibazzi, N.; Porter, T.; Lorenzoni, V.; Pontone, G.; De Santis, D.; De Rosa, A.; Guaricci, A.I. Effect of Coronary Revascularization on the Prognostic Value of Stress Myocardial Contrast Wall Motion and Perfusion Imaging. *J. Am. Heart Assoc.* **2017**, *6*, e006202. [CrossRef] [PubMed]
14. Muscogiuri, G.; Martini, C.; Gatti, M.; Dell'Aversana, S.; Ricci, F.; Guglielmo, M.; Baggiano, A.; Fusini, L.; Bracciani, A.; Scafuri, S.; et al. Feasibility of late gadolinium enhancement (LGE) in ischemic cardiomyopathy using 2D-multisegment LGE combined with artificial intelligence reconstruction deep learning noise reduction algorithm. *Int. J. Cardiol.* **2021**, *343*, 164–170. [CrossRef] [PubMed]
15. Merlo, M.; Gagno, G.; Baritussio, A.; Bauce, B.; Biagini, E.; Canepa, M.; Cipriani, A.; Castelletti, S.; Dellegrottaglie, S.; Guaricci, A.I.; et al. Clinical application of CMR in cardiomyopathies: Evolving concepts and techniques: A position paper of myocardial and pericardial diseases and cardiac magnetic resonance working groups of Italian society of cardiology. *Heart Fail. Rev.* **2023**, *28*, 77–95. [CrossRef] [PubMed]
16. Neglia, D.; Liga, R.; Gimelli, A.; Podlesnikar, T.; Cvijić, M.; Pontone, G.; Miglioranza, M.H.; Guaricci, A.I.; Seitun, S.; Clemente, A.; et al. Use of cardiac imaging in chronic coronary syndromes: The EURECA Imaging registry. *Eur. Heart J.* **2022**, *44*, 142–158. [CrossRef] [PubMed]
17. Connolly, H.M.; Click, R.L.; Schattenberg, T.T.; Seward, J.B.; Tajik, A.J. Congenital absence of the pericardium: Echocardiography as a diagnostic tool. *J. Am. Soc. Echocardiogr.* **1995**, *8*, 87–92. [CrossRef] [PubMed]
18. Walmsley, J.; Huntjens, P.R.; Prinzen, F.W.; Delhaas, T.; Lumens, J. Septal flash and septal rebound stretch have different underlying mechanisms. *Am. J. Physiol. Heart Circ. Physiol.* **2016**, *310*, H394–H403. [CrossRef] [PubMed]
19. Klein, A.L.; Abbara, S.; Agler, D.A.; Appleton, C.P.; Asher, C.R.; Hoit, B.; Hung, J.; Garcia, M.J.; Kronzon, I.; Oh, J.K.; et al. American Society of Echocardiography clinical recommendations for multimodality cardiovascular imaging of patients with pericardial disease: Endorsed by the Society for Cardiovascular Magnetic Resonance and Society of Cardiovascular Computed Tomography. *J. Am. Soc. Echocardiogr.* **2013**, *26*, 965–1012.e1015. [CrossRef]
20. Feneley, M.; Kearney, L.; Farnsworth, A.; Shanahan, M.; Chang, V. Mechanisms of the development and resolution of paradoxical interventricular septal motion after uncomplicated cardiac surgery. *Am. Heart J.* **1987**, *114*, 106–114. [CrossRef]
21. Lehmann, K.G.; Lee, F.A.; McKenzie, W.B.; Barash, P.G.; Prokop, E.K.; Durkin, M.A.; Ezekowitz, M.D. Onset of altered interventricular septal motion during cardiac surgery. Assessment by continuous intraoperative transesophageal echocardiography. *Circulation* **1990**, *82*, 1325–1334. [CrossRef] [PubMed]
22. Giubbini, R.; Rossini, P.; Bertagna, F.; Bosio, G.; Paghera, B.; Pizzocaro, C.; Canclini, S.; Terzi, A.; Germano, G. Value of gated SPECT in the analysis of regional wall motion of the interventricular septum after coronary artery bypass grafting. *Eur. J. Nucl. Med. Mol. Imaging* **2004**, *31*, 1371–1377. [CrossRef] [PubMed]
23. Rubenson, D.S.; Tucker, C.R.; London, E.; Miller, D.C.; Stinson, E.B.; Popp, R.L. Two-dimensional echocardiographic analysis of segmental left ventricular wall motion before and after coronary artery bypass surgery. *Circulation* **1982**, *66*, 1025–1033. [CrossRef] [PubMed]
24. Kang, M.K.; Chang, H.J.; Cho, I.J.; Shin, S.; Shim, C.Y.; Hong, G.R.; Yu, K.J.; Chang, B.C.; Chung, N. Echocardiographic investigation of the mechanism underlying abnormal interventricular septal motion after open heart surgery. *J. Cardiovasc. Ultrasound* **2014**, *22*, 8–13. [CrossRef] [PubMed]
25. Wranne, B.; Pinto, F.J.; Siegel, L.C.; Miller, D.C.; Schnittger, I. Abnormal postoperative interventricular motion: New intraoperative transesophageal echocardiographic evidence supports a novel hypothesis. *Am. Heart J.* **1993**, *126*, 161–167. [CrossRef] [PubMed]
26. Joshi, S.B.; Salah, A.K.; Mendoza, D.D.; Goldstein, S.A.; Fuisz, A.R.; Lindsay, J. Mechanism of paradoxical ventricular septal motion after coronary artery bypass grafting. *Am. J. Cardiol.* **2009**, *103*, 212–215. [CrossRef] [PubMed]
27. Buckberg, G.D.; The RESTORE Group. The ventricular septum: The lion of right ventricular function, and its impact on right ventricular restoration. *Eur. J. Cardiothorac. Surg.* **2006**, *29* (Suppl. S1), S272–S278. [CrossRef]
28. Korshin, A.; Gronlykke, L.; Holmgaard, F.; Kjoller, S.M.; Gustafsson, F.; Nilsson, J.C.; Ravn, H.B. Right ventricular transverse displacement increases following cardiac surgery: Possibly compensating loss in tricuspid annular plane systolic excursion (TAPSE). *J. Clin. Monit. Comput.* **2020**, *34*, 1139–1148. [CrossRef]
29. Ozdemir, S.; Yener, A.U.; Barutcu, A.; Tan, Y.Z.; Celik, F. The assessment of septal wall motion in patients undergoing CABG by myocardial perfusion-gated SPECT. *Nucl. Med. Commun.* **2015**, *36*, 738–746. [CrossRef]
30. Gourdier, M.; Jouannot, P.; Hatt, P.Y. Echocardiographic anomaly of septal contraction after open heart surgery. *Arch. Mal. Coeur Vaiss.* **1982**, *75*, 73–83.

31. Schroeder, E.; Marchandise, B.; Schoevaerdts, J.C.; Kremer, R. Paradoxical ventricular septal motion after cardiac surgery. Analysis of M-mode echocardiograms and follow-up in 324 patients. *Acta Cardiol.* **1985**, *40*, 315–324. [PubMed]
32. Kerber, R.E.; Litchfield, R. Postoperative abnormalities of interventricular septal motion: Two-dimensional and M-mode echocardiographic correlations. *Am. Heart J.* **1982**, *104*, 263–268. [CrossRef] [PubMed]
33. Okada, R.D.M.J.; Boucher, C.A.; Pohost, G.M.; Strauss, H.W.; Johnson, G., 3rd; Daggett, W.M. Relationship between septal perfusion, viability, and motion before and after coronary artery bypass surgery. *Am. Heart J.* **1992**, *124*, 1190–1195. [CrossRef] [PubMed]
34. van der Wall, E.E.; Kasim, M.; Camps, J.A.; van Rijk-Zwikker, G.; Voogd, P.J.; Pauwels, E.K.; Bruschke, A.V. Abnormal septal motion after aortic valve replacement for chronic aortic regurgitation: No evidence for myocardial ischaemia by exercise radionuclide angiography. *Eur. J. Nucl. Med.* **1990**, *17*, 252–256. [CrossRef] [PubMed]
35. De Nardo, D.C.Q.; Mercanti, C.; Alessandri, N.; Scibilia, G.; Chiavarelli, R.; Antolini, M.; Pitucco, G.; Caputo, V.; Marino, B. Effects of Uncomplicated Coronary Artery Bypass Graft Surgery on Global and Regional Left Ventricular Function at Rest Study by Equilibrium Radionuclide Angiocardiography. *Cardiology* **1989**, *76*, 285–292. [CrossRef] [PubMed]
36. Roshanali, F.; Yousefnia, M.A.; Mandegar, M.H.; Rayatzadeh, H.; Alinejad, S. Decreased right ventricular function after coronary artery bypass grafting. *Tex. Heart Inst. J.* **2008**, *35*, 250–255. [PubMed]
37. Moya Mur, J.L.; Garcia Martin, A.; Garcia Lledo, A.; Lazaro Rivera, C.; Rincon Diaz, L.M.; Miguelena Hycka, J.; Boretti, I.; Gimaraes, C.; Casas Rojo, E.; Jimenez Nacher, J.J.; et al. Geometrical and functional cardiac changes after cardiac surgery: A phisiopatological explanation based on speckle tracking. *Int. J. Cardiovasc. Imaging* **2018**, *34*, 1905–1915. [CrossRef] [PubMed]
38. Waggoner, A.D.; Shah, A.A.; Schuessler, J.S.; Crawford, E.S.; Nelson, J.G.; Miller, R.R.; Quinones, M.A. Effect of cardiac surgery on ventricular septal motion: Assessment by intraoperative echocardiography and cross-sectional two-dimensional echocardiography. *Am. Heart J.* **1982**, *104*, 1271–1278. [CrossRef] [PubMed]
39. Force, T.; Bloomfield, P.; O'Boyle, J.E.; Pietro, D.A.; Dunlap, R.W.; Khuri, S.F.; Parisi, A.F. Quantitative two-dimensional echocardiographic analysis of motion and thickening of the interventricular septum after cardiac surgery. *Circulation* **1983**, *68*, 1013–1020. [CrossRef]
40. Akins, C.W.; Boucher, C.A.; Pohost, G.M. Preservation of interventricular septal function in patients having coronary artery bypass grafts without cardiopulmonary bypass. *Am. Heart J.* **1984**, *107*, 304–309. [CrossRef]
41. Schnittger, I.; Keren, A.; Yock, P.G.; Allen, M.D.; Modry, D.L.; Zusman, D.R.; Mitchell, R.S.; Miller, D.C.; Popp, R.L. Timing of abnormal interventricular septal motion after cardiopulmonary bypass operations. Lack of injury proved by preoperative, intraoperative, and postoperative echocardiography. *J. Thorac. Cardiovasc. Surg.* **1986**, *91*, 619–623. [CrossRef] [PubMed]
42. Gigli, G.; Maffei, S.; Picano, E.; Paterni, M.; Baroni, M.; Terrazzi, M.; Rovai, D.; Biagini, A. Cardiac cycle-dependent gray-level variation is not distorted by abnormal septal motion after cardiac surgery: A transesophageal videodensitometric study in humans. *J. Am. Soc. Echocardiogr.* **1995**, *8*, 475–481. [CrossRef] [PubMed]
43. Hedman, A.; Alam, M.; Zuber, E.; Nordlander, R.; Samad, B.A. Decreased right ventricular function after coronary artery bypass grafting and its relation to exercise capacity: A tricuspid annular motion-based study. *J. Am. Soc. Echocardiogr.* **2004**, *17*, 126–131. [CrossRef] [PubMed]
44. Toyoda, T.; Akasaka, T.; Watanabe, N.; Akiyama, M.; Neishi, Y.; Kume, T.; Komuro, I.; Yoshida, K. Evaluation of abnormal motion of interventricular septum after coronary artery bypass grafting operation: Assessment by ultrasonic strain rate imaging. *J. Am. Soc. Echocardiogr.* **2004**, *17*, 711–716. [CrossRef] [PubMed]
45. Choi, S.H.; Choi, S.I.; Chun, E.J.; Chang, H.J.; Park, K.H.; Lim, C.; Kim, S.J.; Kang, J.W.; Lim, T.H. Abnormal motion of the interventricular septum after coronary artery bypass graft surgery: Comprehensive evaluation with MR imaging. *Korean J. Radiol.* **2010**, *11*, 627–631. [CrossRef] [PubMed]
46. Codreanu, I.; Pegg, T.J.; Selvanayagam, J.B.; Robson, M.D.; Rider, O.J.; Dasanu, C.A.; Jung, B.A.; Taggart, D.P.; Clarke, K.; Holloway, C.J. Details of left ventricular remodeling and the mechanism of paradoxical ventricular septal motion after coronary artery bypass graft surgery. *J. Invasive Cardiol.* **2011**, *23*, 276–282. [PubMed]
47. Michaux, I.; Filipovic, M.; Skarvan, K.; Bolliger, D.; Schumann, R.; Bernet, F.; Seeberger, M.D. A randomized comparison of right ventricular function after on-pump versus off-pump coronary artery bypass graft surgery. *J. Thorac. Cardiovasc. Surg.* **2011**, *141*, 361–367. [CrossRef] [PubMed]
48. Buckberg, G.; Hoffman, J.I. Right ventricular architecture responsible for mechanical performance: Unifying role of ventricular septum. *J. Thorac. Cardiovasc. Surg.* **2014**, *148*, 3166–3171.e4. [CrossRef]
49. Azhari, H.; Beyar, R.; Sideman, S. On the human left ventricular shape. *Comput. Biomed. Res.* **1999**, *32*, 264–282. [CrossRef]
50. Clancy, D.J.; McLean, A.; Slama, M.; Orde, S.R. Paradoxical septal motion: A diagnostic approach and clinical relevance. *Australas. J. Ultrasound Med.* **2018**, *21*, 79–86. [CrossRef]
51. Thygesen, K.; Alpert, J.S.; Jaffe, A.S.; Chaitman, B.R.; Bax, J.J.; Morrow, D.A.; White, H.D.; Executive Group on behalf of the Joint European Society of Cardiology/American College of Cardiology/American Heart Association/World Heart Federation Task Force for the Universal Definition of Myocardial Infarction. Fourth Universal Definition of Myocardial Infarction (2018). *Circulation* **2018**, *138*, e618–e651. [CrossRef] [PubMed]

52. Malik, V.; Kale, S.C.; Chowdhury, U.K.; Ramakrishnan, L.; Chauhan, S.; Kiran, U. Myocardial injury in coronary artery bypass grafting: On-pump versus off-pump comparison by measuring heart-type fatty-acid-binding protein release. *Tex. Heart Inst. J.* **2006**, *33*, 321–327. [PubMed]
53. Khan, N.E.; De Souza, A.; Mister, R.; Flather, M.; Clague, J.; Davies, S.; Collins, P.; Wang, D.; Sigwart, U.; Pepper, J. A randomized comparison of off-pump and on-pump multivessel coronary-artery bypass surgery. *N. Engl. J. Med.* **2004**, *350*, 21–28. [CrossRef] [PubMed]
54. Lengyel, M. Abnormal septal motion after coronary bypass surgery. *Am. J. Cardiol.* **1978**, *41*, 619–620. [CrossRef] [PubMed]
55. Gunday, M.; Alpaslan, M.; Ciftci, O.; Ozulku, M.; Copur, G.; Aslamaci, S. Is off-pump coronary artery bypass surgery superior to on-pump coronary artery bypass surgery on postoperative paradoxical ventricular septal motion? *Heart Surg. Forum* **2014**, *17*, E191–E195. [CrossRef] [PubMed]
56. Diviggiano, E.E.; Rosi, S.; Landra, F.; Marallo, C.; Scoppa, C.; Castellani, D.; Mandoli, G.E.; Pastore, M.C.; Cavigli, L.; D'Ascenzi, F.; et al. Reverse Septal Movement: A Step Forward in the Comprehension of the Underlying Causes. *J. Clin. Med.* **2024**, *13*, 928. [CrossRef] [PubMed]
57. Humbert, M.; Kovacs, G.; Hoeper, M.M.; Badagliacca, R.; Berger, R.M.F.; Brida, M.; Carlsen, J.; Coats, A.J.S.; Escribano-Subias, P.; Ferrari, P.; et al. 2022 ESC/ERS Guidelines for the diagnosis and treatment of pulmonary hypertension. *Eur. Respir. J.* **2023**, *61*, 2200879. [CrossRef] [PubMed]
58. Donauer, M.; Schneider, J.; Jander, N.; Beyersdorf, F.; Keyl, C. Perioperative Changes of Right Ventricular Function in Cardiac Surgical Patients Assessed by Myocardial Deformation Analysis and 3-Dimensional Echocardiography. *J. Cardiothorac. Vasc. Anesth.* **2020**, *34*, 708–718. [CrossRef] [PubMed]
59. Guaricci, A.I.; Chiarello, G.; Gherbesi, E.; Fusini, L.; Soldato, N.; Siena, P.; Ursi, R.; Ruggieri, R.; Guglielmo, M.; Muscogiuri, G.; et al. Coronary-specific quantification of myocardial deformation by strain echocardiography may disclose the culprit vessel in patients with non-ST-segment elevation acute coronary syndrome. *Eur. Heart J. Open* **2022**, *2*, oeac010. [CrossRef]
60. Pontone, G.; Andreini, D.; Baggiano, A.; Bertella, E.; Mushtaq, S.; Conte, E.; Beltrama, V.; Guaricci, A.I.; Pepi, M. Functional relevance of coronary artery disease by cardiac magnetic resonance and cardiac computed tomography: Myocardial perfusion and fractional flow reserve. *BioMed Res. Int.* **2015**, *2015*, 297696. [CrossRef]
61. Muscogiuri, G.; Chiesa, M.; Baggiano, A.; Spadafora, P.; De Santis, R.; Guglielmo, M.; Scafuri, S.; Fusini, L.; Mushtaq, S.; Conte, E.; et al. Diagnostic performance of deep learning algorithm for analysis of computed tomography myocardial perfusion. *Eur. J. Nucl. Med. Mol. Imaging* **2022**, *49*, 3119–3128. [CrossRef] [PubMed]
62. Al'Aref, S.J.; Altibi, A.M.; Malkawi, A.; Mansour, M.; Baskaran, L.; Masri, A.; Rahmouni, H.; Abete, R.; Andreini, D.; Aquaro, G.; et al. Cardiac magnetic resonance for prophylactic implantable-cardioverter defibrillator therapy international study: Prognostic value of cardiac magnetic resonance-derived right ventricular parameters substudy. *Eur. Heart J. Cardiovasc. Imaging* **2022**, *24*, 472–482. [CrossRef] [PubMed]
63. Barutcu, A.; Ozdemir, S.; Tan, Y.Z.; Yener, A.U.; Ozcan, S.; Gazi, E. Relationship between fragmented QRS and paradoxical septal motion in coronary artery bypass graft patients. *Ann. Nucl. Med.* **2015**, *29*, 825–832. [CrossRef] [PubMed]
64. Aljaroudi, W.; Alraies, M.C.; Brunken, R.; Cerquiera, M.; Jaber, W.A. Paradoxical septal motion from prior coronary artery bypass graft surgery does not impact left ventricular mechanical dyssynchrony by gated myocardial perfusion imaging. *J. Nucl. Cardiol.* **2012**, *19*, 1190–1197. [CrossRef] [PubMed]
65. Payvandi, M.N.; Kerber, R.E. Echocardiography in congenital and acquired absence of the pericardium. An echocardiographic mimic of right ventricular volume overload. *Circulation* **1976**, *53*, 86–92. [CrossRef] [PubMed]
66. Eslami, B.; Roitman, D.; Karp, R.B.; Sheffield, L.T. The echocardiogram after pericardiectomy. *Jpn. Heart J.* **1979**, *20*, 1–5. [CrossRef]
67. Lindqvist, P.; Holmgren, A.; Zhao, Y.; Henein, M.Y. Effect of pericardial repair after aortic valve replacement on septal and right ventricular function. *Int. J. Cardiol.* **2012**, *155*, 388–393. [CrossRef] [PubMed]
68. Starr, I.J.W.; Meade, R.H. The absence of conspicuous increments of venous pressure after severe damage to the right ventricle of the dog, with a discussion of the relation between clinical congestive failure and heart disease. *Am. Heart J.* **1943**, *26*, 291–301. [CrossRef]
69. Sanz, J.; Sanchez-Quintana, D.; Bossone, E.; Bogaard, H.J.; Naeije, R. Anatomy, Function, and Dysfunction of the Right Ventricle: JACC State-of-the-Art Review. *J. Am. Coll. Cardiol.* **2019**, *73*, 1463–1482. [CrossRef]
70. Giusca, S.; Dambrauskaite, V.; Scheurwegs, C.; D'Hooge, J.; Claus, P.; Herbots, L.; Magro, M.; Rademakers, F.; Meyns, B.; Delcroix, M.; et al. Deformation imaging describes right ventricular function better than longitudinal displacement of the tricuspid ring. *Heart* **2010**, *96*, 281–288. [CrossRef]
71. Rosner, A.; Avenarius, D.; Malm, S.; Iqbal, A.; Schirmer, H.; Bijnens, B.; Myrmel, T. Changes in Right Ventricular Shape and Deformation Following Coronary Artery Bypass Surgery-Insights from Echocardiography with Strain Rate and Magnetic Resonance Imaging. *Echocardiography* **2015**, *32*, 1809–1820. [CrossRef] [PubMed]
72. Stanley, A.; Athanasuleas, C.; Nanda, N. Paradoxical Septal Motion after Uncomplicated Cardiac Surgery: A Consequence of Altered Regional Right Ventricular Contractile Patterns. *Curr. Cardiol. Rev.* **2022**, *18*, e060122200068. [CrossRef] [PubMed]

73. Gaudino, M.; Dangas, G.D.; Angiolillo, D.J.; Brodt, J.; Chikwe, J.; DeAnda, A.; Hameed, I.; Rodgers, M.L.; Sandner, S.; Sun, L.Y. et al. Considerations on the Management of Acute Postoperative Ischemia After Cardiac Surgery: A Scientific Statement from the American Heart Association. *Circulation* **2023**, *148*, 442–454. [CrossRef] [PubMed]
74. Keyl, C.; Schneider, J.; Beyersdorf, F.; Ruile, P.; Siepe, M.; Pioch, K.; Schneider, R.; Jander, N. Right ventricular function after aortic valve replacement: A pilot study comparing surgical and transcatheter procedures using 3D echocardiography. *Eur. J Cardiothorac. Surg.* **2016**, *49*, 966–971. [CrossRef]

Journal of
Clinical Medicine

MDPI

Review

Coronary Artery Anomalies: A Computed Tomography Angiography Pictorial Review

Radu Octavian Baz [1,2], Deria Refi [1], Cristian Scheau [3,4,*], Ilinca Savulescu-Fiedler [5,6], Radu Andrei Baz [1] and Cosmin Niscoveanu [1,2]

1 Clinical Laboratory of Radiology and Medical Imaging, "Sf. Apostol Andrei" County Emergency Hospital, 900591 Constanta, Romania
2 Department of Radiology and Medical Imaging, Faculty of Medicine, "Ovidius" University, 900527 Constanta, Romania
3 Department of Physiology, The "Carol Davila" University of Medicine and Pharmacy, 050474 Bucharest, Romania
4 Department of Radiology and Medical Imaging, "Foisor" Clinical Hospital of Orthopaedics, Traumatology and Osteoarticular TB, 021382 Bucharest, Romania
5 Department of Internal Medicine, The "Carol Davila" University of Medicine and Pharmacy, 050474 Bucharest, Romania
6 Department of Internal Medicine and Cardiology, Coltea Clinical Hospital, 030167 Bucharest, Romania
* Correspondence: cristian.scheau@umfcd.ro

Abstract: Coronary arteries have a wide range of anatomical variability, and their spectrum ranges from asymptomatic cases to those predisposed to hemodynamic compromise or even sudden cardiac death. This paper aims to review the classification of coronary artery anomalies (CAAs) and illustrate their imaging characteristics by highlighting the important role of CT coronary angiography. Some of the coronary anomalies usually met in current practice are the high origin coronary artery, multiple ostia, aberrant origin from the opposite/non-coronary Valsalva sinus, single coronary artery, ALCAPA syndrome, duplications of the left anterior descending artery, coronary fistulas, and extracardiac terminations. CT coronary angiography is a non-invasive diagnostic modality for CAAs. The complex anatomy of these anomalies can be accurately described by employing 3D reconstructions and post-processing techniques. Knowledge of the imaging characteristics and potential functional impact of these anomalies is essential for accurate diagnosis and therapeutic planning of patients.

Keywords: coronary arteries; anomalies; variants; anatomy; CT coronary angiography

1. Introduction

The frequency of coronary artery anomalies in the general population ranges from 1% (identified by classic coronary angiography) to 5.8% (incidental findings on CT coronary angiography) [1]. Besides supplying various anatomic details of coronary anatomy, computed tomography angiography can detect myocardial bridging, which involves identifying the partial intramyocardial course of a coronary artery, an aspect that cannot always be delineated on invasive coronary angiography [2]. CT coronary angiography (CTCA) has become the primary examination used for the diagnosis of these anomalies, providing data regarding the origin of the arteries, their course, and their anatomical relationships with the adjacent cardiac and mediastinal structures [3–5].

2. Embryology

The process of coronary artery development is highly complex and involves elaborate mechanisms of signaling, cell differentiation, and tissue development. The coronary vessels develop initially in the form of a vascular plexus that further matures into a vascular bed. During the first stages of embryogenesis, the heart does not require distinct vessels due to the myocardial thickness, which allows for luminal blood to oxygenate the cells.

However, with a thicker muscular layer, coronary arteries develop to allow for adequate vascularization, growing, and branching throughout the myocardial layer. The expansion is finalized by fusing with the aorta and a subsequent remodeling process transforms the vascular plexus into a vascular coronary system capable of addressing the oxygenation of the entire heart [6].

The pathophysiology of coronary artery anomalies has been thoroughly researched; a specific reason causing each type of anomaly is yet to be established, given the intricate mechanisms of development.

Coronary artery (CA) anomalies of origin: These anomalies stem from a shared defect: the capillary plexus cells around the aorta and pulmonary artery fail to reach and infiltrate their intended sites on these vessels. Multiple molecular mechanisms are involved in CA anomalies. Studies have shown that a deficiency in vascular endothelial growth factor C (VEGF-C) can lead to a scarcity of aortic cardiomyocytes at the aortic root, reduced peritruncal vessels, and malpositioned coronary ostia [7]. Similarly, T-box transcription factor (Tbx1) mutant mice exhibit abnormal coronary ostial development, with either the left ostium forming at the right ventral sinus or the left coronary artery originating from a single ectopic trunk with a proximal intramural course [8]. Connexin43 (Cx43) mutations disrupt proper CA development, causing abnormal origin, course, and intramural tunneling [9]. Regarding the aberrant origin of coronary arteries from the pulmonary artery, this anomaly is frequently seen in the aortopulmonary window, probably as a failure to close the embryonic aortopulmonary foramen [10].

Single coronary artery: The absence of a major coronary vessel might be explained by the failure of one of the two coronary arteries to undergo complete muscularization. Embryonic coronary artery remodeling is followed by a crucial stabilization step mediated by arterial muscularization and disruption of this process could lead to the absence of a major vessel [11].

Mechanisms underlying myocardial bridges and fistulae remain elusive: Vangl2 mutant models, exhibiting disrupted cell polarity, display coronary anomalies such as myocardial bridges and fistulae [12]. Moreover, anomalies in the distribution of myocardial growth factors or signaling molecules across the myocardial wall, from epicardial to endocardial layers, could also be involved. Disruptions in these pathways might influence the growth patterns of the ventricular wall, ultimately compromising the precise positioning of embryonic coronary vessels relative to the ventricular cavity [11]. Persistence of sinusoids has also been associated with coronary artery fistulae [13].

Further understanding of coronary vessel development holds promise for breakthroughs in reparative treatments, cardiac revascularization, and stem cell therapies for coronary artery disease [14–16]. In general, arterial vascularization variants become clinically significant when the luminal flow is altered due to local or systemic conditions, or when surgical procedures are indicated and there is an inarguably high risk of bleeding in critical regions where hemostasis may be difficult and the hemodynamic impact is severe [17–21].

3. Anatomy of the Coronary Arteries

The coronary arteries originate at the level of the coronary sinuses (or Valsalva sinuses), represented by three main vessels: the right coronary artery, the left anterior descending artery, and the circumflex artery. The latter two arteries arise from a common trunk: the left coronary artery or left coronary trunk.

Emerging from the right Valsalva sinus of the ascending aorta, *the right coronary artery* (RCA) (Figure 1) descends vertically through the right atrioventricular groove to reach the heart's diaphragmatic surface. It consists of three segments: proximal, middle, and distal. Its collaterals are represented by the conus, acute marginal, and posterior descending branches. The posterior descending artery is located in the posterior interventricular groove and its origin from the right coronary artery or circumflex artery will determine the type of cardiac dominance [22].

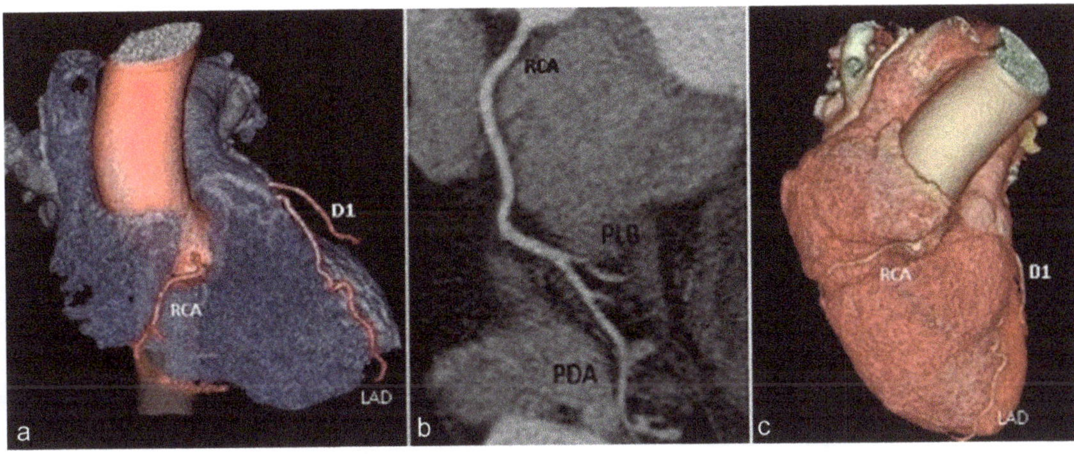

Figure 1. Volume rendered (**a**,**c**) and curved multiplanar reformat (**b**) images showing the right coronary artery (RCA) course from its origin from the right Valsalva sinus, through the right atrioventricular groove, dividing distally into the postero-lateral branch (PLB) and posterior descending artery (PDA). RCA—Right coronary artery. D1—first diagonal branch. LAD—Left anterior descending artery. PLB—postero-lateral branch. PDA—posterior descending artery.

Arising from the left Valsalva sinus, the *left main coronary artery* (LMCA) courses for a variable length of 2 to 4 mm [23], before bifurcating into the left anterior descending artery and the circumflex artery.

The left anterior descending (LAD) artery (Figure 2) has an oblique course descending towards the cardiac apex through the anterior interventricular groove. It divides into three segments and gives rise to diagonal branches (that supply blood to the left ventricular myocardium) and to septal branches (tributary to the interventricular septum).

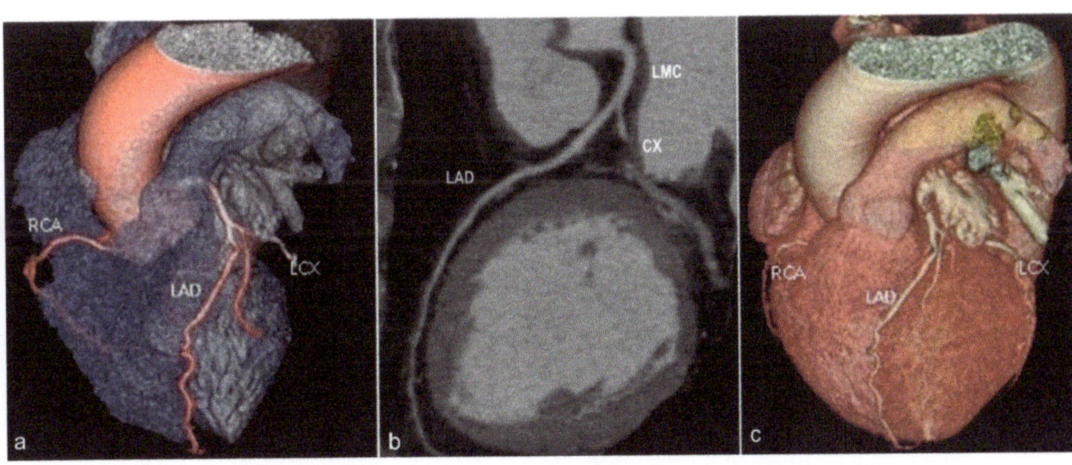

Figure 2. Volume rendered (**a**,**c**) and curved multiplanar reformat (**b**) images demonstrating the left main coronary artery (LMC) arising from the left aortic coronary sinus, with subsequent bifurcation into the left circumflex (LCX) and left anterior descending (LAD) arteries. The left anterior descending artery courses towards the cardiac apex within the anterior interventricular groove. RCA—right coronary artery. LMC—left main coronary artery. LAD—left anterior descending artery. LCX—circumflex artery.

The circumflex artery (LCX) (Figure 3) has a course along the left atrioventricular groove towards the diaphragmatic surface of the heart. The circumflex artery, unlike the right coronary artery and anterior descending artery, has only two segments—proximal and distal—separated by the first obtuse marginal branch's origin. The collateral branches emerging from the circumflex artery are the left marginal artery, obtuse marginal branches, and, sometimes, the postero-lateral branch.

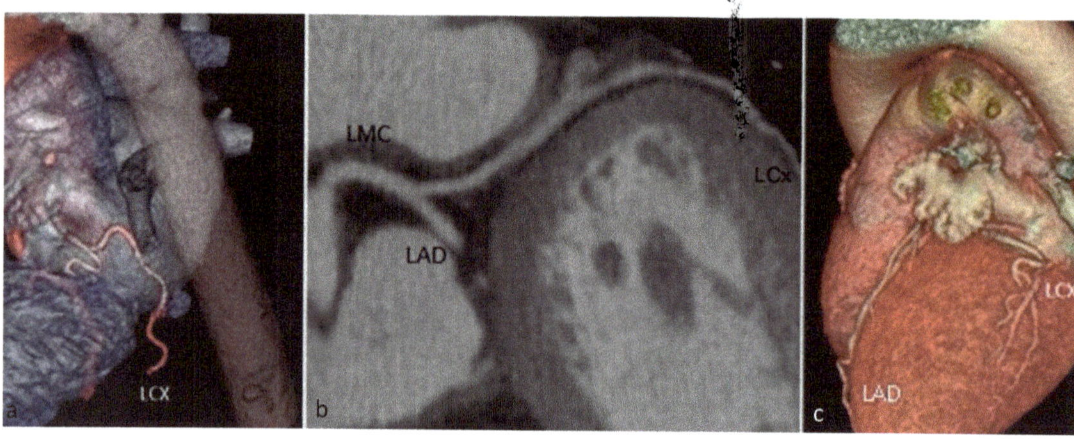

Figure 3. Volume rendered (**a**,**c**) and curved multiplanar reformat (**b**) images demonstrating the origin of the circumflex artery (LCX) as a branch of the left main coronary artery (LMC) and its course within the left atrioventricular sulcus towards the diaphragmatic surface of the heart. LMC—left main coronary artery. LAD—left anterior descending artery. LCX—circumflex artery.

The left main coronary artery may exhibit variations such as trifurcation and quadrifurcation. *The intermediate branch* is an inconstant branch that arises from the trifurcation of the left coronary trunk and has a distribution similar to that of a diagonal or obtuse marginal branch [24] (Figure 4a).

Quadrifurcation of LMCA is a rare anatomic variant of left main coronary artery distribution with an incidence of approximately 5% in cadaveric studies [25]. The left main coronary artery gives rise to the left anterior descending artery, the circumflex artery, and two additional vessels that are usually referred to as diagonal, median, or intermediate branches (Figure 4b). While the presence of additional branches can complicate percutaneous coronary interventions, they also contribute to the formation of collateral circulation, which is essential for maintaining blood flow to the heart in the presence of coronary artery disease [26].

Even though a wide range of variability was described regarding the vasculature of the heart muscle via coronary arteries, the AHA recommends using a standardized numbering system to describe each coronary artery segment and its associated territory (Figure 5). The anterior descending artery, for instance, supplies the basal and middle segments of the anterior and anteroseptal walls, together with the apical, apical anterior, and apical septal segments. The right coronary artery supplies the inferior and infero-septal basal and mid segments, as well as the apical inferior segment. The circumflex artery, meanwhile, supplies the anterolateral and inferolateral basal and mid segments, along with the apical lateral segment [27].

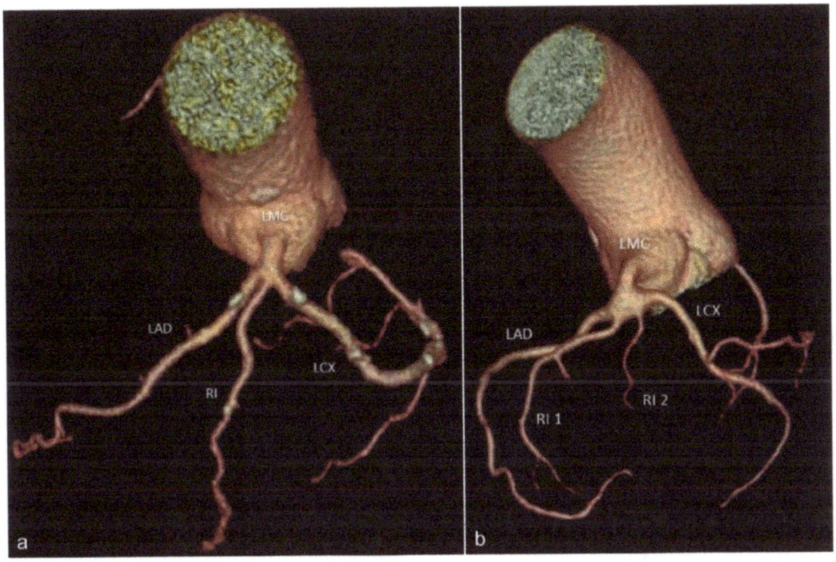

Figure 4. Volume rendering images showing variants of left main coronary artery (LMC) branching: (**a**) trifurcation of LMC into LAD, LCX, and RI; (**b**) quadrifurcation of LMC into LAD, LCX, and two intermediate branches. LMC—left main coronary artery. LAD—left anterior descending artery. LCX—circumflex artery. RI—intermediate branch (ramus intermedius). RI 1—first intermediate branch. RI 2—second intermediate branch.

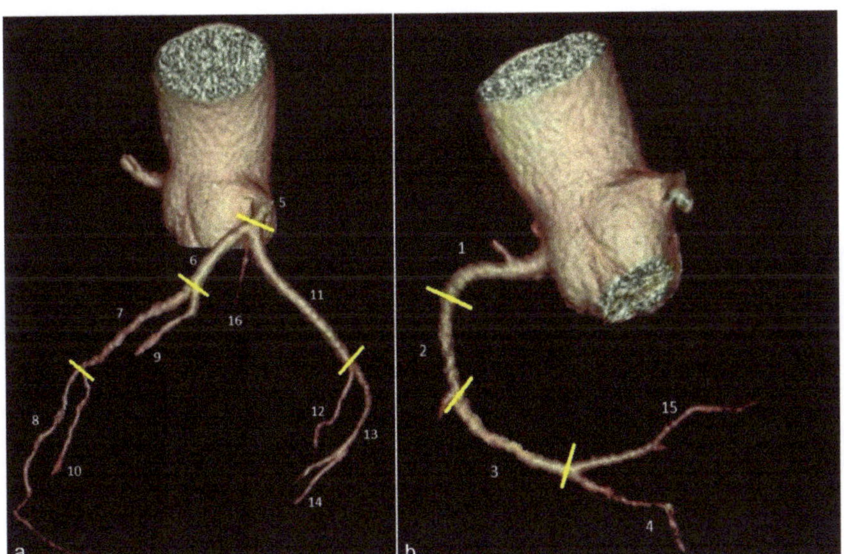

Figure 5. (**a**,**b**) Volume rendering images used for depicting the segmental anatomy of the coronary arteries. (**a**) 5: left main coronary artery; 6, 7, and 8: proximal, mid, and distal left anterior descending artery; 9 and 10: first and second diagonal branches; 11: proximal left circumflex artery; 12: first obtuse marginal branch; 13: mid and distal circumflex artery; 14: second marginal branch; and 16: intermediate branch. (**b**) 1, 2, and 3: proximal, mid, and distal right coronary artery; 4: posterior descending artery; and 15: postero-lateral branch. Yellow lines separate adjacent segments.

The pattern of *coronary arterial dominance* is determined by the vessel of origin for the posterior descending artery (PDA) and postero-lateral branch (PLB). This pattern can manifest in three distinct forms: right dominance (70% of cases), left dominance (10% of cases), and codominance (20% of cases) [28].

Right dominance is characterized by the posterior descending artery (PDA) and postero-lateral branch (PLB) both originating from the right coronary artery (Figure 6a), whereas left dominance involves the two vessels arising from the circumflex artery (Figure 6b). In the case of codominance, the PDA is supplied by the right coronary artery, while the postero-lateral branch arises from the left circumflex artery (Figure 6c).

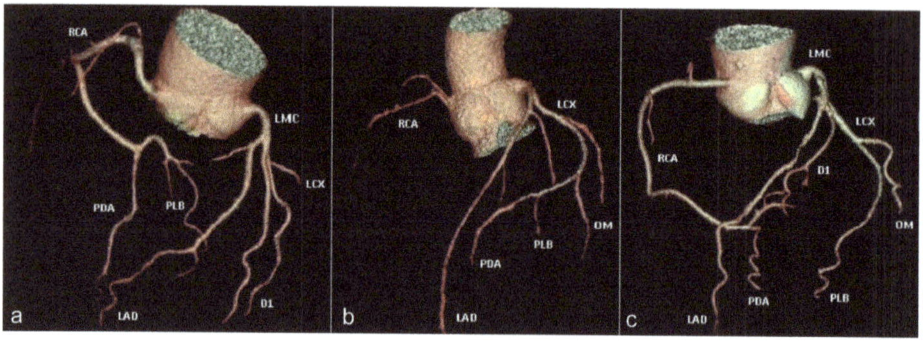

Figure 6. Volume-rendered images illustrating coronary arterial dominance. (**a**) Right dominance: with the posterior descending artery (PDA) and postero-lateral branch (PLB) arising from the right coronary artery (RCA). (**b**) Left dominance: both the posterior descending artery (PDA) and postero-lateral branch (PLB) originate from the distal segment of the circumflex artery (LCX). (**c**) Codominance: the right coronary artery (RCA) gives rise to the posterior descending artery (PDA), whereas the circumflex artery (LCX) supplies the postero-lateral branch (PLB). RCA—right coronary artery. PDA—posterior descending artery. PLB—postero-lateral branch. LMC—left main coronary artery. LAD—left anterior descending artery. LCX—circumflex artery. D1—first diagonal branch. OM—obtuse marginal branch.

4. Considerations of the Scanning Protocol

While each medical center follows specific guidelines to obtain high-quality images in conditions of patient safety and comfort, there are certain common features of the scanning protocol approach.

If there are no contraindications for beta-blockers, patients with a heart rate (HR) greater than 70 beats per minute (bpm) may receive beta-blockers to lower their heart rate. In order to familiarize patients with the procedure, breathing exercises should be performed immediately before the CTCA.

The examinations should be performed on imaging platforms that are recommended for cardiology applications, using CT scanners with a higher number of detector rows that allow for significantly improved images. A 512-slice CT scanner acquires the images in a single breath-hold using ECG-modulated acquisition.

A dose of iodinated contrast agent ranging from 60 to 100 mL is usually injected intravenously at a rate of 4.5 to 5 mL per second, followed by a saline flush of 20 to 30 mL injected at the same rate.

The scan is performed in the systolic phase of the cardiac cycle, followed by retrospective reconstruction to generate ECG-modulated images of the cardiac cycle at 10% intervals.

3D processing and post-processing are commonly employed methods and generate the following images:

- Maximum intensity projections (MIP): these images highlight the most intense areas of contrast.
- Curved multiplanar reformats (cMPRs): allowing for visualization of the coronary arteries in any plane.
- Volume rendering technique (VRT): images provide a three-dimensional view of the coronary arteries (Videos S1–S3).

The quality of post-processing is dependent on slice thickness and pitch, so it is recommended to obtain a thickness of 0.6 mm or lower with very low pitch values (0.2–0.4) allowing for high-quality reconstructions and further processing of data for other applications such as 3D printing or segmentation [29–31].

5. Pictorial Review of Coronary Artery Anomalies

There is a broad range in the reported frequency of coronary artery anomalies in the literature. The rise in non-invasive diagnostic methods has resulted in more incidental detections, with some studies citing an incidence of about 2–3%. [32–36].

There are multiple proposed classifications for coronary artery anomalies, but no single standard approach is universally adopted. Most authors advocate for an anatomically based system, based on the vessel's origin, course, and termination [37–40]. Within the context of origin anomalies, several types of courses of the aberrant artery have been described, prepulmonic, retroaortic, trans-septal, or interarterial, the latter being able to predispose to a decrease in blood flow by compression between the pulmonary trunk and the aortic root.

Very few authors focus on a distinct classification, based on the hemodynamic impact of the coronary artery anomalies, more or less dividing them into "major" or "minor", "malignant" or "benign", and hemodynamically significant or insignificant [41–44].

Hemodynamically significant anomalies can cause myocardial perfusion disturbances with increased risk of myocardial ischemia or sudden cardiac death [45] and include the following:

- Ectopic origin of a coronary artery arising from the pulmonary trunk or directly from the right or left pulmonary arteries;
- Anomalous proximal course with the vessel running between the aorta and the pulmonary trunk (interarterial course), when arising from the opposite or non-coronary sinus of Valsalva;
- Coronary artery fistulae; however, only when resulting in a steal phenomenon (impaired myocardial perfusion due to the diversion of blood flow) or a substantial shunt.

Anomalies of origin from the pulmonary artery: Anomalous origin of the left coronary artery from the pulmonary artery is nearly always fatal within the first year of life if left untreated, with 90% of the cases resulting in death [46]. Treatment typically involves either reimplantation of the left main coronary artery into the aorta (Figure 7) or ligation of the artery followed by an aorto-coronary bypass graft.

The abnormal origin of a coronary artery from the opposite coronary sinus or non-coronary sinus, following one of the four described trajectories, depends on the anatomical relationships with the aorta and the pulmonary trunk—interarterial, retroaortic, prepulmonic, or trans-septal (Figure 8). Aberrant origin of a coronary artery from the opposite coronary sinus has an incidence reported in the literature of approximately 1% [47].

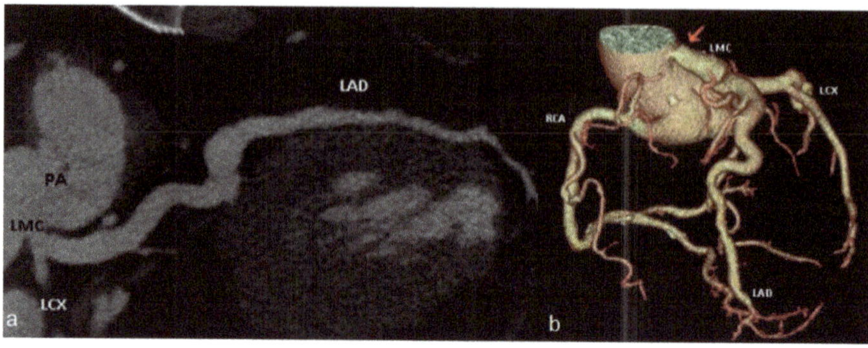

Figure 7. (**a**) cMPR image of the left main coronary artery (LMC) originating from the main pulmonary artery (PA). (**b**) Volume rendering reconstruction of post-operative imaging, following reimplantation of left main coronary artery (LMC) into the aorta (red arrow). PA—pulmonary artery. LMC—left main coronary artery. LAD—left anterior descending artery. LCX—left circumflex artery. RCA—right coronary artery.

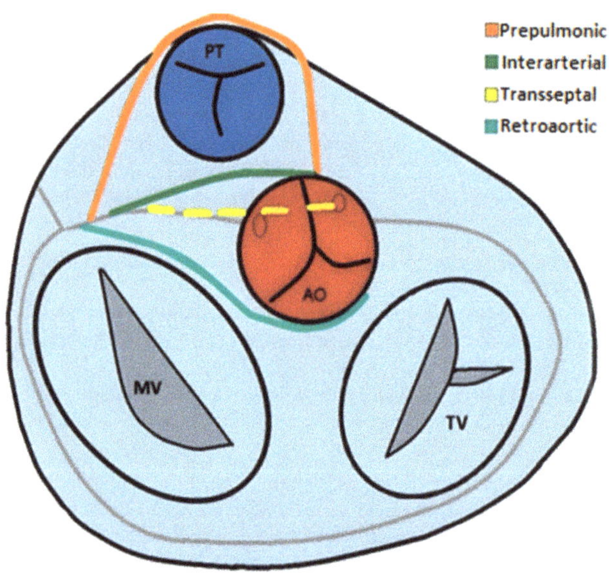

Figure 8. Schematic representation illustrating variants of arterial course in case of aberrant origin of the coronary arteries. PT—pulmonary trunk. AO—aorta. MV—mitral valve. TV—tricuspid valve.

The most common anomalies of origin of a coronary artery from the opposite sinus of Valsalva are as follows:

Origin of the circumflex artery from the right coronary sinus (Figure 9c,d), with an incidence reported to be 0.37% to 0.7% [48] and the retroaortic course having no hemodynamic implications [49].

Origin of the right coronary artery from the left sinus of Valsalva with an incidence of 0.23% [50], where the interaortic–pulmonary course (Figure 9a) can result in diminished blood supply to the myocardial territory served by this artery [47].

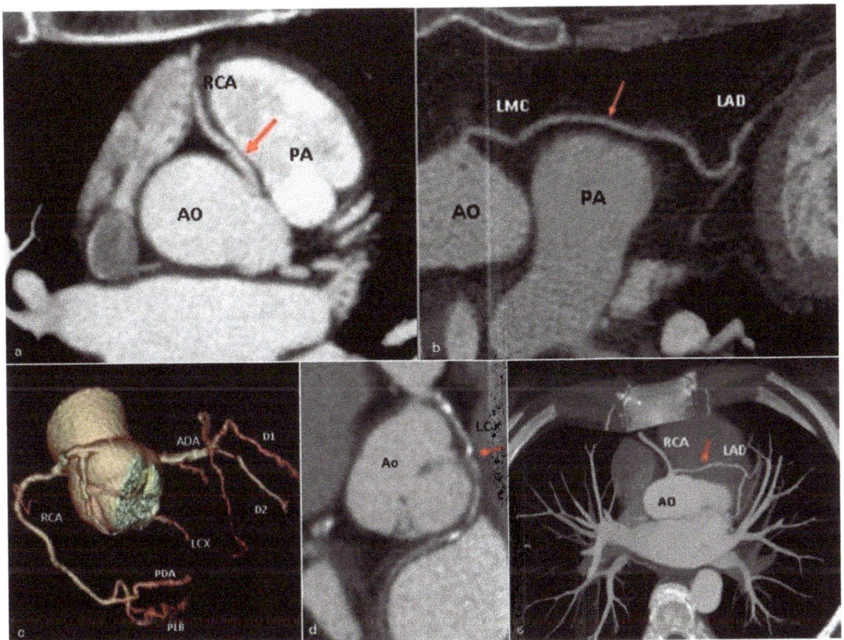

Figure 9. (**a**) The maximum intensity projection image shows the right coronary artery (RCA) originating from the left sinus of Valsalva and its interarterial course (arrow). (**b**) Curved multiplanar reformat image depicting the left main coronary artery (LMC) arising from the right coronary sinus with a prepulmonic course, passing anteriorly to the pulmonary artery (PA) (arrow). Volume rendering (**c**) and curved multiplanar reformat (**d**) image illustrating the origin of the circumflex artery (LCX) emerging from the right coronary sinus and its retroaortic course, posterior to the aortic root (arrow). (**e**) Maximum intensity projection image demonstrating left main coronary artery (LMC) originating from the right coronary sinus with a proximal trans-septal (or subpulmonic) course (arrow). AO—aorta. PA—pulmonary artery. RCA—right coronary artery. LMC—left main coronary artery. LAD—left anterior descending artery. PDA—posterior descending artery. PLB—postero-lateral branch. D1—first diagonal branch. D2—second diagonal branch. ADA—anterior descendent artery.

The interarterial course is considered to be a particularly dangerous anomaly, especially when it involves the origin of the left main coronary artery from the right coronary sinus. This anomaly has been implicated in approximately 33% of sudden cardiac death cases [51].

Hemodynamically insignificant coronary artery anomalies are, for the most part, incidental findings that do not require treatment and do not expose patients to the risk of any adverse effects. However, they can lead to complications of coronary catheterization or surgical interventions involving the aortic root or ascending aorta. They can also make it difficult to clamp the aorta below the origin of a high-origin coronary artery, thus resulting in the unsuccessful induction of cardioplegia. For these reasons, their recognition is of particular importance [41,52–54]. Additional anomalies of origin, course, and termination without hemodynamic relevance include the following:

I. Anomalies of origin

Presence of multiple ostia: can be caused by congenital absence of the left main coronary artery. In this case, the left anterior descending artery and circumflex artery can have a common or separate origin from the left coronary sinus (Figure 10d). It is considered a benign anomaly, usually discovered incidentally through invasive coronary angiography or

CT coronary angiography. Rarely, patients may experience exertional angina, palpitations, syncope, and arrhythmias [45]. Another situation is generated by the separate origin of the conus artery from the right sinus of Valsalva (Figure 10e). The conus artery is responsible for the vascularization of the right ventricular infundibulum and plays an important role in the formation of collateral circulation in proximal obstructions of the right coronary artery. When it has a separate emergence from the right coronary sinus, it can be injured in ventriculostomies or other surgical maneuvers [55].

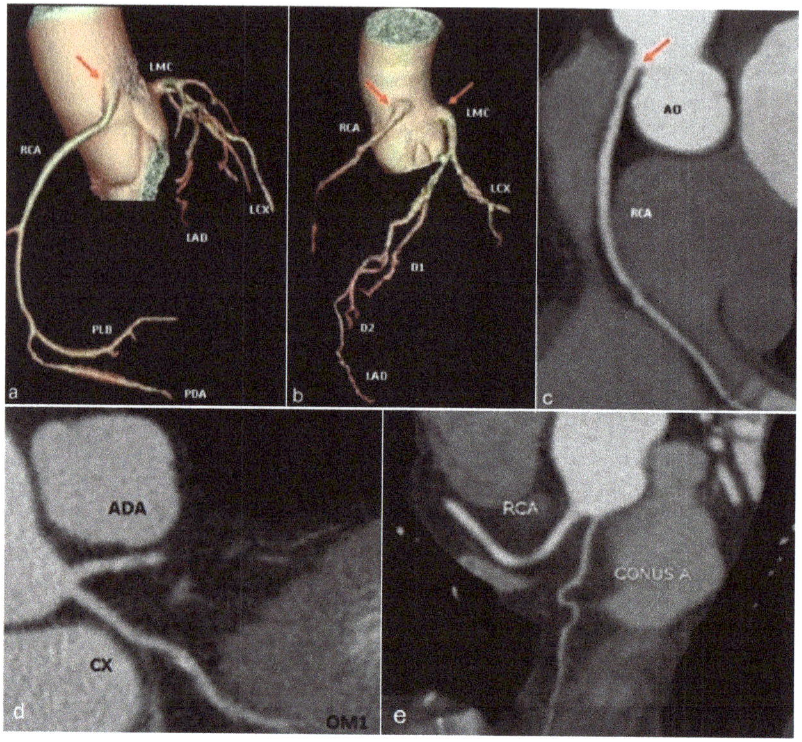

Figure 10. Volume rendering (**a**,**b**) and curved multiplanar reformat (**c**) images showing high origin of the right coronary (RCA) and left main coronary (LMC) arteries (arrows). (**d**) Curved multiplanar image illustrating the absence of the left main coronary artery (LMC), with separate origins of left anterior descending (LAD) and circumflex (LCX) arteries from the left coronary sinus. (**e**) Curved multiplanar reformat image demonstrating separate origin of the conus branch from the right sinus of Valsalva. RCA—right coronary artery. LMC—left main coronary artery. LAD—left anterior descending artery. LCX—left circumflex artery. PDA—posterior descending artery. PLB—postero-lateral branch. D1—first diagonal branch. D2—second diagonal branch. AO—aorta. OM1—first marginal obtuse branch. Conus A.—conus branch. ADA—anterior descendent artery.

Regarding the *high origin of the coronary arteries*, the right coronary artery is the most commonly affected vessel [32] (Figure 10a–c). Even if hemodynamically insignificant, it is important because it can complicate coronary catheterization and should be identified prior to surgical interventions [39].

The separate emergence of the three coronary arteries through distinct ostia from the right coronary sinus is extremely rare (Figure 11a). The right coronary artery usually follows its trajectory along the right atrioventricular groove despite common variation in the course of the coronary arteries [56].

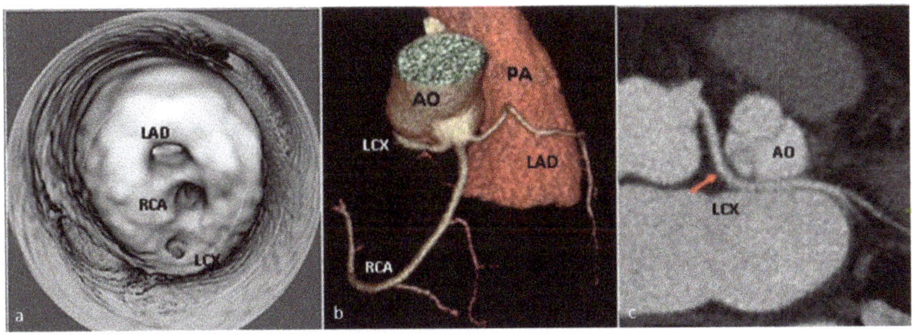

Figure 11. (**a**) Virtual endoluminal navigation image identifying the three separate ostia of the left anterior descending artery (LAD), right coronary artery (RCA), and left circumflex artery (LCX) from the right coronary sinus. (**b**) Virtual rendering image showing the prepulmonic course of the left anterior descending artery (LAD). (**c**) Curved multiplanar reformat image depicting the retroaortic course of left circumflex artery (LCX)—red arrow. LAD—left anterior descending artery. RCA—right coronary artery. LCX—left circumflex artery. AO—aorta. PA—pulmonary artery.

The circumflex artery often has a retroaortic course (Figure 11c), but it can also lie anterior to the pulmonary trunk. The left anterior descending artery may exhibit prepulmonic (Figure 11b), trans-septal, or interarterial courses. In terms of their hemodynamic significance, patients with coronary arteries with an interaortic course may experience myocardial ischemia, while variants with prepulmonic or retroaortic courses are generally benign [57].

A single coronary artery is a rare congenital anomaly in which there is a single main coronary artery stemming from either the right, left, or non-coronary sinus. This anomaly is estimated to occur in less than 0.04% of the population [58,59]. There are several subtypes, depending on the sinus from which the artery branches off and its path, one of the rarest being L II A-V2 (Figures 12 and 13), where the right coronary artery arises from the proximal segment of the left anterior descending artery and arches over the pulmonary trunk. This subtype is infrequently observed in the medical literature, with fewer than 50 reported cases [60]. There might be other congenital cardiovascular malformations associated, such as transposition of the great vessels, coronary fistulas, bicuspid aortic valve, and tetralogy of Fallot [47,61].

II. Anomalies of course

Myocardial bridging is a congenital anomaly in which a segment of a coronary artery is embedded in the myocardium (Figure 14) [62]. The most commonly affected segment is the second segment of the left anterior descending artery [63,64]. Typically, coronary arteries are surrounded by epicardial fat. However, in some cases, they may have an atypical intramyocardial course that can lead to extrinsic compression of the vessel during systole. Most patients with myocardial bridges are asymptomatic. Nonetheless, some individuals may experience atypical symptoms of angina, depending on the length of the embedded segment and the thickness of the overlying myocardium. Because the initial scan acquisition is performed in diastole, it is necessary to reconstruct the images in the systolic phase and the radiologic report should mention the following information: the involved coronary arterial segment, its length and depth, and, additionally, the hemodynamic significance, determined by comparing the vascular diameter during systole and diastole. In symptomatic cases, surgical de-bridging or stent implantation should be considered [65].

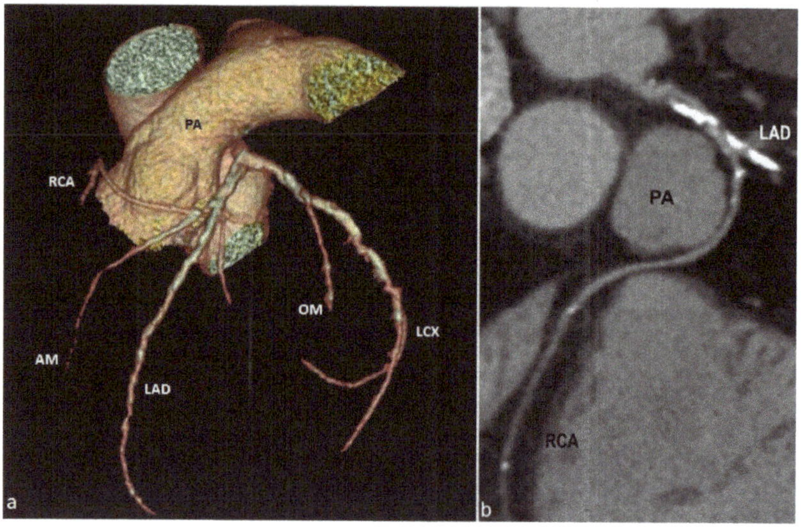

Figure 12. Volume rendering (**a**) and curved multiplanar reformat (**b**) images depicting single coronary artery type LII A—V2, with the right coronary artery (RCA) originating from the proximal segment of the left anterior descending artery (LAD), following a prepulmonic course towards the right atrioventricular groove. PA—pulmonary artery. RCA—right coronary artery. AM—acute marginal branch. LAD—left anterior descending artery. OM—obtuse marginal branch. LCX—left circumflex artery.

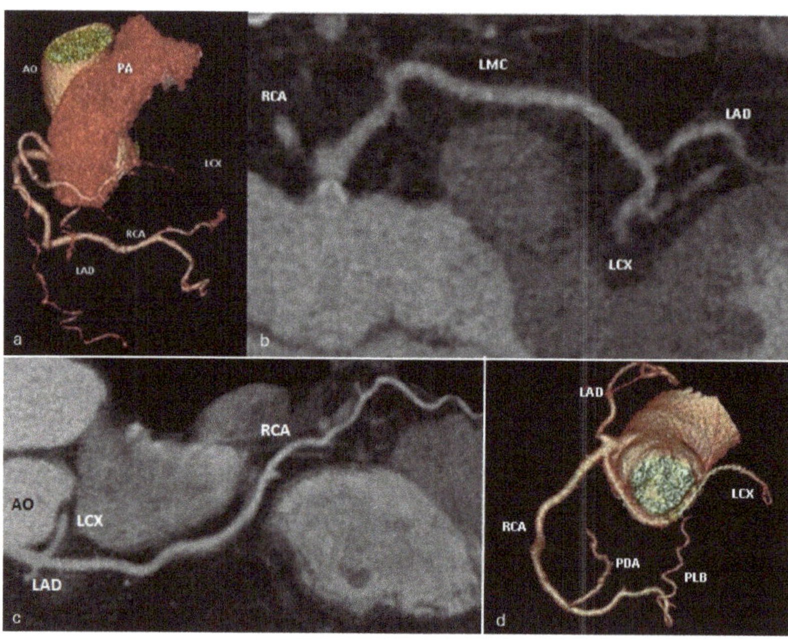

Figure 13. Virtual rendering (**a**) and curved multiplanar reformat (**b**) images showing Type R II A single coronary artery, emerging from the right sinus of Valsalva, bifurcating in its proximal segment

into the right coronary (RCA) and left main coronary (LMC) arteries, the latter with a proximal prepulmonic course, branching afterward into left anterior descending (LAD) and left circumflex (LCX) arteries. Curved multiplanar reformat (**c**) and volume rendering (**d**) images demonstrating a type R III LAD-A, LCX-P single coronary artery, originating from the right sinus of Valsalva, branching after a short course into the right coronary (RCA), left anterior descending (LAD—with a prepulmonic course), and left circumflex (LCX—with a retroarotic course) arteries. PA—pulmonary artery. AO—aorta. RCA—right coronary artery. LAD—left anterior descending artery. LCX—left circumflex artery. PDA—posterior descending artery. PLB—postero-lateral branch.

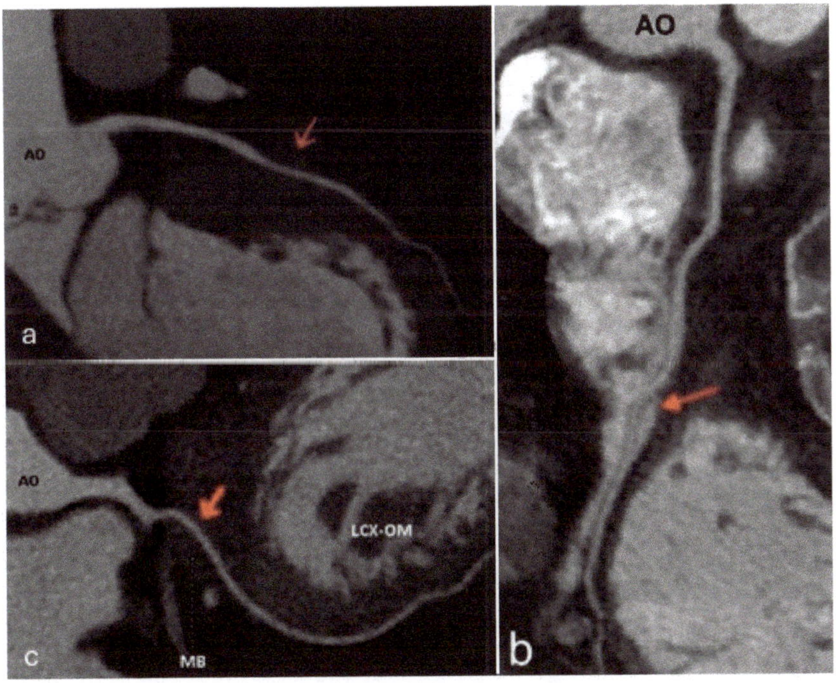

Figure 14. Curved multiplanar reformat images showing (red arrows) myocardial bridging of left anterior descending artery (LAD) (**a**), right coronary artery (RCA) (**b**), and left circumflex artery (LCX) (**c**). AO—aorta. LAD—left anterior descending artery. LCX-OM—left circumflex artery and obtuse marginal branch. MB—myocardial bridging.

Duplication of the left anterior descending artery (LAD) includes a group of anomalies subdivided into 10 types, in which the LAD either originates from the left main coronary artery (LMCA) and bifurcates into two branches, both with the same distribution territory, or with separate origins from two different sources (LMCA and, respectively, the right coronary artery or the right coronary sinus) but vascularize the same myocardial territory [66]. Type 1 duplication is the most common type found in the literature [67]. In this case, both branches originate from a common trunk of the LAD, the short branch having a course towards the proximal third of the interventricular septum, and the long branch lying on the left ventricular side of the interventricular septum, re-entering the distal portion of it (Figure 15a,b). Adequate identification of this anomaly is crucial to prevent misinterpretation of segmental occlusion, especially for patients seeking revascularization procedures [51]. The differential diagnosis with a diagonal branch should be considered, which is recognized by the fact that the former does not re-enter the distal portion of the anterior interventricular groove [68].

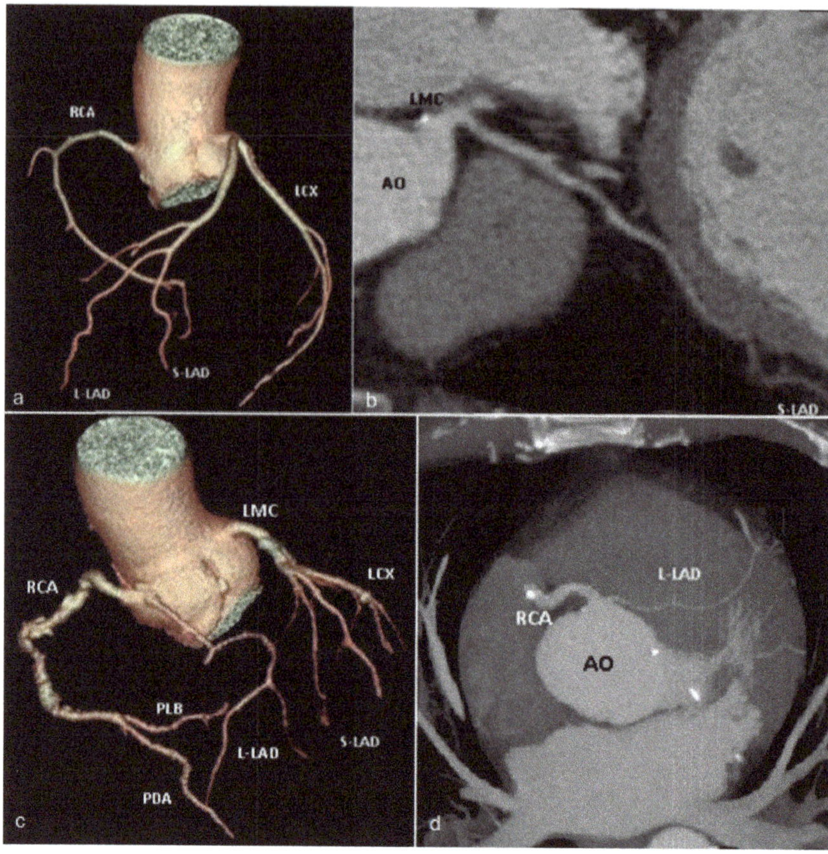

Figure 15. Volume rendering (**a**) and curved multiplanar reformat (**b**) images showing Type I LAD duplication: two branches of LAD originating from a common trunk, short-LAD inserting into the interventricular septum, while long-LAD has an epicardial course on the left ventricular side of the proximal anterior interventricular groove, re-entering its distal portion. Volume rendering (**c**) and maximum intensity projection (**d**) images showing Type V LAD duplication: short-LAD originated as a branch of the left main coronary artery, while the long-LAD arose from the right coronary sinus and followed an intramyocardial course before reaching the distal interventricular groove. RCA—right coronary artery. L-LAD—long branch of left anterior descending artery. S-LAD—short branch of left anterior descending artery. LCX—left circumflex artery. AO—aorta. LMC—left main coronary artery. PDA—posterior descending artery. PLB—postero-lateral branch.

III. Anomalies of termination

Coronary fistulas have a reported prevalence of approximately 0.002% [69] and represent abnormal communication between a coronary artery and the pulmonary arteries, superior vena cava, coronary sinuses, or the left atrium (Figure 16a,b), most with a right-to-left vascular shunt. Patients with small coronary fistulas remain asymptomatic, while in the case of fistulas of considerable size, myocardial ischemia may occur due to arterial steal phenomena [70]. The location of the fistula's drainage point rather than the origin artery plays a more significant role in determining the artery's vascular caliber and tortuosity. Cases with symptomatic coronary fistulas are indicated for surgical correction by ligation of the aberrant vascular branch at the drainage site [41,54,71,72].

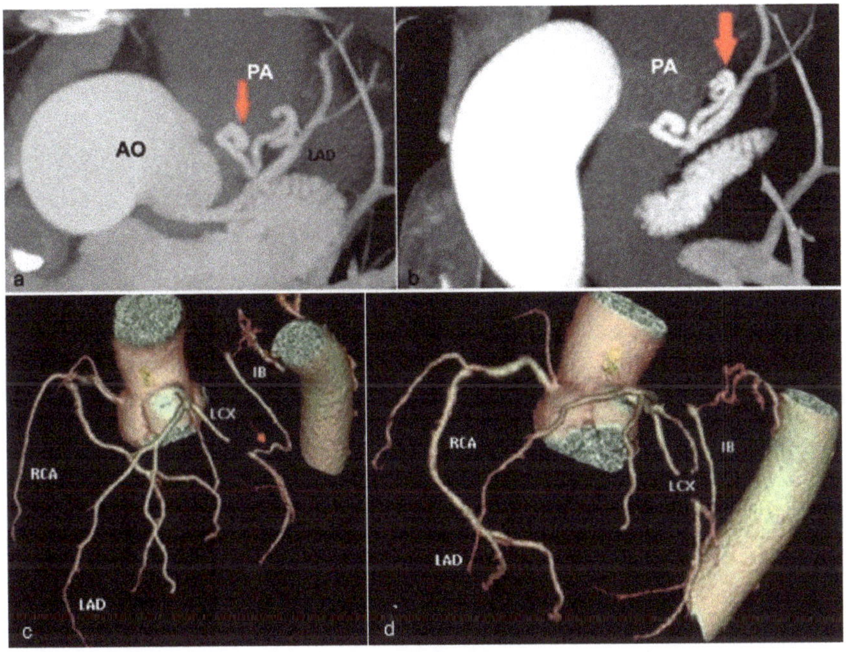

Figure 16. Maximum intensity projection images (**a**,**b**) illustrating coronary fistula: an aberrant vascular branch (red arrows in images **a**,**b**) connects the middle third of the left anterior descending artery (LAD) to the pulmonary artery (PA). Virtual rendering images (**c**,**d**) depicting extracardiac termination—aberrant communication between the circumflex artery (LCX) and an intercostal branch (IB) arising from the descending thoracic aorta (red arrow in image **c**). AO—aorta. PA—pulmonary artery. LAD—left anterior descending artery. RCA—right coronary artery. LCX—left circumflex artery. IB—intercostal branch.

Extracardiac termination of the coronary arteries is an abnormal coronary connection with extracardiac vessels—bronchial, internal mammary, pericardial, anterior mediastinal, diaphragmatic, intercostal (Figure 16c,d), and esophageal [73]. These are functionally significant in the case of different pressure gradients between the two arterial systems [74]. In the circumstances where extracardiac termination is suspected, it is advised to expand the scanning field to encompass the aortic arch and the entire thoracic descending aorta to facilitate accurate diagnosis.

The coronary arcade is an extremely rare termination anomaly, with a prevalence of approximately 0.02% in the general population [41,75,76]. It consists of a wide arterial communication between the right and left coronary arteries, in the absence of significant coronary stenoses. These intercoronary communications manifest as prominent, linear collaterals between the two unobstructed arteries, usually formed in the vicinity of the crux cordis. The differential diagnosis includes tortuous collaterals developed between a patent and an obstructed vessel [73,77].

Recognizing the heterogeneity of the coronary artery anomaly spectrum and understanding that the correct diagnosis implies both anatomical and functional characterization, the authors of this review propose a combined approach for a more effective evaluation, as illustrated in Table 1.

Table 1. Proposed combined classification of the coronary artery anomalies.

Hemodynamically Significant	Hemodynamically Insignificant
Anomalies of origin	
Anomalous origin of the left coronary artery from the pulmonary artery (ALCAPA)	Multiple ostia
Abnormal origin of a coronary artery from the opposite coronary sinus or non-coronary sinus with an interarterial course	High take-off
	Abnormal origin of a coronary artery from the opposite coronary sinus or non-coronary sinus with: • Retroaortic; • Trans-septal/subpulmonic; • Prepulmonic course.
	Separate emergence of the three coronary arteries through distinct ostia from the right coronary sinus
	Single coronary artery
Anomalies of course	
Myocardial bridging *	
	Duplication
Anomalies of termination	
Coronary artery fistula *	
	Coronary arcade
	Extracardiac systemic termination

* Coronary artery anomalies that may have hemodynamical significance.

6. Conclusions

Classical coronary angiography has long been the gold standard method for evaluating coronary arteries. However, CT coronary angiography has proven its usefulness in the diagnosis of coronary artery anomalies.

The identification of hemodynamically significant (or malignant) anomalies, including ALCAPA syndrome, the single coronary artery anomaly, coronary fistulae, and the interarterial course in the case of aberrant origin from the opposite or non-coronary sinus, highlights the importance of CT coronary angiography as a non-invasive diagnostic tool for coronary artery anomalies. The intricate anatomy can be rendered with remarkable clarity using 3D reconstructions and advanced post-processing techniques.

A comprehensive understanding of the imaging characteristics and potential functional implications of these vascular anatomical variations serves as the foundation for accurate diagnosis and informed therapeutic decision-making for patients.

Supplementary Materials: The following supporting information can be downloaded at: https://www.mdpi.com/article/10.3390/jcm13133920/s1, Video S1: VRT of the heart and major vessels with a clear view of the emergence and course of the coronary arteries on the cardiac surface; Video S2: VRT of the proximal aorta and coronary origins with increased transparency of the heart for better clarity; Video S3: cut-out VRT of the proximal aorta and emergence of the coronary arteries.

Author Contributions: Conceptualization: R.O.B. and C.N.; Protocol development: R.O.B., D.R., R.A.B. and C.N.; Data collection: D.R. and R.A.B.; Data analysis: D.R., C.S., I.S.-F. and C.N. Manuscript writing: R.O.B., D.R., C.S., I.S.-F., R.A.B. and C.N.; Manuscript editing: R.O.B., C.S., I.S.-F. and C.N. All authors have read and agreed to the published version of the manuscript.

Funding: This research received no external funding.

Institutional Review Board Statement: This study was conducted in accordance with the Declaration of Helsinki, approved by the Ethics Committee for approval of clinical trials and research studies of the "Sf. Apostol Andrei" County Emergency Hospital, Constanta, Romania (no. 11/28 December 2023).

Informed Consent Statement: Informed consent was obtained from all subjects involved in the study. Written informed consent has been obtained from the patients to publish this paper.

Data Availability Statement: The data that support the findings of this study are not openly available due to reasons of sensitivity but are available from the corresponding author upon reasonable request.

Conflicts of Interest: The authors declare no conflicts of interest. All the figures and videos were prepared and created by the authors.

Abbreviations

ALCAPA	Anomalous left coronary artery from the pulmonary artery
AM	Acute marginal branch
AO	Aorta
CAA	Coronary artery anomalies
cMPR	Curved multiplanar reformat
CONUS A	Conus artery
CTCA	CT coronary angiography
D1	First diagonal branch
D2	Second diagonal branch
IB	Intercostal branch
LAD	Left anterior descending
LCX	Left circumflex artery
L-LAD	Long branch of left anterior descending
LMC	Left main coronary artery
LPA	Left pulmonary artery
MIP	Maximum intensity projections
OM	Obtuse marginal branch
PA	Pulmonary artery
PDA	Posterior descending artery
PLB	Postero-lateral branch
RCA	Right coronary artery
RI	Ramus intermedius
RPA	Right pulmonary artery
S-LAD	Short branch of left anterior descending
VEGF	Vascular endothelial growth factor
VR	Volume rendering

References

1. Agarwal, P.P.; Dennie, C.; Pena, E.; Nguyen, E.; LaBounty, T.; Yang, B.; Patel, S. Anomalous Coronary Arteries That Need Intervention: Review of Pre- and Postoperative Imaging Appearances. *Radiographics* **2017**, *37*, 740–757. [CrossRef]
2. Beecham, R.; Prater, S.; Batlle, J. Coronary Artery Anomalies. In *StatPearls*; StatPearls Publishing: Treasure Island, FL, USA, 2024.
3. Chen, Q.; Pan, T.; Wang, Y.N.; Schoepf, U.J.; Bidwell, S.L.; Qiao, H.; Feng, Y.; Xu, C.; Xu, H.; Xie, G.; et al. A Coronary CT Angiography Radiomics Model to Identify Vulnerable Plaque and Predict Cardiovascular Events. *Radiology* **2023**, *307*, e221693. [CrossRef]
4. Baz, R.O.; Gherghescu, G.; Mustafa, A.; Enyedi, M.; Scheau, C.; Baz, R.A. The Role of CT Imaging in a Fractured Coronary Stent with Pseudoaneurysm Formation. *Diagnostics* **2024**, *14*, 840. [CrossRef]
5. Cademartiri, F.; Casolo, G.; Clemente, A.; Seitun, S.; Mantini, C.; Bossone, E.; Saba, L.; Sverzellati, N.; Nistri, S.; Punzo, B.; et al. Coronary CT angiography: A guide to examination, interpretation, and clinical indications. *Expert Rev. Cardiovasc. Ther.* **2021**, *19*, 413–425. [CrossRef]
6. Sharma, B.; Chang, A.; Red-Horse, K. Coronary Artery Development: Progenitor Cells and Differentiation Pathways. *Annu. Rev. Physiol.* **2017**, *79*, 1–19. [CrossRef]
7. Ramai, D.; Lai, J.; Monzidelis, C.; Reddy, S. Coronary Artery Development: Origin, Malformations, and Translational Vascular Reparative Therapy. *J. Cardiovasc. Pharmacol. Ther.* **2018**, *23*, 292–300. [CrossRef]

8. Tomanek, R.; Angelini, P. Embryology of coronary arteries and anatomy/pathophysiology of coronary anomalies. A comprehensive update. *Int. J. Cardiol.* **2019**, *281*, 28–34. [CrossRef]
9. Walker, D.L.; Vacha, S.J.; Kirby, M.L.; Lo, C.W. Connexin43 deficiency causes dysregulation of coronary vasculogenesis. *Dev. Biol.* **2005**, *284*, 479–498. [CrossRef]
10. Spicer, D.E.; Henderson, D.J.; Chaudhry, B.; Mohun, T.J.; Anderson, R.H. The anatomy and development of normal and abnormal coronary arteries. *Cardiol. Young* **2015**, *25*, 1493–1503. [CrossRef]
11. Pérez-Pomares, J.M.; de la Pompa, J.L.; Franco, D.; Henderson, D.; Ho, S.Y.; Houyel, L.; Kelly, R.G.; Sedmera, D.; Sheppard, M.; Sperling, S.; et al. Congenital coronary artery anomalies: A bridge from embryology to anatomy and pathophysiology—A position statement of the development, anatomy, and pathology ESC Working Group. *Cardiovasc. Res.* **2016**, *109*, 204–216. [CrossRef]
12. Phillips, H.M.; Rhee, H.J.; Murdoch, J.N.; Hildreth, V.; Peat, J.D.; Anderson, R.H.; Copp, A.J.; Chaudhry, B.; Henderson, D.J. Disruption of Planar Cell Polarity Signaling Results in Congenital Heart Defects and Cardiomyopathy Attributable to Early Cardiomyocyte Disorganization. *Circ. Res.* **2007**, *101*, 137–145. [CrossRef]
13. Kiefer, T.L.; Crowley, A.L.; Jaggers, J.; Harrison, J.K. Coronary arteriovenous fistulae: The complexity of coronary artery-to-coronary sinus connections. *Tex. Heart Inst. J.* **2012**, *39*, 218–222.
14. Díez-Villanueva, P.; Gutiérrez-Ibañes, E.; Cuerpo-Caballero, G.P.; Sanz-Ruiz, R.; Abeytua, M.; Soriano, J.; Sarnago, F.; Elízaga, J.; González-Pinto, A.; Fernández-Avilés, F. Direct injury to right coronary artery in patients undergoing tricuspid annuloplasty. *Ann. Thorac. Surg.* **2014**, *97*, 1300–1305. [CrossRef]
15. Berezin, A.E.; Berezin, A.A. Adverse Cardiac Remodelling after Acute Myocardial Infarction: Old and New Biomarkers. *Dis. Markers* **2020**, *2020*, 1215802. [CrossRef]
16. Aggarwal, R.; Potel, K.N.; Shao, A.; So, S.W.; Swingen, C.; Reyes, C.P.; Rose, R.; Wright, C.; Hocum Stone, L.L.; McFalls, E.O.; et al. An Adjuvant Stem Cell Patch with Coronary Artery Bypass Graft Surgery Improves Diastolic Recovery in Porcine Hibernating Myocardium. *Int. J. Mol. Sci.* **2023**, *24*, 5475. [CrossRef]
17. Chen, J.; Ceholski, D.K.; Liang, L.; Fish, K.; Hajjar, R.J. Variability in coronary artery anatomy affects consistency of cardiac damage after myocardial infarction in mice. *Am. J. Physiol. Heart Circ. Physiol.* **2017**, *313*, H275–H282. [CrossRef]
18. Baz, R.A.; Jurja, S.; Ciuluvica, R.; Scheau, C.; Baz, R. Morphometric study regarding ophthalmic and internal carotid arteries utilizing computed tomography angiography. *Exp. Ther. Med.* **2022**, *23*, 112. [CrossRef]
19. Baquero, G.A.; Azarrafiy, R.; de Marchena, E.J.; Carrillo, R.G. Hybrid off-pump coronary artery bypass grafting surgery and transaortic transcatheter aortic valve replacement: Literature review of a feasible bailout for patients with complex coronary anatomy and poor femoral access. *J. Card. Surg.* **2019**, *34*, 591–597. [CrossRef]
20. Enyedi, M.; Scheau, C.; Baz, R.O.; Didilescu, A.C. Circle of Willis: Anatomical variations of configuration. A magnetic resonance angiography study. *Folia Morphol.* **2023**, *82*, 24–29. [CrossRef]
21. Baz, R.A.; Scheau, C.; Niscoveanu, C.; Bordei, P. Morphometry of the Entire Internal Carotid Artery on CT Angiography. *Medicina* **2021**, *57*, 832. [CrossRef]
22. Shahoud, J.S.; Ambalavanan, M.; Tivakaran, V.S. Cardiac Dominance. In *StatPearls*; StatPearls Publishing: Treasure Island, FL, USA, 2024.
23. Angelini, P. Normal and anomalous coronary arteries: Definitions and classification. *Am. Heart J.* **1989**, *117*, 418–434. [CrossRef]
24. Chiribiri, A.; Ishida, M.; Nagel, E.; Botnar, R.M. Coronary Imaging With Cardiovascular Magnetic Resonance: Current State of the Art. *Prog. Cardiovasc. Dis.* **2011**, *54*, 240–252. [CrossRef]
25. Khalid, N.; Chhabra, L.; Ahmad, S.A.; Sareen, P. A Large-Sized Left Main Coronary Artery with Quadfurcation: A Rare Anatomy. *Conn. Med.* **2015**, *79*, 211–212.
26. Tyczyński, P.; Pręgowski, J.; Skowroński, J.; Wojtkowska, I.; Brutkiewicz, A.; Witkowski, A. Left main coronary artery quadrifurcation and acute coronary syndrome. *Pol. Heart J.* **2017**, *75*, 398. [CrossRef]
27. Cerqueira, M.D.; Weissman, N.J.; Dilsizian, V.; Jacobs, A.K.; Kaul, S.; Laskey, W.K.; Pennell, D.J.; Rumberger, J.A.; Ryan, T.; Verani, M.S. Standardized Myocardial Segmentation and Nomenclature for Tomographic Imaging of the Heart. *Circulation* **2002**, *105*, 539–542. [CrossRef]
28. Ispas, V.; Iliescu, D.; Baz, R.; Bordei, P. Specific morphological characteristics of the coronary arteries. *ARS Medica Tomitana* **2013**, *2*, 112–116. [CrossRef]
29. Sun, Z.; Choo, G.H.; Ng, K.H. Coronary CT angiography: Current status and continuing challenges. *Br. J. Radiol.* **2012**, *85*, 495–510. [CrossRef]
30. Timofticiuc, I.-A.; Călinescu, O.; Iftime, A.; Dragosloveanu, S.; Caruntu, A.; Scheau, A.-E.; Badarau, I.A.; Didilescu, A.C.; Caruntu, C.; Scheau, C. Biomaterials Adapted to Vat Photopolymerization in 3D Printing: Characteristics and Medical Applications. *J. Funct. Biomater.* **2024**, *15*, 7. [CrossRef]
31. Sun, Z.; Ng, K.H. Multislice CT angiography in cardiac imaging. Part II: Clinical applications in coronary artery disease. *Singap. Med. J.* **2010**, *51*, 282–289.
32. Graidis, C.; Dimitriadis, D.; Karasavvidis, V.; Dimitriadis, G.; Argyropoulou, E.; Economou, F.; George, D.; Antoniou, A.; Karakostas, G. Prevalence and characteristics of coronary artery anomalies in an adult population undergoing multidetector-row computed tomography for the evaluation of coronary artery disease. *BMC Cardiovasc. Disord.* **2015**, *15*, 112. [CrossRef]

33. Gräni, C.; Benz, D.C.; Schmied, C.; Vontobel, J.; Possner, M.; Clerc, O.F.; Mikulicic, F.; Stehli, J.; Fuchs, T.A.; Pazhenkottil, A.P.; et al. Prevalence and characteristics of coronary artery anomalies detected by coronary computed tomography angiography in 5634 consecutive patients in a single centre in Switzerland. *Swiss Med. Wkly.* **2016**, *146*, w14294. [CrossRef]
34. Ilić, D.S.; Stojanov, D.; Koraćević, G.; Petrović, S.; Radovanović, Z.; Arsić, S. The prevalence of coronary artery anomalies in adults: Studied with computed tomography coronary angiography. *Vojnosanit. Pregl.* **2018**, *75*, 16–22. [CrossRef]
35. Schmitt, R.; Froehner, S.; Brunn, J.; Wagner, M.; Brunner, H.; Cherevatyy, O.; Gietzen, F.; Christopoulos, G.; Kerber, S.; Fellner, F. Congenital anomalies of the coronary arteries: Imaging with contrast-enhanced, multidetector computed tomography. *Eur. Radiol.* **2005**, *15*, 1110–1121. [CrossRef]
36. Onciu, M.; Baz, R.; Onciu, C. Particularités de distribution des branches des artères coronnaires. *Morphologie* **2005**, *89*, 189. [CrossRef]
37. Greenberg, M.A.; Fish, B.G.; Spindola-Franco, H. Congenital anomalies of the coronary arteries. Classification and significance. *Radiol. Clin. N. Am.* **1989**, *27*, 1127–1146. [CrossRef]
38. Angelini, P. Coronary Artery Anomalies: An entity in search of an identity. *Circulation* **2007**, *115*, 1296–1305. [CrossRef]
39. Villa, A.D.; Sammut, E.; Nair, A.; Rajani, R.; Bonamini, R.; Chiribiri, A. Coronary artery anomalies overview: The normal and the abnormal. *World J. Radiol.* **2016**, *8*, 537–555. [CrossRef]
40. Gentile, F.; Castiglione, V.; Caterina, R.D. Coronary Artery Anomalies. *Circulation* **2021**, *144*, 983–996. [CrossRef]
41. Yamanaka, O.; Hobbs, R.E. Coronary artery anomalies in 126,595 patients undergoing coronary arteriography. *Catheter. Cardiovasc. Diagn.* **1990**, *21*, 28–40. [CrossRef]
42. Ogden, J.A. Congenital anomalies of the coronary arteries. *Am. J. Cardiol.* **1970**, *25*, 474–479. [CrossRef]
43. Levin, D.C.; Fellows, K.E.; Abrams, H.L. Hemodynamically significant primary anomalies of the coronary arteries. Angiographic aspects. *Circulation* **1978**, *58*, 25–34. [CrossRef] [PubMed]
44. Rigatelli, G.; Docali, G.; Rossi, P.; Bandello, A.; Rigatelli, G. Validation of a Clinical-Significance-Based Classification of Coronary Artery Anomalies. *Angiology* **2005**, *56*, 25–34. [CrossRef] [PubMed]
45. Reagan, K.; Boxt, L.M.; Katz, J. Introduction to Coronary Arteriography. *Radiol. Clin. N. Am.* **1994**, *32*, 419–433. [CrossRef] [PubMed]
46. Peña, E.; Nguyen, E.T.; Merchant, N.; Dennie, C. ALCAPA Syndrome: Not Just a Pediatric Disease. *Radiographics* **2009**, *29*, 553–565. [CrossRef] [PubMed]
47. Roberts, W.C.; Siegel, R.J.; Zipes, D.P. Origin of the right coronary artery from the left sinus of Valsalva and its functional consequences: Analysis of 10 necropsy patients. *Am. J. Cardiol.* **1982**, *49*, 863–868. [CrossRef] [PubMed]
48. Çitaku, H.; Kamberi, L.; Gorani, D.; Koçinaj, D.; Krasniqi, X. Anomalous Origin of Left Circumflex Artery. *Med. Arch.* **2015**, *69*, 423–424. [CrossRef] [PubMed]
49. Bhattad, P.B.; Ramsaran, E. Anomalous Origin of the Left Circumflex Coronary Artery: Approach in Acute Coronary Syndrome. *Cureus* **2022**, *14*, e29330. [CrossRef] [PubMed]
50. Cheezum, M.K.; Liberthson, R.R.; Shah, N.R.; Villines, T.C.; O'Gara, P.T.; Landzberg, M.J.; Blankstein, R. Anomalous Aortic Origin of a Coronary Artery From the Inappropriate Sinus of Valsalva. *J. Am. Coll. Cardiol.* **2017**, *69*, 1592–1608. [CrossRef] [PubMed]
51. Agarwal, P.P.; Kazerooni, E.A. Dual Left Anterior Descending Coronary Artery: CT Findings. *Am. J. Roentgenol.* **2008**, *191*, 1698–1701. [CrossRef]
52. Frescura, C.; Basso, C.; Thiene, G.; Corrado, D.; Pennelli, T.; Angelini, A.; Daliento, L. Anomalous origin of coronary arteries and risk of sudden death: A study based on an autopsy population of congenital heart disease. *Hum. Pathol.* **1998**, *29*, 689–695. [CrossRef]
53. Menke, D.M.; Waller, B.F.; Bless, J.E. Hypoplastic Coronary Arteries and High Takeoff Position of the Right Coronary Ostium: A Fatal Combination of Congenital Coronary Artery Anomalies in an Amateur Athlete. *Chest* **1985**, *88*, 299–301. [CrossRef] [PubMed]
54. Shriki, J.E.; Shinbane, J.S.; Rashid, M.A.; Hindoyan, A.; Withey, J.G.; DeFrance, A.; Cunningham, M.; Oliveira, G.R.; Warren, B.H.; Wilcox, A. Identifying, Characterizing, and Classifying Congenital Anomalies of the Coronary Arteries. *Radiographics* **2012**, *32*, 453–468. [CrossRef]
55. Van Geuns, R.J.M.; Cademartiri, F. Anatomy of the Coronary Arteries and Veins in CT Imaging. In *CT of the Heart: Principles and Applications*; Schoepf, U.J., Ed.; Humana Press: Totowa, NJ, USA, 2005; pp. 219–227. [CrossRef]
56. Ispas, V.; Bordei, P.; Iliescu, D.; Baz, R. Coronary arteries morphometry and their vascular territories. *ARS Medica Tomitana* **2013**, *3*, 130–135. [CrossRef]
57. Al-Mohaissen, M.; Heilbron, B.; Leipsic, J.; Ignaszewski, A. Anomalous origin of the entire coronary system by three separate ostia within the right coronary sinus—A rarely observed coronary anomaly. *Can. J. Cardiol.* **2010**, *26*, e206–e208. [CrossRef] [PubMed]
58. Al Umairi, R.; Al-khouri, M. Prevalence, Spectrum, and Outcomes of Single Coronary Artery Detected on Coronary Computed Tomography Angiography (CCTA). *Radiol. Res. Pract.* **2019**, *2019*, 2940148. [CrossRef] [PubMed]
59. Zeina, A.R.; Blinder, J.; Sharif, D.; Rosenschein, U.; Barmeir, E. Congenital coronary artery anomalies in adults: Non-invasive assessment with multidetector CT. *Br. J. Radiol.* **2014**, *82*, 254–261. [CrossRef] [PubMed]
60. Salih, M.; Abdel-Hafez, O.; Ibrahim, R.; Halabi, A.R.; Aloka, F. A Single Coronary Artery Anomaly: Right Coronary Artery as a Branch From the Left Anterior Descending Artery. *Cureus* **2020**, *12*, e9801. [CrossRef] [PubMed]

61. Yurtdaş, M.; Gülen, O. Anomalous origin of the right coronary artery from the left anterior descending artery: Review of the literature. *Cardiol. J.* **2012**, *19*, 122–129. [CrossRef] [PubMed]
62. Bordei, P.; Iliescua, D.M.; Dina, C.; Niţu, R.; Baz, R. Particularités morphologiques des ponts myocardiques diagnostiqués par coronarographie CT. *Morphologie* **2016**, *100*, 135–136. [CrossRef]
63. Nakanishi, R.; Rajani, R.; Ishikawa, Y.; Ishii, T.; Berman, D.S. Myocardial bridging on coronary CTA: An innocent bystander or a culprit in myocardial infarction? *J. Cardiovasc. Comput. Tomogr.* **2012**, *6*, 3–13. [CrossRef]
64. Rajendran, R.; Hegde, M. The prevalence of myocardial bridging on multidetector computed tomography and its relation to coronary plaques. *Pol. J. Radiol.* **2019**, *84*, 478–483. [CrossRef]
65. Sternheim, D.; Power, D.A.; Samtani, R.; Kini, A.; Fuster, V.; Sharma, S. Myocardial Bridging: Diagnosis, Functional Assessment and Management: JACC State-of-the-Art Review. *J. Am. Coll. Cardiol.* **2021**, *78*, 2196–2212. [CrossRef] [PubMed]
66. Celik, T.; Bozlar, U.; Ozturk, C.; Balta, S.; Verim, S.; Demir, M.; Demirkol, S.; Iyisoy, A. A new anomaly of the left anterior descending artery: Type X dual LAD. *Indian Heart J.* **2015**, *67*, S14–S17. [CrossRef]
67. Bozlar, U.; Uğurel, M.; Sarı, S.; Akgün, V.; Örs, F.; Taşar, M. Prevalence of dual left anterior descending artery variations in CT angiography. *Diagn. Interv. Radiol.* **2015**, *21*, 34–41. [CrossRef]
68. Jariwala, P.; Jadhav, K.P.; Koduganti, S. Dual left anterior descending artery: Diagnostic criteria and novel classification. *Indian J Thorac. Cardiovasc. Surg.* **2021**, *37*, 285–294. [CrossRef] [PubMed]
69. Nepal, S.; Annamaraju, P. Coronary Arteriovenous Fistula. In *StatPearls*; StatPearls Publishing: Treasure Island, FL, USA, 2024.
70. Zenooz, N.A.; Habibi, R.; Mammen, L.; Finn, J.P.; Gilkeson, R.C. Coronary Artery Fistulas: CT Findings. *Radiographics* **2009**, *29*, 781–789. [CrossRef]
71. Angelini, P. Coronary artery anomalies--current clinical issues: Definitions, classification, incidence, clinical relevance, and treatment guidelines. *Tex. Heart Inst. J.* **2002**, *29*, 271–278. [PubMed]
72. Young, P.M.; Gerber, T.C.; Williamson, E.E.; Julsrud, P.R.; Herfkens, R.J. Cardiac Imaging: Part 2, Normal, Variant, and Anomalous Configurations of the Coronary Vasculature. *Am. J. Roentgenol.* **2011**, *197*, 816–826. [CrossRef]
73. Pleva, L.; Jonszta, T.; Kukla, P. Congenital coronary anomalies. *Cor Et Vasa* **2014**, *56*, e27–e36. [CrossRef]
74. Kim, S.Y.; Seo, J.B.; Do, K.-H.; Heo, J.-N.; Lee, J.S.; Song, J.-W.; Choe, Y.H.; Kim, T.H.; Yong, H.S.; Choi, S.I.; et al. Coronary Artery Anomalies: Classification and ECG-gated Multi–Detector Row CT Findings with Angiographic Correlation. *Radiographics* **2006**, *26*, 317–333. [CrossRef]
75. Abreu, G.; Nabais, S.; Enes, V.; Marques, J.; Costa, J.; Correia, A. Arcada coronária—Uma anomalia rara da circulação coronária. *Rev. Port. Cardiol.* **2014**, *33*, 241.e1. [CrossRef] [PubMed]
76. Carangal, V.P.; Dehmer, G.J. Intercoronary communication between the circumflex and right coronary arteries. *Clin. Cardiol.* **2000**, *23*, 125–126. [CrossRef] [PubMed]
77. Gan, X.D.; Tu, P.; Gong, Y.; Song, W.H.; Zhang, L.; Wang, H.R. Two cases of intercoronary communication between circumflex artery and right coronary artery. *J. Geriatr. Cardiol.* **2019**, *16*, 384–386. [CrossRef] [PubMed]

Journal of
Clinical Medicine

MDPI

Article

Stress Echocardiography in the Follow-Up of Young Patients with Repaired Aortic Coarctation

Giovanni Di Salvo [1,2,*], Jennifer Fumanelli [1,2], Serena Graziano [1], Alice Pozza [1,2], Irene Cattapan [1,2], Sara Moscatelli [1,2], Biagio Castaldi [1] and Domenico Galzerano [2,3]

1 Pediatric Cardiology and Adult Congenital Unit, Department of Women's and Child's Health, University of Padua, 35121 Padova, Italy; jennifer.fumanelli@aopd.veneto.it (J.F.); serena.graziano@studenti.unipd.it (S.G.); irene.cattapan@aopd.veneto.it (I.C.); b.castaldi@yahoo.it (B.C.)
2 Working Group on Congenital Heart Disease and Cardiovascular Prevention of the Italian Society of Cardiology, 00136 Roma, Italy; dgalzerano@kfshrc.edu.sa
3 Heart Center, King Faisal Specialist Hospital and Research Center, Riyadh 12611, Saudi Arabia
* Correspondence: giovanni.disalvo@unipd.it

Abstract: Background: Aortic coarctation (CoA) is a congenital heart disease affecting 5–8% of patients, with long-term complications persisting despite successful correction. Stress echocardiography (SE) is increasingly used for evaluating cardiac function under stress, yet its role in repaired CoA remains under-explored. **Objective:** This study aimed to assess the predictive value of SE and myocardial strain in repaired CoA patients with a history of hypertension without significant gradients or with borderline gradients at rest. **Methods:** Between June 2020 and March 2024, we enrolled 35 consecutive CoA patients with successful repairs and either a history of hypertension or borderline Doppler gradients. Baseline and peak exercise echocardiographic measurements, including left ventricular mass index (LVMi) and global longitudinal strain (LVGLS), were recorded. Patients were followed for up to 4 years. **Results:** At baseline, the positive SE group had higher systolic blood pressure (SBP) and diastolic blood pressure (DBP) compared to the negative SE group. The positive SE group also exhibited significantly higher basal and peak trans-isthmic gradients. Positive SE was found in 45.7% of patients, with 68.7% of these requiring re-intervention during follow-up. A peak trans-isthmic gradient > 61 mmHg during exercise predicted recoarctation with 100% sensitivity and 71% specificity (AUC = 0.836, $p < 0.004$). **Conclusions:** SE identifies at-risk patients post-CoA repair, aiding in early intervention. A peak trans-isthmic gradient > 61 mmHg during exercise is a strong predictor of recoarctation. These findings support incorporating SE into routine follow-up protocols for CoA patients, particularly those with a history of hypertension and borderline gradients, to improve long-term outcomes and quality of life.

Keywords: coarctation; stress echocardiography; hypertension

1. Introduction

Aortic coarctation (CoA) is a well-known congenital heart disease (CHD), representing approximately 5–8% of all congenital heart diseases, with a higher prevalence in males [1]. Despite successful correction, this population experiences reduced life expectancy due to mid- and long-term complications [1]. CoA is also considered a general arteriopathy due to modifications to aortic wall elastic properties since the fetal period [2]. Even with early repair, hypertension remains a frequent complication [3], and aortic elastic abnormalities persist into adulthood despite neonatal correction [4]. Recoarctation is one of the most feared complications, often necessitating re-intervention to reduce left ventricular (LV) pressure overload [5]. Abnormal myocardial deformation indices, such as strain and strain rate, are reduced even in patients with successful CoA repair [6]. Recoarctation is defined as: hypertension with a clinical gradient between upper and lower limbs > 20 mmHg confirmed with invasive measurement (peak to peak > 20 mmHg) [6]. However, in clinical practice, CoA patients who are hypertensive but without a significant gradient, or with a borderline gradient without hypertension, are frequent [7]. The decision-making in this borderline situation is unclear and the role of non-invasive tests is debated [7].

Stress echocardiography (SE) is a widely used tool to assess various cardiac diseases in the adult population [8–10]. Recently, it has gained consensus as part of the diagnostic–prognostic work-up in adult congenital heart diseases [10]. SE allows for simultaneous assessment of myocardial function and hemodynamics under physiological or pharmacological conditions, including in CoA patients. However, data on cardiac function and on trans-isthmic gradient during exercise in repaired CoA patients remain limited.

Thus, the aim of our study is to assess the predictive value of SE and myocardial strain in repaired CoA patients with a history of hypertension without a significant gradient or with a borderline gradient at rest.

2. Methods

2.1. Study Population

Between June 2020 and March 2024, we prospectively enrolled 35 consecutive CoA patients, regularly followed at our pediatric cardiology and adult congenital heart disease tertiary center. Inclusion criteria included isolated coarctation and successful repair (surgical or interventional), defined as a post-procedure invasive gradient $\leq$ 20 mmHg, with no significant valvular heart disease (only mild cases were included), either a history of hypertension in the presence of a trans-isthmic Doppler mean gradient $\leq$ 20 mmHg, or without hypertension but with a borderline Doppler gradient at rest > 20 mmHg and $\leq$40 mmHg, without diastolic drugs and without clinical gradient. Exclusion criteria included arrhythmias, paced rhythm, valvulopathy more than mild, and a height below 130 cm (required to use the semi-supine bicycle).

Anthropometrical and clinical data were collected at the time of stress echocardiography evaluation, including age, gender, body surface area (BSA), systolic and diastolic arterial pressure at rest and during exercise, history of systolic hypertension, type and timing of correction (surgical vs. endovascular), and symptoms at rest and during physical activity. The definition of systolic hypertension at rest and at peak exercise in children and adults is based on the respective current guidelines.

The study was performed in line with the principles of the Declaration of Helsinki and was approved by the institutional ethics committee. As this study involved the retrospective analysis of data collected during clinical activity, the institutional review board waived the need for patients to provide written informed consent.

2.2. Baseline Echocardiography and Stress Echocardiography Study

All patients underwent a basal transthoracic echocardiography using a GE Vivid E95 machine (GE Healthcare, Wauwatosa, WI, USA) with an M5S ultrasound transducer. Standard parasternal short- and long-axis, apical 2-3-4-dimensional chambers, suprasternal view of the arch, and color-guided pulsed- and continuous-wave Doppler images were acquired at rest in the left lateral decubitus or supine position. Blood pressure at rest was measured at pre- and post-ductal sites before performing the basal echocardiography.

Stored images were analyzed and post-processed using EchopacTM software (EchoPac version 204, GE Healthcare). Measurements included LV wall thicknesses, LV mass index, LV systolic function through Simpson's biplane method, LV diastolic function (E/A and E/E′ index), aortic valve gradient and/or regurgitation, and peak and mean gradient across the descending aorta, following European Association of Echocardiography and European Association of Cardiovascular Imaging (EACVI) guidelines. An expert operator performed speckle tracking echocardiography (STE) on stored DICOM echo clips using the EchoPac software (EchoPac version 206, GE Healthcare). LV GLS was analyzed on standard gray-scale images in the apical 2-chamber, 3-chamber, and 4-chamber views with a frame rate of 50–80/s. Echocardiographic measurements were repeated at peak effort.

Patients underwent an exercise test according to the Bruce protocol to study cardiac performance during maximal exercise. This protocol involves using a semi-supine bicycle with increasing cycling power of 25 watts every 2 min. During the exam, a 12-lead ECG and blood pressure were continuously monitored non-invasively. Systolic–diastolic pressure values were detected every two minutes by a sphygmomanometer connected to a cuff positioned at the right arm (pre-ductal site), and heart rates were recorded simultaneously.

We defined a positive stress echocardiographic exam [8] as an average trans-isthmic gradient under stress $\geq$ 30 mmHg (major criterion), associated with at least one of the minor criteria: hypertensive response to effort, appearance of diastolic run-off at the descending aorta, and/or abdominal level.

2.3. Follow-Up

Patients were followed for up to 4 years (range 6–48 months). Recoarctation was defined according to ESC guidelines [6] as: hypertension with a clinical gradient between upper and lower limbs > 20 mmHg confirmed with invasive measurement (peak to peak > 20 mmHg).

2.4. Statistical Analysis

Statistical analysis was performed using MedCalc® Statistical Software version 22.023 (MedCalc Software Ltd., Ostend, Belgium; https://www.medcalc.org; 2024).

Categorical variables were reported as percentages (%), while continuous variables were presented as mean ± standard deviation. The Shapiro–Wilk test and histogram were used to verify normality for each variable. Student's t-test was performed for normally distributed continuous variables, while the Mann–Whitney U test was used for nonparametric continuous variables. The chi-square test was used for categorical variables to test for significant differences between groups. ROC analysis was performed to identify the best cut-off value. Statistical significance was attributed to p-values < 0.05.

3. Results

3.1. Baseline Characteristics

The study population consisted of 35 children and young adults with an average age of 23.8 ± 12.8 years, of which 24 (68.6%) were male (Table 1). The average body surface area (BSA) was 1.69 ± 0.24 m^2. Baseline systolic blood pressure (SBP) was 127.63 ± 14.99 mmHg, and baseline diastolic blood pressure (DBP) was 72.17 ± 8.8 mmHg. Common associated defects included bicuspid aortic valve in 24 (68.6%) patients, ventricular septal defect (VSD) in 12 (34.3%) patients, and various mitral valve anomalies. Mitral dysplasia was observed in three (8.6%) patients. The average age at correction was 2.36 ± 4.19 years. The primary types of correction were end-to-end anastomosis in 23 (65.7%) patients, percutaneous dilation with stent in 6 (17.1%), and percutaneous aortoisthmoplasty in 3 (8.6%).

Table 1. General Characteristics of the Studied Sample.

	Patients = 35
Age at Evaluation (years)	23.8 ± 12.8
Sex (male)	24 (68.6%)
Height (cm)	169.3 ± 11.6
Weight (kg)	61.8 ± 15
BSA (m^2)	1.69 ± 0.24
BMI (kg/m^2)	21.5 ± 4.3
SBP Basal (mmHg)	127.6 ± 14.9
DBP Basal (mmHg)	72.2 ± 8.8

Table 1. *Cont.*

	Patients = 35
Associated Defects	Bicuspid Aortic Valve 24 (68.6%)
	Aortic Subvalvar Membrane 3 (8.6%)
	VSD 12 (34.3%)
	Mitral Valve Anomalies
	Parachute Mitral Valve 2 (5.7%)
	Mitral Arcade 1 (3.5%)
	Mitral Dysplasia 3 (8.6%)
	Isolated Cleft 1 (3.5%)
	Tricuspid Dysplasia 1
Age at Correction (Years)	2.4 ± 4.2

A history of systolic hypertension was present in 20 (57%) patients, with anti-hypertensive therapy including beta-blockers (n = 4), ACE inhibitors (n = 2), ARI (n = 5), and calcium channel blockers (n = 1), or life-style recommendations (n = 9). None of the studied patients had a clinical gradient between right arm and right leg > 20 mmHg.

3.2. Baseline Echocardiographic Measurements

The baseline echocardiographic characteristics of the studied sample are presented in Table 2.

Table 2. The Baseline and Peak Exercise Echocardiographic Characteristics of the Studied Sample.

	Basal (n = 35)	Peak-Exercise (n = 35)	*p* Value
SBP (mmHg)	127.6 ± 15	168.5 ± 31.5	**<0.0001**
DBP (mmHg)	72.2 ± 8.8	87.4 ± 19.4	**<0.0001**
HR (bpm)	73.8 ± 17.7	141.0 ± 21.6	**<0.0001**
Trans-Isthmic Gradient Mean (mmHg)	17.9 ± 9.2	34.5 ± 15.5	**<0.0001**
Trans-Isthmic Gradient Peak (mmHg)	30.6 ± 9.9	64.9 ± 27.2	**<0.0001**
Olo-Diastolic Run-Off at Descending Aorta	0	17 (48.6%)	**0.0001**
LVEDD (mm)	46.6 ± 5.2		
IVSDD (mm)	9.8 ± 2.9		
PWDD (mm)	8.6 ± 1.6		
LVMi (g\m^2)	88.5 ± 26.5		
E\E′average	8.1 ± 4.9	NA	
LVEF (%)	62.5 ± 5.7	65 ± 5.1	0.05
LVGLS (−%)	−18.5 ± 1.7	−18.8 ± 1.9	0.30

Legend: SBP: Systolic Blood Pressure; DBP: Diastolic Blood Pressure; HR: Heart Rate; LVEDD: Left Ventricular End Diastolic Diameter; IVSD: Interventricular Septum Diastolic Diameter; Posterior Wall Diastolic Diameter; PWDD: Posterior Wall Diastolic Diameter; LVMi: Left Ventricular Mass Index; LVEF: Left Ventricular Ejection Fraction; LVGLS: Left Ventricular Global Longitudinal Strain.

The left ventricular mass index (LVMI), as per the ASE guidelines, was increased (88.54 ± 26.92 g/m^2). Twenty patients (55%) showed left ventricular hypertrophy. All patients presented normal systolic function at rest. Diastolic function at rest was within the normal range (8.1 ± 4.9). The baseline mean trans-isthmic gradient was 17.9 ± 9.2 mmHg, no patient had a olodiastolic drag at rest.

3.3. Echocardiographic Findings at Peak Exercise (Table 2)

Twenty-two patients reached at least 80% of the target heart rate (220-age), while in the remaining 13 patients the exam was stopped because of leg pain. None of the studied patients had symptoms like angina, dyspnea, or palpitations. ECG did not show any significant modification in the ST-T segment. No arrythmias, other than sporadic premature atrial beats, occurred during the exam.

In the studied sample, blood pressure and trans-isthmic gradient significantly increased at peak exercise (64.9 ± 27.2 mmHg, $p < 0.0001$). At peak exercise, diastolic run-off in the descending aorta became apparent in 48.6% of the population, while no run-off was seen in the abdominal aorta. Global systolic function, as assessed by LVEF, significantly increased at peak exercise. No changes were observed in LV GLS.

According to the guidelines, in our studied sample, 16 (45.7%) patients had a positive stress echocardiographic (PSE) evaluation [8]. Comparing baseline clinical and echocardiographic characteristics (Table 3), PSE patients showed higher basal SBP, were more frequently under hypertensive therapy (50% vs. 21%, $p = 0.03$). Left ventricular mass index (LVMi) was similar between groups (88.1 ± 28.8 g/m^2 vs. 88.9 ± 24.4 g/m^2, $p = 0.93$). The basal trans-isthmic gradient was significantly higher in the PSE group (22.6 ± 8.6 mmHg) compared to the NSE group (12.6 ± 6.2 mmHg, $p = 0.002$).

Table 3. Comparison of Clinical and Echocardiographic Data Between Patients with a Positive Stress Echo (PSE) and Patients with a Negative Stress Echo (NSE).

	PSE (n = 16)	NSE (n = 19)	p Value
Age at Study (Years)	25.5 ± 14.1	22.4 ± 11.1	0.489
Age at Correction (Years)	2.26 ± 3.0	2.44 ± 4.9	0.905
Basal SBP mmHg	133.6 ± 12.7	122.6 ± 14.6	**0.03**
Basal DBP mmHg	72.9 ± 6.4	76.6 ± 19.1	**0.03**
Basal HR bpm	70.4 ± 14.3	76.6 ± 19.1	0.34
Hypertensive Therapy (%)	8 (50%)	4 (21%)	**0.03**
Peak SBP mmHg	178.9 ± 25.9	159.8 ± 32.3	0.07
Peak DBP mmHg	94.1 ± 18.2	81.2 ± 17.9	0.05
Peak HR bpm	142.3 ± 20.5	139.9 ± 21.8	0.77
LVMi g\m^2	88.1 ± 28.8	88.9 ± 24.4	0.93
Rest-Trans-Isthmic Gradient (Peak) mmHg	43.3 ± 19.1	24.6 ± 8.5	**0.003**
Rest-Trans-Isthmic Gradient (Mean) mmHg	22.6 ± 8.6	12.6 ± 6.2	**0.002**
Peak-Exercise Trans-Isthmic Gradient (peak) mmHg	81.7 ± 24.9	45.8 ± 13.9	**<0.0001**
Peak-Exercise Trans-Isthmic Gradient (mean) mmHg	45.1 ± 12.1	22.4 ± 7.3	**<0.0001**
Basal LVEF (%)	63.2 ± 6.4	61.6 ± 4.2	0.37
Peak LVEF (%)	66.1 ± 5.4	64.1 ± 4.4	0.279
Basal LVGLS (−%)	−17.6 ± 1.9	−18.1 ± 2.1	0.63
Peak LVGLS (−%)	−18.7 ± 2.3	−18.9 ± 1.9	0.75

Legends: SBP: Systolic Blood Pressure; DBP: Diastolic Blood Pressure; HR: Heart Rate; LVMi: Left Ventricular Mass Index; LVEF: Left Ventricular Ejection Fraction; LVGLS: Left Ventricular Global Longitudinal Strain.

Peak SBP and DBP tended to be higher in the PSE group compared to the NSE group, although this difference was not statistically significant ($p = 0.05$).

Similarly, the peak trans-isthmic gradient was significantly higher in the PSE group (45.1 ± 12.1 mmHg) compared to the NSE group (22.4 ± 7.3 mmHg, $p < 0.0001$).

There were no significant differences in basal left ventricular ejection fraction (LVEF) between the PSE (63.2 ± 6.4%) and NSE groups (61.6 ± 4.2%, $p = 0.37$), nor in peak

LVEF (66.1 ± 5.4% for PSE vs. 64.1 ± 4.4% for NSE, p = 0.279). Basal left ventricular global longitudinal strain (LVGLS) was also similar between the PSE (−17.6 ± 1.9%) and NSE groups (−18.1 ± 2.1%, p = 0.63), as was peak LVGLS (−18.7 ± 2.3% for PSE vs. −18.9 ± 1.9% for NSE, p = 0.75). Diastolic function (E\E′average) was not included in the analysis because at peak exercise the pattern was frequently fused.

Among the 35 studied patients, there were 11 cases (31.4%) of recoarctation during follow-up, (mean duration (18 ± 14 months)) requiring percutaneous stent implantation (Figure 1). Two cases refused treatment and were left on anti-hypertensive medications and close follow-up. All 11 cases belonged to the PSE group (68.7%).

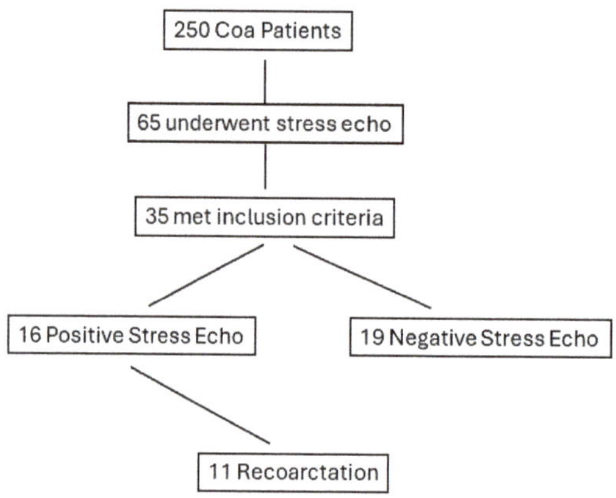

Figure 1. Flow chart displaying the stratification of patients based on positive response to stress echocardiography. CoA, coarctation of the aorta.

A peak trans-isthmic gradient at peak exercise > 61 mmHg showed a sensitivity of 100% and specificity of 71% (AUC of 0.836, $p < 0.004$) in terms of predicting recoarctation (Figure 2). A mean trans-isthmic gradient > 34 mmHg showed a sensitivity of 77.8% and specificity of 71% (AUC of 0.765, $p < 0.006$) in terms of predicting recoarctation.

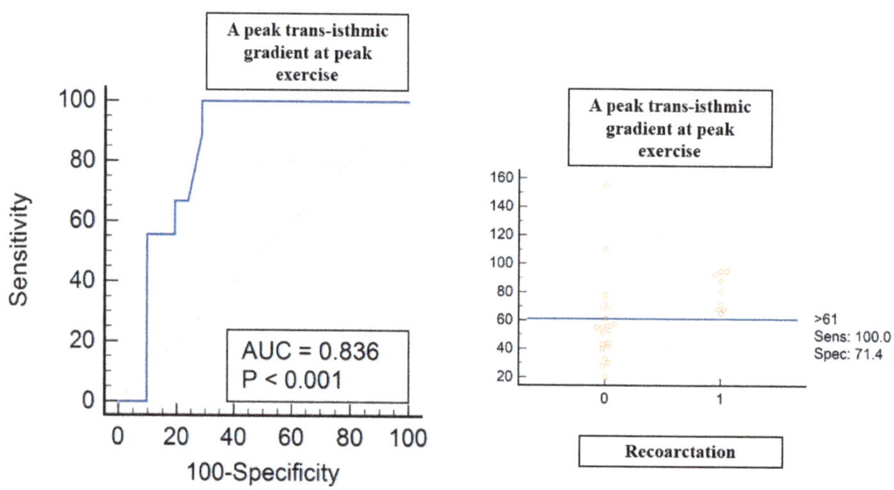

Figure 2. ROC curve analysis for peak trans-isthmic gradient at peak exercise and recoarctation. Red circles are coa patients, 0 without recoarctation, 1 with recoarctation.

4. Discussion

Our study demonstrates that approximately 45% of children or young adults with apparently successfully repaired CoA have a positive stress echocardiographic evaluation. Notably, 68.7% of the patients with a positive stress echo required percutaneous intervention. Stress echocardiography plays a crucial role in the long-term monitoring of patients with various cardiac diseases [6]. However, its role in the follow-up of patients who have undergone successful repair of CoA remains unclear [7]. CoA patients, despite initial successful intervention, are at risk for complications such as recoarctation, hypertension, and heart failure, affecting long-term survival [1–5]. Thus, a better non-invasive test to identify at-risk groups could be beneficial.

The gradient observed during exercise is predictive of recoarctation [6]. This finding is critical as it provides a quantifiable measure that can be monitored over time, allowing for timely identification and management of recoarctation, preventing adverse outcomes and preserving long-term cardiovascular health in these young patients. At rest, an isthmus gradient may be absent due to collaterals, but during exercise, the increased cardiac output may overwhelm the collaterals, revealing the isthmus gradient.

Our findings of a mean trans-isthmic gradient at peak exercise > 34 mmHg predictive of recoarctation are in keeping with guidelines that suggest a cut-off of 30 mmHg [6]. However, in our study, a peak trans-isthmic gradient at peak exercise > 61 mmHg showed a better accuracy. However, measurements of peak velocity, especially at peak exercise, can be challenging and more subjective.

Patients with a history of hypertension and higher baseline isthmus gradient were more frequently positive at stress echo. Previous studies using pharmacological or physical stress echo have demonstrated a positive correlation between systolic blood pressure and trans-isthmic gradient in CoA patients [10,11].

A recent study demonstrated that hypertensive response to exercise in CoA patients is not predictive of cardiovascular events [12]. Interestingly, in our study, a positive stress echo was found in all patients who developed during follow-up an indication for percutaneous treatment. These findings suggest that it is not the hypertensive response per se, but the combination between peak exercise trans-isthmic gradient and hypertensive response, that may hold a prognostic value.

At peak exercise, LV GLS was not different between PSE and NSE patients. This finding is somehow surprising since several papers demonstrated LV GLS to be able to early detect subclinical dysfunction [5]. This is likely due to technical limitations in measuring LV GLS at peak exercise. The speckle-tracking software processes video at a frame rate between 50 and 100 bpm, which is suitable for resting heart rates but inadequate for peak exercise heart rates, leading to under-sampling and less accurate measurements [13]. However, LV GLS in both groups did not show a physiological increase at peak exercise in both groups. This finding may suggest an early subclinical endocardial damage affecting longitudinally oriented fibers. The value of LV GLS, even in the presence of normal or recovered LVEF, in terms of predicting the deterioration of LV EF over time or cardiovascular events, has been consistently observed in several studies on congenital heart disease, regardless of whether patients had right or left heart lesions, suggesting LV GLS is a robust imaging tool for risk stratification [14]. The use of advanced echocardiography could be beneficial to also predict outcomes in CoA patients; however, some technical limitations for its application at higher heart rates need to be implemented [15,16].

Limitations of the study. This study carries several limitations. First, the sample size may seem small; however, it is in the range of previous studies on the same topic [7,17,18] and it reflects the selection criteria. Some of the results (LV GLS at peak exercise) may be influenced by technical challenges, but this reflects the limits of the current technology.

In conclusion, stress echocardiography in our experience has an important role in the follow-up of young patients with repaired CoA. It helps identify patients at higher risk for recurrence. This proactive approach may ensure timely intervention and improve long-term outcomes and quality of life for these patients. Our findings support the inclusion of stress echo in routine follow-up protocols for patients with repaired CoA, especially those with a history of hypertension and borderline baseline gradients.

Author Contributions: Conceptualization, G.D.S., S.M., B.C. and D.G.; Methodology, A.P. and B.C.; Software, S.G. and I.C.; Validation, B.C. and D.G.; Formal analysis, D.G.; Resources, J.F. and S.G.; Data curation, J.F. and S.G.; Writing—original draft, G.D.S.; Writing—review & editing, A.P. and D.G.; Supervision, I.C. and S.M. All authors have read and agreed to the published version of the manuscript.

Funding: This research received no external funding.

Institutional Review Board Statement: Ethical review and approval were waived for this study due to the retrospective analysis of anonymized data collected during clinical activity.

Informed Consent Statement: Patient written informed consent was waived due to the retrospective analysis of anonymized data collected during clinical activity.

Data Availability Statement: Data will be available upon motivated request to the Authors.

Conflicts of Interest: The authors declare no conflicts of interest.

References

1. Meijs, T.A.; Minderhoud, S.C.S.; Muller, S.A.; de Winter, R.J.; Mulder, B.J.M.; van Melle, J.P.; Hoendermis, E.S.; van Dijk, A.P.J.; Zuithoff, N.P.A.; Krings, G.J.; et al. Cardiovascular Morbidity and Mortality in Adult Patients with Repaired Aortic Coarctation *J. Am. Heart Assoc.* **2021**, *10*, e023199. [CrossRef] [PubMed] [PubMed Central]
2. Saengsin, K.; Gauvreau, K.; Prakash, A. Comparison of aortic stiffness and hypertension in repaired coarctation patients with a bicuspid versus a tricuspid aortic valve. *J. Cardiovasc. Magn. Reson.* **2023**, *25*, 31. [CrossRef] [PubMed] [PubMed Central]
3. Kenny, D.; Hijazi, Z.M. Coarctation of the aorta: From fetal life to adulthood. *Cardiol. J.* **2011**, *18*, 487–495. [CrossRef] [PubMed]
4. Kenny, D.; Polson, J.W.; Martin, R.P.; Paton, J.F.; Wolf, A.R. Hypertension and coarctation of the aorta: An inevitable consequence of developmental pathophysiology. *Hypertens. Res.* **2011**, *34*, 543–547. [CrossRef] [PubMed]
5. di Salvo, G.; Pacileo, G.; Limongelli, G.; Verrengia, M.; Rea, A.; Santoro, G.; Gala, S.; Castaldi, B.; D'Andrea, A.; Caso, P.; et al. Abnormal regional myocardial deformation properties and increased aortic stiffness in normotensive patients with aortic coarctation despite successful correction: An ABPM, standard echocardiography and strain rate imaging study. *Clin. Sci.* **2007**, *113*, 259–266. [CrossRef] [PubMed]
6. Baumgartner, H.; De Backer, J.; Babu-Narayan, S.V.; Budts, W.; Chessa, M.; Diller, G.-P.; Bernard, L.; Kluin, J.; Lang, I.M.; Meijboom, F.; et al. 2020 ESC Guidelines for the management of adult congenital heart disease: The Task Force for the management of adult congenital heart disease of the European Society of Cardiology (ESC). Endorsed by: Association for European Paediatric and Congenital Cardiology (AEPC), International Society for Adult Congenital Heart Disease (ISACHD). *Eur. Heart J.* **2021**, *42*, 563–645. [CrossRef] [PubMed]
7. Patel, N.D.; Sullivan, P.M.; Takao, C.M.; Badran, S.; Ahdoot, J.; Ing, F.F. Unmasking the borderline coarctation: The utility of isoproterenol in the paediatric cardiac catheterisation laboratory. *Cardiol. Young* **2018**, *28*, 804–810. [CrossRef] [PubMed]
8. Lancellotti, P.; Pellikka, P.A.; Budts, W.; Chaudhry, F.A.; Donal, E.; Dulgheru, R.; Edvardsen, T.; Garbi, M.; Ha, J.W.; Kane, G.C.; et al. The Clinical Use of Stress Echocardiography in Non-Ischaemic Heart Disease: Recommendations from the European Association of Cardiovascular Imaging and the American Society of Echocardiography. *J. Am. Soc. Echocardiogr.* **2017**, *30*, 101–138. [CrossRef] [PubMed]
9. Pergola, V.; Previtero, M.; Lorenzoni, G.; Ocagli, H.; Simeti, G.; Aruta, P.; Baritussio, A.; Cecchetto, A.; Leoni, L.; Mancuso, D.; et al. Feasibility and Role of Right Ventricular Stress Echocardiography in Adult Patients. *J. Cardiovasc. Echogr.* **2021**, *31*, 68–72. [CrossRef] [PubMed] [PubMed Central]
10. Araujo, J.J. Stress Echocardiography in Pediatric and Adult Congenital Heart Disease: A Complement in Anatomical and Functional Assessment. *Curr. Probl. Cardiol.* **2021**, *46*, 100762. [CrossRef] [PubMed]
11. Foulds, H.J.A.; Giacomantonio, N.B.; Bredin, S.S.D.; Warburton, D.E.R. A systematic review and meta-analysis of exercise and exercise hypertension in patients with aortic coarctation. *J. Hum. Hypertens.* **2017**, *31*, 768–775. [CrossRef] [PubMed]
12. Meijs, T.A.; Muller, S.A.; Minderhoud, S.C.S.; de Winter, R.J.; Mulder, B.J.M.; van Melle, J.P.; Hoendermis, E.S.; van Dijk, A.P.J.; Zuithoff, N.P.A.; Krings, G.J.; et al. Hypertensive response to exercise in adult patients with repaired aortic coarctation. *Heart* **2022**, *108*, 1121–1128. [CrossRef] [PubMed]
13. Di Salvo, G.; Pergola, V.; Fadel, B.; Bulbul, Z.A.; Caso, P. Strain Echocardiography and Myocardial Mechanics: From Basics to Clinical Applications. *J. Cardiovasc. Echogr.* **2015**, *25*, 1–8. [CrossRef] [PubMed] [PubMed Central]
14. Egbe, A.C.; Miranda, W.R.; Anderson, J.H.; Pellikka, P.A.; Connolly, H.M. Prognostic Value of Left Ventricular Global Longitudinal Strain in Patients with Congenital Heart Disease. *Circ. Cardiovasc. Imaging* **2022**, *15*, e014865. [CrossRef] [PubMed] [PubMed Central]

15. Galzerano, D.; Pergola, V.; Eltayeb, A.; Ludovica, F.; Arbili, L.; Tashkandi, L.; Michele, S.D.; Barchitta, A.; Parato, M.V.; Salvo, G.D. Echocardiography in Simple Congenital Heart Diseases: Guiding Adult Patient Management. *J. Cardiovasc. Echogr.* **2023**, *33*, 171–182. [CrossRef] [PubMed] [PubMed Central]
16. Sperlongano, S.; D'Andrea, A.; Mele, D.; Russo, V.; Pergola, V.; Carbone, A.; Ilardi, F.; Di Maio, M.; Bottino, R.; Giallauria, F.; et al. Left Ventricular Deformation and Vortex Analysis in Heart Failure: From Ultrasound Technique to Current Clinical Application. *Diagnostics* **2021**, *11*, 892. [CrossRef] [PubMed] [PubMed Central]
17. Banaszak, P.; Szkutnik, M.; Kusa, J.; Banaszak, B.; Białkowski, J. Utility of the dobutamine stress echocardiography in the evaluation of the effects of a surgical repair of aortic coarctation in children. *Cardiol. J.* **2009**, *16*, 20–25. [PubMed]
18. Runte, K.; Brosien, K.; Salcher-Konrad, M.; Schubert, C.; Goubergrits, L.; Kelle, S.; Schubert, S.; Berger, F.; Kuehne, T.; Kelm, M. Hemodynamic Changes during Physiological and Pharmacological Stress Testing in Healthy Subjects, Aortic Stenosis and Aortic Coarctation Patients—A Systematic Review and Meta-Analysis. *Front. Cardiovasc. Med.* **2019**, *6*, 43. [CrossRef] [PubMed] [PubMed Central]

Journal of
Clinical Medicine

MDPI

Review

Transforming Heart Failure Management: The Power of Strain Imaging, 3D Imaging, and Vortex Analysis in Echocardiography

Domenico Galzerano [1,2,*], Maria Teresa Savo [3], Biagio Castaldi [4], Naji Kholaif [1,2], Feras Khaliel [2], Alice Pozza [4], Saif Aljheish [2], Irene Cattapan [4], Marika Martini [3], Eleonora Lassandro [3], Gabriele Cordoni [3], Donatella Tansella [3], Dan Alexandru Cozac [5], Bandar Alamro [1,2] and Giovanni Di Salvo [4]

1 College of Medicine, Alfaisal University, Riyadh 11533, Saudi Arabia; dr.kholaif@gmail.com (N.K.); b.alamro@hotmail.com (B.A.)
2 Heart Centre, King Faisal Specialist Hospital & Research Centre, Riyadh 11564, Saudi Arabia; fekhaliel@ksfhrc.edu.sa (F.K.); saif.aljheish@gmail.com (S.A.)
3 Cardiology Unit, Cardio-Thoraco-Vascular and Public Health Department, Padova University Hospital, 35121 Padova, Italy; mariateresa.savo@studenti.unipd.it (M.T.S.); marika.martini.1@phd.unipd.it (M.M.); eleonora.lassandro@studenti.unipd.it (E.L.); gabriele.cordoni@studenti.unipd.it (G.C.); donatella.tansella@studenti.unipd.it (D.T.)
4 Division of Pediatric Cardiology, Department for Women's and Children's Health, University of Padua, 35128 Padua, Italy; biagio.castaldi@unipd.it (B.C.); irene.cattapan@phd.unipd.it (I.C.); giovanni.disalvo@unipd.it (G.D.S.)
5 Emergency Institute for Cardiovascular Diseases and Transplantation of Targu Mures, 540136 Targu Mures, Romania; dan.alexandru03@yahoo.com
* Correspondence: domenicogalzerano@libero.it; Tel.: +39-3284157343

Abstract: Heart failure (HF) remains a critical global health challenge, necessitating advancements in diagnostic and therapeutic strategies. This review explores the evolution of imaging technologies and their impact on HF management, focusing on three-dimensional echocardiography (3DE), myocardial strain imaging, and vortex dynamics imaging. Three-dimensional echocardiography enhances traditional echocardiography by providing more accurate assessments of cardiac structures, while myocardial strain imaging offers the early detection of subclinical myocardial dysfunction, crucial in conditions such as chemotherapy-induced cardiotoxicity and ischemic heart disease. Vortex dynamics imaging, a novel technique, provides insights into intracardiac flow patterns, aiding in the evaluation of left ventricular function, valve diseases, and congenital heart anomalies. The integration of these advanced imaging modalities into clinical practice facilitates personalized treatment strategies, enabling the earlier diagnosis and more precise monitoring of disease progression. The ongoing refinement of these imaging techniques holds promise for improving patient outcomes and advancing the field of precision medicine in HF care.

Keywords: heart failure; advanced cardiac imaging; three-dimensional echocardiography; myocardial strain imaging; vortex dynamics

1. Introduction

Heart failure (HF) remains a critical global health issue, affecting millions of patients worldwide. The evolution of imaging technologies has significantly impacted HF management, providing clinicians with advanced tools to assess cardiac function and tailor treatment strategies. Two-dimensional echocardiography (2DE) uses sound waves to create images of the heart. It is widely available and provides essential information about the cardiac structures and function. However, it has limitations in detecting subtle myocardial changes and complex flow dynamics [1,2]. Despite these limitations, 2DE remains a cornerstone for the initial cardiac assessment [3,4]. Cardiac magnetic resonance imaging (MRI) utilizes magnetic fields to produce detailed images of the heart. It offers excellent structural and tissue characterizations, making it invaluable for diagnosing various cardiac conditions. However, the cost and limited availability can restrict its use [1,2]. Traditional imaging techniques have been complemented by innovations such as three-dimensional echocardiography (3DE), myocardial strain imaging, and vortex analysis, which offer deeper insights into cardiac function and dysfunction (Table 1) [5,6]. This review explores these advancements and their implications for HF management.

Table 1. Overview of traditional and advanced echocardiography techniques.

Imaging Technique	Description	Key Benefits
2D Echocardiography	Sound waves to create 2D images of the heart	Widely available, provides basic structural information.
3D Echocardiography	Provides three-dimensional images of cardiac structures	Enhanced visualization and accurate volumetric measurements.
Myocardial Strain Imaging	Measures myocardial deformation during the cardiac cycle	Sensitive to subtle myocardial changes, useful for the early detection of dysfunction.
Vortex Analysis	Analyzes swirling patterns of blood flow in the heart	Offers insights into cardiac flow dynamics and function.

MRI: magnetic resonance imaging.

2. Three-Dimensional Echocardiography

Three-dimensional echocardiography has expanded the capabilities of traditional 2DE by providing a presentation of the cardiac structure from any spatial point of view. To create larger volumetric data, multiple beat 3DE acquisition acquires narrow volumes of information over several heartbeats that are then stitched together. This compensates for the poor temporal resolution of single beat full volumetric real-time 3DE acquisition but has the disadvantage of having a stitch artifact. The presence of respiratory motion or irregular cardiac rhythms can create artifacts [7].

2.1. Clinical Applications

1. **Left ventricular function:** This technology allows for a more accurate evaluation of the left ventricle (LV) function, avoiding geometric assumptions regarding the LV shape. It provides faster, more accurate, and reproducible measurements of ventricular volumes, compared to traditional 2DE (Figure 1).

The accuracy of 3DE is comparable to a cardiac MRI; however, the variability in the results may be greater due to differences in the image quality and operator expertise. Two primary approaches can be used: the first one utilizes a "full-volume" data set to generate standard 2DE images, with the careful optimization of the cut planes to ensure they are aligned "on axis" (Figure 2). This method is particularly effective for assessing the segmental wall motion and for tracing the LV borders to calculate the volumes. In segmental imaging, obtaining orthogonal views offers the advantage of confirming wall motion abnormalities in any given segment. This is important in conditions such as HF, cardiomyopathies, and cardio-oncology, where the precise quantification of the cardiac function is essential for guiding treatment decisions and monitoring disease progression. The second approach involves the visualization of rendered 3DE images, which provide a comprehensive impression of cardiac structures, such as the LV mass [7].

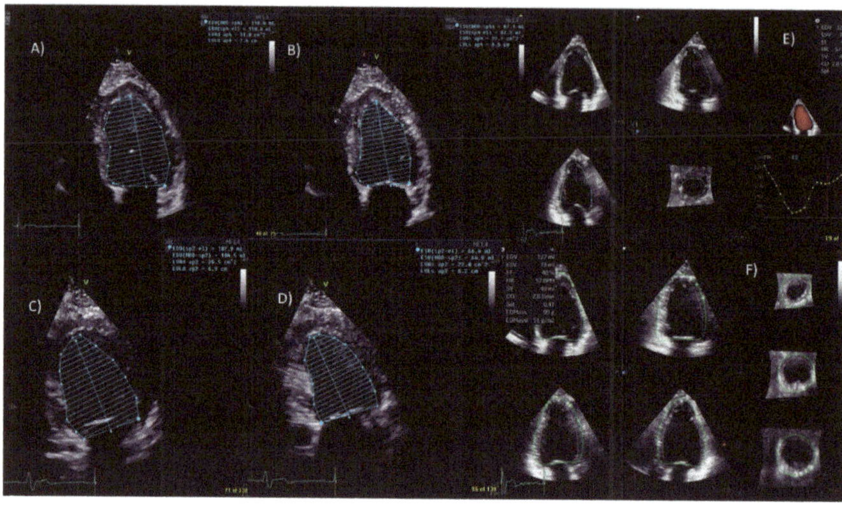

Figure 1. Two-dimensional and three-dimensional LVEF valuation. In presence ofminimal differences in the ejection fraction measurement, the indications for medical therapy or possible resynchronization therapy can shift. In this case, the volumes were measured both with the 2D and 3D Simpson's methods of disks (MODs). Panels (**A**,**B**): the left ventricular (LV) ejection fraction is 38%, measured with the MODs. The volumes in diastole and systole are 110 mL and 67 mL. Panels (**C**,**D**): the MODs in the two-chamber view. In diastole and systole, the volumes are, respectively, 107 mL and 66 mL. Panels (**E**,**F**): LV ejection fraction of 40% with volumes of 73 mL and 122 mL. Although the ejection fraction was similar, there was a difference in the volumes, underscoring a likely systematic error in measuring the volumes in two-dimensional method.

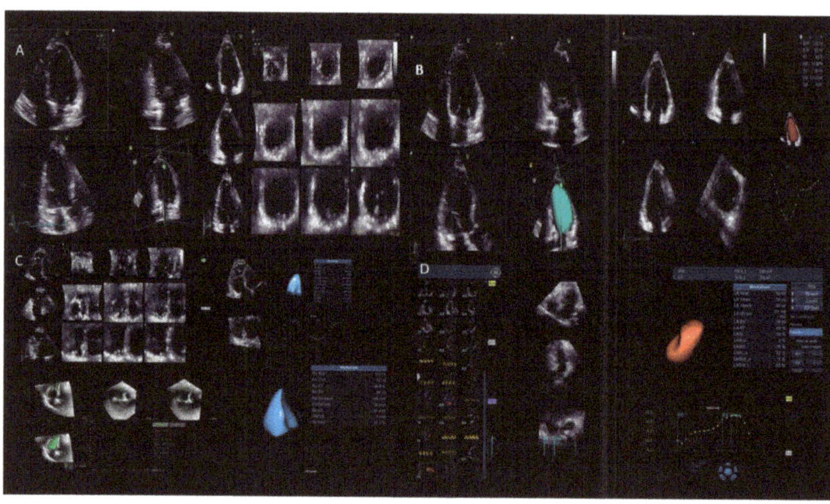

Figure 2. Possible applications of 3DE. Panel (**A**) shows a 3DE image "full volume" for the left ventricular volume; the orthogonal views confirm wall motion abnormalities in any given segment. Panel (**B**) shows the 3D left ventricular volume and function. Panel (**C**) shows the 3D right ventricular volume and function. Panel (**D**) shows the 3D left atrium volume and function.

2. **LV desynchrony:** For this assessment, the segmental LV volumes are tracked throughout the cardiac cycle. This temporal analysis allows for the identification of differences

in the timing of each segment reaching its minimal volume, which corresponds to the maximal contraction. Under normal physiological conditions, all the LV segments reach their minimal volume simultaneously during ventricular systole. However, in the presence of dyssynchrony, there is a temporal dispersion, with diseased segments achieving the minimal volume later in systole. The systolic dyssynchrony index (SDI) quantifies dyssynchrony by calculating the standard deviation of the times to the regional minimal volume across all the segments. Studies have demonstrated that the SDI is a strong predictor of cardiac resynchronization therapy (CRT) response, with significant predictive power observed at 48 h [8], as well as at 6-month and 1-year follow-ups [9]. Additionally, the importance of the optimal LV pacing lead placement has been highlighted in studies using 3DE. Patients with pacing leads positioned at the site of the maximal mechanical delay experienced significantly greater improvements in the LV function, reverse remodeling, and peak oxygen consumption compared to those with leads placed distal to the optimal site [10].

3. **Valve assessment:** Three-dimensional echocardiography offers detailed visualization of the heart valves, which is crucial for diagnosing and planning surgical interventions in patients with valve diseases, such as stenosis or regurgitation (Figure 3). The ability to visualize the valves in three dimensions allows clinicians to measure the exact size and shape of the valve orifice, the extent of leaflet prolapse, and the severity of regurgitation or stenosis. This detailed assessment helps in selecting the most appropriate treatment strategy, whether it be surgical repair, valve replacement, or percutaneous interventions.

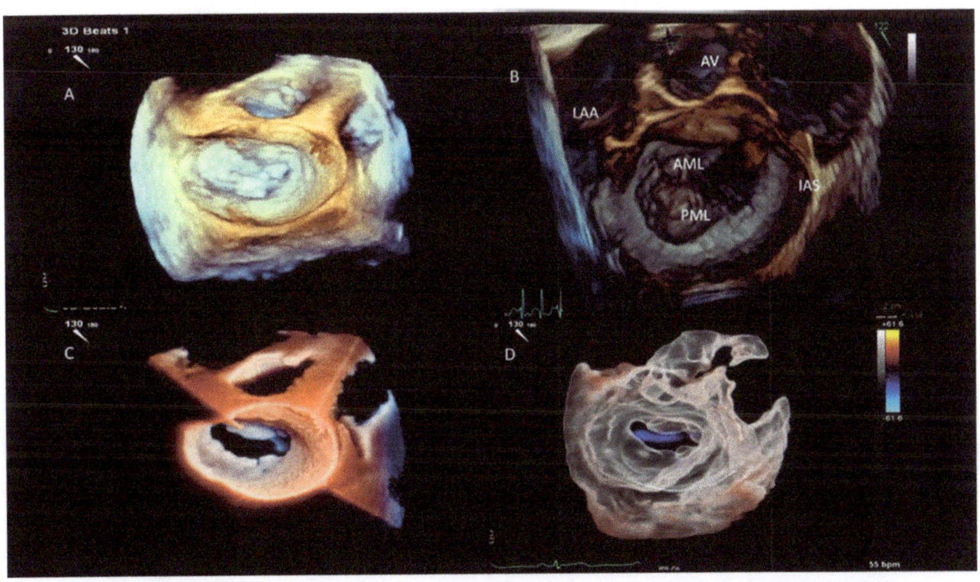

Figure 3. Three-dimensional image of mitral valve surgical atrial view. Panel (**A**) shows normal mitral valve with 3D echocardiography evaluation; panel (**B**) showsprolapse of mitral valve scallop P2; panel (**C**) shows normal mitral valve with TrueVue view modality; and panel (**D**) GlassVue view of normal mitral valve (LAA, left atrial appendage; AV, aortic valve; IAS, interatrial septum; AML, anterior mitral leaflet; and PML, posterior mitral leaflet).

4. **Interventional procedure and cardiac surgery:** It is used for intraoperative monitoring during complex cardiac surgeries, providing real-time visual guidance that can improve surgical outcomes. In procedures such as transcatheter aortic and mitral valve replacements, mitral valve repairs, or the closure of atrial septal defects, real-

time 3DE imaging provides invaluable guidance. It allows for the accurate positioning of catheters and devices, ensuring optimal procedural outcomes and reducing the risk of complications. The ability to visualize the heart and the devices in three dimensions enhances the precision of these interventions and improves patient safety.

5. **Assessment of atrial function:** It allows for the detailed evaluation of the atrial size, shape, and function, which is important in conditions such as atrial fibrillation and atrial septal defects. The ability to visualize the atria in three dimensions provides a better understanding of their pathophysiology and helps in planning interventions such as catheter ablation or the surgical closure of defects [11–13].

2.2. Limitations

One of the main limitations of 3D echocardiography, in addition to being an operator-dependent technique, is the trade-off between spatial and temporal resolutions. Achieving a higher spatial resolution requires the acquisition of a greater number of scan lines per volume, which in turn increases the time required for the image acquisition and processing, ultimately reducing the temporal resolution. To maintain an adequate temporal resolution, it is often necessary to compromise by acquiring smaller volumes. Additionally, the presence of arrhythmias poses another significant challenge, because they complicate reliable recording R-R intervals. In such cases, increasing the number of cardiac cycles while reducing the acquisition volume can serve as a feasible compromise to enhance the temporal resolution. Lastly, optimal 3D imaging relies on high-quality 2D images, with efforts to minimize respiratory artifacts during acquisition. In 3D color Doppler imaging, it can be difficult to strike an optimal balance between spatial and temporal resolutions with existing technology. Opting for a smaller acquisition volume can be a beneficial strategy to overcome this limitation.

3. Myocardial Strain Imaging

Strain imaging is an advanced echocardiographic technique that has greatly improved the assessment of myocardial function. By measuring the deformation of the cardiac muscle during the cardiac cycle, strain imaging provides detailed insights into the myocardial mechanics (Table 2) that traditional measures of cardiac function, such as the ejection fraction, cannot provide [11,14]. In clinical practice, myocardial deformation is typically described using three orthogonal components: longitudinal, radial, and circumferential. The circumferential–longitudinal LV shear strain is expressed as rotation, twist, or torsion, though, like other shear strain components, it is rarely applied in clinical settings. Myocardial fibers contribute to both longitudinal and circumferential shortening, depending on their orientation. Radial deformation results from fiber shortening across all layers, enhanced by the thickening and inward movement of the myocardium. Due to the intricate architecture of the LV, a fiber shortening of just 15% can translate into a 60% reduction in the LV volume. This structure also means that regional pathology often affects all three strain components, allowing clinicians to select the most reliable component for measurement. Longitudinal strain is the most commonly used deformation measure, as it is relatively uniform along the LV wall and enables the comprehensive assessment of the entire LV from just three apical views, making it simple and reliable to use [15]. Global strain, most often assessed as global longitudinal strain (GLS), evaluates only one of the deformation components. Studies have demonstrated that strain imaging is more effective at identifying subtle systolic dysfunction than the left ventricular ejection fraction (LVEF). This is likely because the heart can compensate for early longitudinal dysfunction by increasing other strain components, allowing the LV to maintain a normal ejection fraction despite early impairment [16].

Table 2. Key applications of myocardial strain imaging.

Application	Description	Clinical Impact
Cardiac Function Assessment	Evaluates myocardial deformation to identify dysfunction	Enhances the early detection of cardiac impairment
Risk Stratification	Uses strain metrics to predict adverse outcomes	Improves risk assessment and management strategies
Treatment Monitoring	Assesses changes in strain to evaluate therapy effectiveness	Provides insights into treatment responses

3.1. Clinical Applications

1. **Left ventricular function:** One of the main uses of strain imaging is to detect early subclinical myocardial dysfunction. For instance, in patients undergoing chemotherapy, strain imaging can detect early signs of heart damage before a significant reduction in the LVEF occurs. This allows for prompt intervention and adjustments to the cancer treatment to prevent further harm to the myocardium [17,18]. The current definitions of cancer therapy-related cardiac dysfunction primarily rely on a reduction in the LVEF and/or a relative decrease in the GLS beyond a specific threshold [19]. As a result, baseline cardiac assessments are recommended for all patients prior to initiating cardiotoxic cancer treatments. GLS assessment using speckle tracking, particularly from three apical views, is strongly advised at the baseline, especially for patients at a moderate-to-high risk. It is important to acknowledge that strain measurements may vary between different vendors. Therefore, to ensure consistency, serial GLS evaluations for each patient should be conducted using the same equipment and software. A median GLS reduction of 13.6% has been identified as a predictor of future LVEF decline, with an upper limit of 15% recommended as the threshold for GLS reduction during cancer therapy to enhance specificity [19,20]. These measurements help stratify the risk of cancer treatment-related cardiovascular toxicity and identify significant changes during therapy. Notably, a normal LVEF does not exclude the presence of cancer treatment-related cardiac dysfunction; GLS, instead, can reliably detect early systolic impairment. For instance, Muckiene et al. demonstrated that a reduction in GLS is significantly linked to early anthracycline-induced cardiotoxicity in patients undergoing anthracycline-based chemotherapy. This finding suggests that GLS could potentially serve as a predictor for any subsequent declines in the LVEF associated with this chemotherapy regimen [21]. In the assessment of ischemic heart disease, strain imaging provides valuable information about regional myocardial function [16]. During an ischemic event, specific areas of the myocardium may show reduced strain, indicating impaired contractility. This technique can help identify a viable but hibernating myocardium, which can benefit from revascularization procedures. Strain imaging is also useful in evaluating the effectiveness of reperfusion therapies following acute myocardial infarction by assessing the recovery of myocardial function in the affected regions [22–24]. Furthermore, the management of HF patients benefits significantly from strain imaging. It offers a more sensitive measure of myocardial function compared to traditional echocardiographic parameters (Figure 4). GLS has been shown to correlate better with outcomes in heart failure patients, providing prognostic information that aids in clinical decision-making. In patients with HF with mildly reduced ejection fraction (HFmrEF), strain imaging can uncover subtle myocardial dysfunction that is often missed by conventional measures. Chang et al. demonstrated that in patients with HFmrEF, a LV GLS cut-off value of −11% effectively differentiated the subsequent risk of cardiovascular death [25]. This enhances the understanding and management of this complex condition [26].

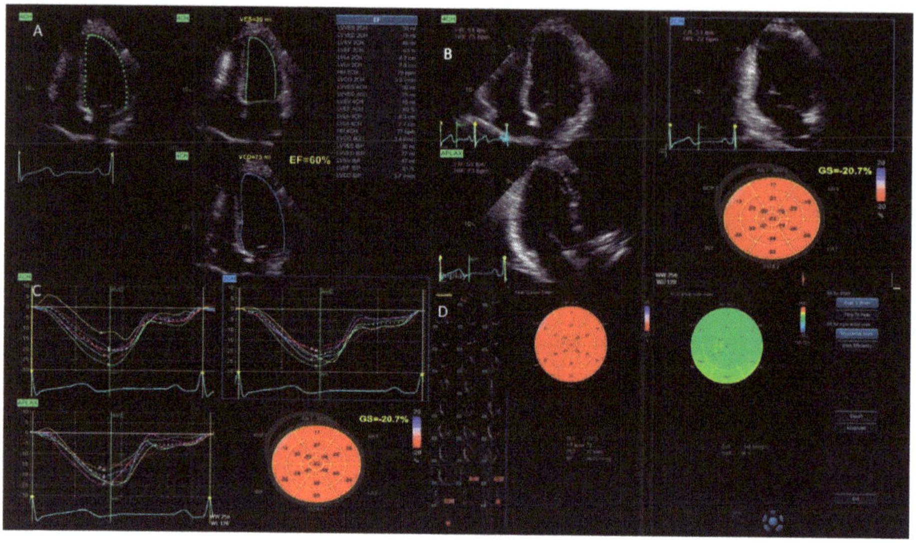

Figure 4. Myocardial strain valuation. Panel (**A**) shows the auto ejection fraction calculation with a good quality apical acoustic window of the endocardial edges with artificial intelligence technology that allows semi-automatic recognition; in this image, the LVEF = 60%. Panels (**B**,**C**) show a 2D left ventricular echocardiography with speckle tracking with a normal global longitudinal strain (GLS) in the range of −21.7%. Panel (**D**) shows a normal global longitudinal strain (GLS) of −20% and a normal myocardial work index of 1548 mm Hg%.

2. **Cardiomyopathies:** In hypertrophic cardiomyopathy (HCM), strain imaging can identify areas of abnormal myocardial mechanics that are indicative of the disease [27,28]. Reduced strain in the thickened segments of the LV, usually correlated with the extent of late gadolinium enhancement in a cardiac MRI, can signal the presence of fibrosis and assist in assessing the risk of sudden cardiac death [29]. Similarly, in dilated cardiomyopathy (DCM), strain imaging allows for a detailed evaluation of the global and regional myocardial function, aiding in the monitoring of disease progression and response to therapy [30]. Moreover, the relative apical sparing of the GLS ratio (the average of the apical longitudinal strain/the average of the combined mid and basal longitudinal strain > 1) is typically presented in cardiac amyloidosis, both associated with light chain and transthyretin deposits [31]. A reduced longitudinal strain with an apical sparing pattern is therefore considered a typical red flag disease [32].
3. **LV dyssynchrony:** This technique evaluates the mechanical function of various segments of the LV to identify patients who are suitable for CRT and to monitor their response to the therapy [33,34]. Although cardiac imaging has not yet been proven to be effective for selecting candidates for CRT, there is emerging evidence supporting the use of strain imaging to identify the optimal placement of the pacing lead on the LV free wall [35]. Several studies have shown that positioning the lead in the area of the latest mechanical activation leads to better clinical outcomes [36]. Additionally, it is crucial to avoid placing the lateral lead over regions of transmural scarring. A peak radial strain value of less than 10% has been suggested as a marker for identifying the scar tissue [37].
4. **Valve assessment:** Strain imaging provides additional insight into the effect of valvular lesions on myocardial function. For example, in aortic stenosis, strain imaging can detect early myocardial dysfunction before the onset of obvious HF symptoms, helping to determine the optimal timing for surgical intervention [38,39]. Likewise, in mitral regurgitation, it assists in evaluating the compensatory mechanisms and

identifying the point at which myocardial function starts to deteriorate, thereby aiding in the decision-making process for valve repair or replacement [40]. Characteristically, the longitudinal strain impairment detected in individuals with mitral valve prolapse is more regional than global, with a distinct involvement of the left ventricular basal inferolateral segments and a relative sparing of the apical region [41].

5. **Congenital heart disease:** Strain imaging is being used more and more in this field. It provides detailed functional assessments that are crucial for managing complex congenital anomalies. In patients with repaired congenital heart defects, strain imaging can monitor long-term myocardial function and detect early signs of dysfunction that may require further intervention [42]. A recent meta-analysis demonstrated that myocardial deformation parameters can be used for risk stratification in congenital heart disease (CHD) follow-ups, with an added clinical value over conventional echocardiography [43]. Indeed, in CHD, the anatomy of the ventricles is frequently distorted by the congenital abnormalities, the different surgeries, and the percutaneous procedures, with abnormal loading conditions related to the disease and surgical sequels, as well as residual lesions. In these conditions, the use of parameters that are independent by geometrical assumption, less affected by loading conditions, and not influenced by tethering provides obvious advantages over any geometric- or volumetric-based functional parameter [44]. Single ventricle strain was predictive of outcomes in hypoplastic left heart syndrome during the interstage period [45].

In Tetralogy of Fallot patients, the use of speckle tracking to assess longitudinal strain in the meta-analysis showed both RV global longitudinal strain and LV longitudinal strain to be prognostic of MACEs, independent of other conventional parameters, including the QRS duration and RV ejection fraction measured by an MRI [43]. This finding is particularly relevant, because the current volumetric cut-offs for pulmonary valve replacements are not well established [46]. Thus, biventricular strain should be included in the current risk stratification criteria, to better identify the proper timing for pulmonary valve implantations. In adult patients with repaired coarctation of the aorta (CoA), myocardial deformation properties of the left ventricle are frequently impaired despite a normal LVEF [47]. It has been demonstrated that this reduced LV GLS has a strong association with all-cause mortality and cardiovascular mortality and provided a superior prognostic performance compared with the LVEF [48]. Of note, in CoA patients with a normal LVEF, the coexistence of a reduced LV GLS is associated with a higher risk of all-cause mortality, compared with CoA patients with a normal LVGLS and LVEF [48].

3.2. Limitations

In clinical practice, speckle-tracking echocardiography has several limitations as it may be suboptimal in patients with poorly defined subendocardial borders, particularly in cases with near-field artifacts. These artifacts can reduce the accuracy of endocardial visualization, leading to errors in the automated tracing of the myocardium by the software. Moreover, automated software packages designed to trace the endocardium can be prone to error and, as a result, the manual verification of automated tracings is often required, which can be time-consuming. The most critical challenge is the variation between different vendors' software, as differences in the algorithms used for the temporal and spatial smoothing can affect the accuracy of the strain measurements. The variability of normal values, assessed through different software packages, complicates the interpretation of the results, especially when comparing the results across different populations or using different software packages.

4. Vortex Dynamics Imaging

Vortex imaging is an innovative echocardiographic technique that provides a detailed visualization of intracardiac blood flow patterns. Unlike conventional Doppler imaging, which focuses on linear velocity measurements, vortex imaging captures the complex, swirling blood flow within the heart chambers, offering a more comprehensive understanding of hemodynamics [49]. The presence of vortices appears to play a key role in preventing the energy loss that would occur with a chaotic distribution of flow within the cardiac chambers [50]. During diastole, two distinct vortices can be observed within the LV. The first vortex, positioned anteriorly, exhibits a clockwise rotation across the LV inflow–outflow region, while the second vortex, located posteriorly, rotates counterclockwise [50]. The geometrical properties of the vortex in the LV are quantified by several key measures. These include the vortex area, which is scaled relative to the overall LV area, and the vortex intensity, which is the integral of the vorticity within the vortex, normalized by the total vorticity of the LV. Additionally, the vortex depth, defined as the distance from the vortex center to the LV base, and the vortex length, measured along the base–apex axis, are both normalized by the total length of the LV. The energy dynamics of the vortex flow are assessed by calculating the total kinetic energy dissipation (KED), which represents the amount of kinetic energy lost through viscous friction during the cardiac cycle. The total KED is integrated across the entire LV and is typically normalized by the average kinetic energy to ensure it is not directly influenced by variations in the LV size. This allows for a more consistent comparison across different heart sizes [50].

The evaluation of intracardiac flow dynamics has traditionally been limited by the need for a phase contrast cardiac MRI or contrast echocardiography with particle imaging velocimetry [51]. These methods are impractical for widespread use in patients. In recent years, color Doppler-based ultrasound techniques such as Vector Flow Mapping (VFM) have been developed to analyze organized vortical structures in the heart more practically [52]. VFM can detect and measure the flow motion in all directions within a scan plane by applying a series of mathematical equations to the color Doppler data [53]. This technique enables the visualization and quantification of complex flow patterns, such as those in cardiac chambers, where the vortices are believed to significantly reduce energy loss and optimize cardiac function. HyperDoppler is another non-invasive advanced echocardiographic technique that enhances the visualization of intracardiac vortices, providing a detailed assessment of the complex blood flow dynamics within the heart chambers, which is crucial for optimizing the understanding of cardiac function and energy efficiency [54]. Vortices appear to contribute to atrioventricular coupling and the redirection of ventricular blood inflow toward the outflow tracts, while maintaining blood motion and preventing the potential effects of stasis [55].

4.1. Clinical Applications

1. **LV function:** Vortex imaging helps clinicians visualize and measure the vortices within the LV, which are crucial for the efficient blood ejection and filling. By analyzing these flow patterns, clinicians can identify early signs of LV dysfunction that might not be obvious using standard measures. Two vortex components were consistently observed following each transmitral filling wave. The anterior vortex was analyzed due to its greater relevance in the cardiac cycle, occurring after early filling and atrial contraction. The vortex generated after early filling appears to aid LV inflow and plays a more prominent role in individuals with impaired relaxation. The vortex formed after atrial contraction seems to store kinetic energy and redirect the flow toward the outflow tract, facilitating ejection and contributing to the mitral valve closure [56]. Diastolic vortices are especially important for assessing the left atrial function and ventricular filling pressures. This is particularly valuable in conditions like heart failure with a preserved ejection fraction, where vortex dynamics can reveal underlying diastolic dysfunction [56]. Moreover, a reduced vortex formation time (VFT), a dimensionless index used to quantify the vortex development, strongly correlates with LV dysfunction and predicts adverse outcomes in patients with HF [57]. As an example, the VFT ranged between 3.3 and 5.5 in healthy subjects, but decreased to values < 2.0 in patients with dilated cardiomyopathy [58].
2. **Valve disease:** In mitral regurgitation, vortex imaging can depict the altered flow patterns caused by the regurgitant jet, helping to quantify the severity of the lesion

and its effect on the LV filling. Restoring normal intracardiac LV flow patterns, as observed primarily after mitral valve replacements, may help preserve kinetic energy momentum, thereby reducing the LV workload and shear stress. A recent study revealed that intracardiac blood flow patterns are restored after mitral valve repairs, regardless of the repair technique used. In contrast, a mitral valve replacement with either biological or mechanical prostheses in non-anatomical orientations is associated with persistent alterations in the blood flow. A transcatheter edge-to-edge repair completely disrupts the LV vortices, while a transcatheter mitral valve replacement with a Tendyne valve has an effect similar to a mitral valve repair in restoring normal flow patterns [59]. Similarly, in aortic stenosis, the technique can illustrate the turbulent flow distal to the stenotic valve, offering a visual representation of the hemodynamic burden on the LV (Figures 5 and 6). This information aids in the decision-making process for valve repairs or replacements by providing a more nuanced understanding of the disease's impact on cardiac function [60,61]. Some studies have reported that aortic stenosis is associated with reduced LV filling efficiency, resulting in decreased VFT values. However, in patients with aortic stenosis and moderate aortic insufficiency, the VFT significantly increases, suggesting that the VFT may be an unreliable index of LV filling efficiency when competitive diastolic flows into the LV are present [62].

3. **Congenital heart** diseases: CHDs often involve complex intracardiac flow abnormalities that can be challenging to assess with traditional imaging techniques. Vortex imaging is particularly effective in this area, providing a detailed visualization of abnormal flow patterns, which is essential for accurate diagnosis and surgical planning. For instance, in conditions such as the Tetralogy of Fallot or the transposition of the great arteries, vortex imaging can depict the intricate flow dynamics and help in understanding the physiological consequences of the defects. In patients with transposition of the great arteries, an increased flow across the pulmonary valve secondary to a large ventricular septal defect may be responsible for a Doppler gradient at the level of the pulmonary valve, mimicking a pulmonary stenosis. In this case, the differentiation between a real valvular stenosis and a gradient secondary to volume overload is extremely important in defining the surgical timing and the type of surgery (arterial switch and ventricular septal defect closure vs. Rastelli operation). These are the kinds of situations where the traditional Doppler and color Doppler techniques demonstrate all their limitations. The use of blood speckle imaging to study flow dynamics has proven to be helpful in formulating the correct diagnosis, especially in this difficult context [63]. Post-surgical follow-ups in CHD patients also benefit from vortex imaging, as it can monitor the restoration or alteration of normal flow patterns [60].
4. **LV dyssynchrony:** Vortex imaging can assess the changes in intracavitary flow patterns before and after the CRT implantation, providing insights into the therapy's effectiveness. Goliasch et al. utilized vortex imaging to assess the impact of an acute interruption and reactivation of the CRT. Deactivating the CRT significantly disrupted the LV filling, resulting in the reduced mitral inflow acceleration and increased total diastolic volume. This, in turn, led to the formation of an underdeveloped diastolic vortex, which impaired the transfer of kinetic energy from diastole to systole, delayed the redirection of the blood flow toward the aorta, and hindered the timely opening of the aortic valve, thereby prolonging the isovolumetric contraction period [64]. Upon the reactivation of the CRT, the LV filling improved immediately, and the total diastolic volume decreased. This restored the optimal timing of the diastolic vortex formation and shortened the isovolumetric interval [64]. By visualizing the improvement in flow efficiency and the reduction in dysfunctional vortices, clinicians can better evaluate the success of a CRT and make adjustments as needed to optimize patient outcomes.
5. **Cardiomyopathies:** In DCM, vortex imaging helps to evaluate the impact of dilated chambers on intracardiac flow and to pinpoint the regions of flow stagnation that may

contribute to thrombus formation. Furthermore, vortex patterns are used to gauge the severity of HF, as fragmented or abnormal patterns are associated with increased cardiac dysfunction [65].

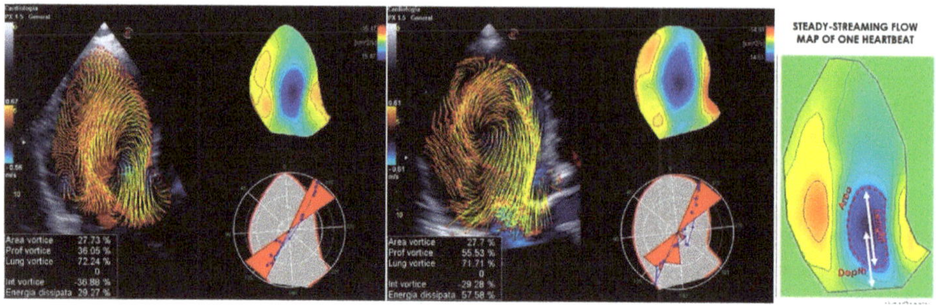

Figure 5. Vortex geometric analysis. A normal (**one the right**) versus a pathological (**on the left**) subject with aortic stenosis. The geometric values to consider are area, depth, and length. The area is identical in both the normal and pathological subjects. The depth varies between the two, with the normal subject having a smaller depth. This suggests that the aortic stenosis pushes the structure towards the tip in the normal subject. The length is the same in both subjects.

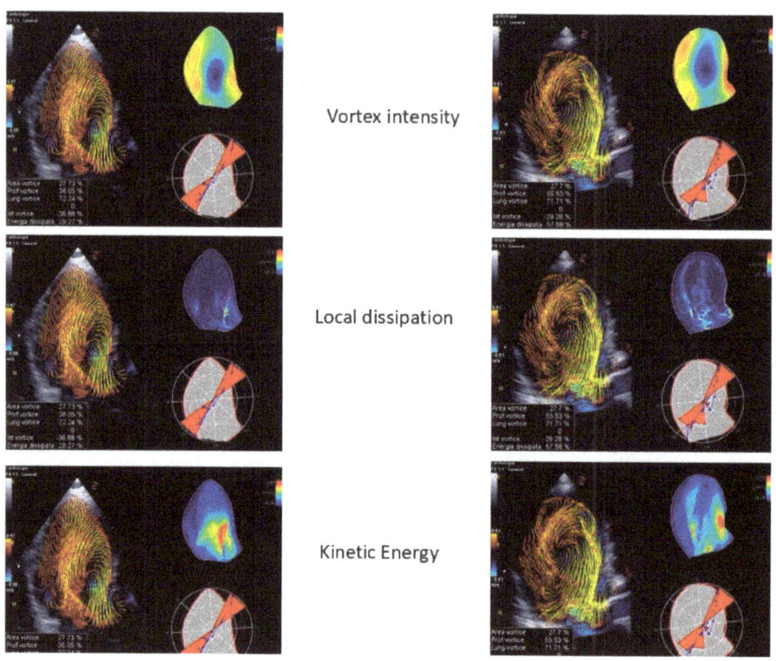

Figure 6. Normal vs. pathological subjects with aortic stenosis. The vortex's energetic values to consider are the following: vortex intensity, local dissipation, and kinetic energy. The vortex intensity varies, with the normal subject exhibiting a higher intensity, compared to the pathological subject, who shows a greater local dissipation.

4.2. Limitations

One of the main limitations of vortex analysis is the need for specialized software, which is often expensive and not always readily available. Furthermore, this technique has not yet been fully validated in large-scale populations, highlighting the need for future studies to confirm its reliability and broader applicability.

5. Multimodality Imaging

5.1. Integrative Approach

Multimodality imaging combines various imaging techniques, such as echocardiography and a cardiac MRI, to provide a comprehensive view of the cardiac structure and function. This integrated approach enhances diagnostic accuracy and treatment planning [1]. By combining different modalities, clinicians achieve a holistic view of cardiac health, which is particularly beneficial in complex HF cases. When used together, strain imaging, 3DE, and vortex analysis provide a comprehensive assessment of cardiac function. Strain imaging identifies early myocardial dysfunction; 3D echocardiography provides more precise volumetric and structural assessments of the cardiac chambers, offering improved accuracy in evaluating heart size, shape, and function; and vortex analysis offers a deeper understanding of intraventricular flow dynamics. This multimodal approach can better define a patient's cardiac condition, allowing for more tailored and accurate clinical decision-making. This approach also aids in monitoring the treatment by observing structural and functional changes over time (Table 3).

Table 3. Specific contributions of each imaging modality across various clinical scenarios, emphasizing their complementary roles in enhancing cardiac diagnosis and treatment.

Clinical Scenario	3D Echocardiography	Myocardial Strain Imaging	Vortex Imaging
Left Ventricular Function	Accurate evaluation of LV function, avoiding geometric assumptions. Reproducible measurements of volumes and ejection fraction. Visualization of rendered 3DE images for comprehensive cardiac structure analysis.	Detects early subclinical myocardial dysfunction, especially in conditions like chemotherapy-induced cardiotoxicity. Offers a sensitive measure of myocardial function, correlating well with outcomes in heart failure.	Visualizes and measures the intracardiac vortices crucial for efficient blood ejection and filling. Diastolic vortices assess left atrial function and ventricular filling pressures, valuable in HFpEF.
LV Dyssynchrony	Tracks segmental LV volumes throughout the cardiac cycle. The SDI predicts response to CRT. Optimal pacing lead placement guided by 3DE improves CRT outcomes.	Assesses desynchrony in CRT patients. Guides optimal pacing lead placement to improve outcomes.	Assesses changes in intracavitary flow patterns before and after CRT implantation. Visualizes improvement in flow efficiency post-CRT.
Valve Assessment	Detailed visualization of heart valves. Measures valve orifice size, leaflet prolapse, and severity of regurgitation or stenosis.	Detects early myocardial dysfunction in valvular diseases like aortic stenosis and mitral regurgitation. Helps determine timing for surgical intervention.	Depicts altered flow patterns in valve diseases like mitral regurgitation and aortic stenosis. Visualizes hemodynamic burden on the LV.
Atrial Function	Detailed evaluation of atrial size, shape, and function. Valuable in atrial fibrillation and atrial septal defects.	Provides global insight into cardiac function, which can include atrial contribution.	Not directly used in assessing atrial function but could offer insights into atrioventricular coupling dynamics.
Cardiomyopathies	Assists in the detailed assessment of LV structure and function in hypertrophic and dilated cardiomyopathy. Important for risk stratification and management.	Identifies abnormal myocardial mechanics in HCM. Assesses global and regional myocardial function in DCM, aiding in disease monitoring. Apical sparing as red flag in cardiac amyloidosis.	Evaluates the impact of dilated chambers on flow in DCM.
Congenital Heart Diseases	Provides comprehensive views essential for surgical planning. Monitors structural changes post-repair.	Monitors myocardial function in repaired congenital heart defects. Detects early signs of dysfunction post-surgery.	Visualizes complex flow abnormalities in congenital heart disease. Monitors restoration of normal flow patterns post-surgery.

CRT: cardiac resynchronization therapy; DCM: dilated cardiomyopathy; HCM: hypertrophic cardiomyopathy; HFpEF: heart failure with a preserved ejection fraction; LV: left ventricle; and SDI: systolic dyssynchrony index.

5.2. Emerging Technologies

Emerging technologies such as video-based artificial intelligence (AI) are revolutionizing HF management. Video-based AI allows for the real-time evaluation of cardiac function, improving early detection and intervention [66]. This technology provides a detailed beat-to-beat assessment, enhancing the precision of cardiac evaluations.

As an example, high frame rate imaging offers the enhanced visualization of intracardiac vortices, providing deeper insights into cardiac flow and function [67]. Blood speckle tracking may be used to understand and quantify intra- and extra-cardiac flow patterns, improving our understanding of cardiac physiology. Compared to conventional Doppler imaging, high frame rate imaging is an ultrafast technique, which generates up to thousands of frames per second and which is independent of the angle of insonation [67]. This advancement improves the analysis of vortex dynamics, contributing to a better understanding of cardiac performance and potentially leading to more effective treatments.

5.3. Advanced Imaging in Clinical Practice

The integration of advanced imaging technologies into clinical practice has enabled more personalized treatment strategies for HF patients. By providing detailed and accurate assessments of cardiac function, these technologies allow for tailored therapeutic approaches, improving patient outcomes. Unfortunately, vortex analysis is not yet in routine clinical practice, as it primarily remains a research tool with ongoing studies to assess its clinical relevance. However, GLS and 3DE have already been integrated into standard clinical use. GLS is particularly valuable in the assessment of cardiomyopathies, where it helps to detect the subclinical dysfunction or fibrosis and to monitor disease progression. Additionally, 3DE has proven beneficial for the more accurate evaluation of valve structures and function, offering a more comprehensive analysis compared to traditional 2DE. These advancements have improved diagnostic accuracy and patient management in daily practice. For instance, myocardial strain imaging can identify patients who would benefit most from CRT, while vortex analysis can pinpoint those at risk for diastolic dysfunction. One of the key benefits of advanced imaging is the ability to detect cardiac abnormalities early, before they manifest as clinical symptoms. Advanced imaging techniques, such as 3DE and high frame rate imaging, provide more detailed views of cardiac structures and flow dynamics, leading to enhanced diagnostic accuracy. This precision is crucial for diagnosing complex cases where traditional methods may fall short. However, difficult cases to interpret, where the risk of false positives or false negatives remains high, often require a collegial evaluation, where the echocardiographer must consult with the radiologist or the hemodynamic specialist who is about to perform or has performed a procedure.

6. Future Directions and Research

As technology continues to evolve, further advancements in imaging techniques are expected. These may include improvements in AI algorithms for better real-time analysis, higher resolution imaging for more detailed assessments, and the development of new modalities that can provide even deeper insights into cardiac function. The integration of advanced imaging technologies with wearable devices holds promise for the continuous monitoring of cardiac function in HF patients. This could enable real-time data collection and analysis, leading to more dynamic and responsive treatment strategies. The future of HF management lies in personalized medicine, where treatment is tailored to the individual patient's genetic makeup, lifestyle, and specific cardiac abnormalities. Advanced imaging will play a pivotal role in this approach, providing the detailed information needed to customize treatments effectively.

7. Conclusions

The integration of advanced imaging technologies, such as 3DE, myocardial strain imaging, and vortex analysis, has significantly transformed HF management. These advancements provide more detailed and accurate assessments of cardiac function, facilitating earlier diagnosis, improved risk stratification, and personalized treatment strategies. As these technologies continue to evolve, they promise to further enhance HF management and patient outcomes. The ability to detect subtle myocardial changes, analyze complex flow dynamics, and integrate various imaging modalities equips clinicians with a comprehensive toolkit to address the multifaceted nature of HF. The continued refinement and development of these technologies will undoubtedly lead to significant improvements in patient care and outcomes.

Author Contributions: Conceptualization, B.C., D.G. and G.D.S.; methodology, M.M., D.T., E.L. and G.C.; investigation, N.K., F.K., S.A. and B.A.; resources, N.K., F.K., S.A., I.C. and A.P.; data curation, B.C.; writing—original draft preparation, D.G. and G.D.S.; writing—review and editing, B.A., M.T.S. and D.A.C.; visualization, A.P., D.A.C. and I.C.; and supervision, D.G., M.M., E.L., G.C. and D.T. All authors have read and agreed to the published version of the manuscript.

Funding: This research received no external funding.

Informed Consent Statement: Not applicable.

Data Availability Statement: Not applicable.

Conflicts of Interest: The authors declare no conflicts of interest.

Abbreviations

AI: artificial intelligence; CoA: coarctation of the aorta; CHD: congenital heart disease; CRT: cardiac resynchronization therapy; DCM: dilated cardiomyopathy; GLS: global longitudinal strain; HCM: hypertrophic cardiomyopathy; HF: heart failure; HFmrEF: HF with mildly reduced ejection fraction; KED: kinetic energy dissipation; LV: left ventricle; LVEF: left ventricle ejection fraction; MACEs: major adverse cardiac events; MRI: magnetic resonance imaging; SDI: systolic dyssynchrony index; RV: right ventricle; VFM: Vector Flow Mapping; VFT: vortex formation time; 2DE: two-dimensional echocardiography; and 3DE: three-dimensional echocardiography.

References

1. Pergola, V.; Cameli, M.; Mattesi, G.; Mushtaq, S.; D'Andrea, A.; Guaricci, A.I.; Pastore, M.C.; Amato, F.; Dellino, C.M.; Motta, R.; et al. Multimodality Imaging in Advanced Heart Failure for Diagnosis, Management and Follow-Up: A Comprehensive Review. *J. Clin. Med.* **2023**, *12*, 7641. [CrossRef]
2. Pergola, V.; D'Andrea, A.; Galzerano, D.; Mantovani, F.; Rizzo, M.; Giannuario, G.D.; Khoury, G.; Polizzi, V.; Rabia, G.; Gimelli, A.; et al. Unveiling the Hidden Chamber: Exploring the Importance of Left Atrial Function and Filling Pressure in Cardiovascular Health. *J. Cardiovasc. Echogr.* **2023**, *33*, 117–124. [CrossRef]
3. Marwick, T.H.; Shah, S.J.; Thomas, J.D. Myocardial Strain in the Assessment of Patients with Heart Failure: A Review. *JAMA Cardiol.* **2019**, *4*, 287–294. [CrossRef] [PubMed]
4. Nagueh, S.F.; Appleton, C.P.; Gillebert, T.C.; Marino, P.N.; Oh, J.K.; Smiseth, O.A.; Waggoner, A.D.; Flachskampf, F.A.; Pellikka, P.A.; Evangelisa, A. Recommendations for the evaluation of left ventricular diastolic function by echocardiography. *Eur. J. Echocardiogr. J. Work. Gr. Echocardiogr. Eur. Soc. Cardiol.* **2009**, *10*, 165–193. [CrossRef] [PubMed]
5. Sperlongano, S.; D'Andrea, A.; Mele, D.; Russo, V.; Pergola, V.; Carbone, A.; Ilardi, F.; Di Maio, M.; Bottino, R.; Giallauria, F.; et al. Left Ventricular Deformation and Vortex Analysis in Heart Failure: From Ultrasound Technique to Current Clinical Application. *Diagnostics* **2021**, *11*, 892. [CrossRef]
6. Pestelli, G.; Pergola, V.; Totaro, G.; Previtero, M.; Aruta, P.; Cecchetto, A.; Fiorencis, A.; Palermo, C.; Iliceto, S.; Mele, D. Value of Left Ventricular Indexed Ejection Time to Characterize the Severity of Aortic Stenosis. *J. Clin. Med.* **2022**, *11*, 1877. [CrossRef]
7. Lang, R.M.; Badano, L.P.; Tsang, W.; Adams, D.H.; Agricola, E.; Buck, T.; Faletra, F.F.; Franke, A.; Hung, J.; de Isla, L.P.; et al. EAE/ASE recommendations for image acquisition and display using three-dimensional echocardiography. *Eur. Heart J. Cardiovasc. Imaging* **2012**, *13*, 1–46. [CrossRef]
8. Marsan, N.A.; Bleeker, G.B.; Ypenburg, C.; Ghio, S.; van de Veire, N.R.; Holman, E.R.; van der Wall, E.E.; Tavazzi, L.; Schalij, M.J.; Bax, J.J. Real-time three-dimensional echocardiography permits quantification of left ventricular mechanical dyssynchrony and predicts acute response to cardiac resynchronization therapy. *J. Cardiovasc. Electrophysiol.* **2008**, *19*, 392–399. [CrossRef]
9. Soliman, O.I.I.; Geleijnse, M.L.; Theuns, D.A.M.J.; van Dalen, B.M.; Vletter, W.B.; Jordaens, L.J.; Metawei, A.K.; Al-Amin, A.M.; ten Cate, F.J. Usefulness of left ventricular systolic dyssynchrony by real-time three-dimensional echocardiography to predict long-term response to cardiac resynchronization therapy. *Am. J. Cardiol.* **2009**, *103*, 1586–1591. [CrossRef] [PubMed]

10. Becker, M.; Hoffmann, R.; Schmitz, F.; Hundemer, A.; Kühl, H.; Schauerte, P.; Kelm, M.; Franke, A. Relation of optimal lead positioning as defined by three-dimensional echocardiography to long-term benefit of cardiac resynchronization. *Am. J. Cardiol.* **2007**, *100*, 1671–1676. [CrossRef]
11. Lang, R.M.; Badano, L.P.; Mor-Avi, V.; Afilalo, J.; Armstrong, A.; Ernande, L.; Flachskampf, F.A.; Foster, E.; Goldstein, S.A. Kuznetsova, T.; et al. Recommendations for cardiac chamber quantification by echocardiography in adults: An update from the American Society of Echocardiography and the European Association of Cardiovascular Imaging. *J. Am. Soc. Echocardiogr. Off. Publ. Am. Soc. Echocardiogr.* **2015**, *28*, 1–39.e14. [CrossRef]
12. Yu, Z.-X.; Yang, W.; Yin, W.-S.; Peng, K.X.; Pan, Y.L.; Chen, W.W.; Du, B.B.; He, Y.Q.; Yang, P. Clinical utility of left atrial strain in predicting atrial fibrillation recurrence after catheter ablation: An up-to-date review. *World J. Clin. Cases* **2022**, *10*, 8063–8075. [CrossRef]
13. Martini, L.; Lisi, M.; Pastore, M.C.; Righini, F.M.; Rubboli, A.; Henein, M.Y.; Cameli, M. The Role of Speckle Tracking Echocardiography in the Evaluation of Advanced-Heart-Failure Patients. *J. Clin. Med.* **2024**, *13*, 4037. [CrossRef] [PubMed]
14. Brady, B.; King, G.; Murphy, R.T.; Walsh, D. Myocardial strain: A clinical review. *Ir. J. Med. Sci.* **2023**, *192*, 1649–1656. [CrossRef] [PubMed]
15. Voigt, J.U.; Cvijic, M. 2- and 3-Dimensional Myocardial Strain in Cardiac Health and Disease. *JACC Cardiovasc. Imaging* **2019**, *12*, 1849–1863. [CrossRef] [PubMed]
16. Stokke, T.M.; Hasselberg, N.E.; Smedsrud, M.K.; Sarvari, S.I.; Haugaa, K.H.; Smiseth, O.A.; Edvardsen, T.; Remme, E.W. Geometry as a Confounder When Assessing Ventricular Systolic Function: Comparison Between Ejection Fraction and Strain. *J. Am. Coll. Cardiol.* **2017**, *70*, 942–954. [CrossRef] [PubMed]
17. Gorgiladze, N.; Shavdia, M.; Gaprindashvili, T.; Gogua, E.; Gachechiladze, L.; Gujabidze, M.; Pagava, Z. Detection of Cardiotoxicity Using Right Ventricular Free Wall Longitudinal Strain in Low Cardiovascular Risk Breast Cancer Patients Receiving Low-Dose Anthracycline Treatment. *Cureus* **2024**, *16*, e63138. [CrossRef] [PubMed]
18. Liu, R.; Xu, L.A.; Zhao, Z.; Han, R. Application of two-dimensional speckle-tracking echocardiography in radiotherapy-related cardiac systolic dysfunction and analysis of its risk factors: A prospective cohort study. *BMC Cardiovasc. Disord.* **2024**, *24*, 328. [CrossRef] [PubMed]
19. Lyon, A.R.; López-Fernández, T.; Couch, L.S.; Asteggiano, R.; Aznar, M.C.; Bergler-Klein, J.; Boriani, G.; Cardinale, D.; Cordoba, R. Cosyns, B.; et al. 2022 ESC Guidelines on cardio-oncology developed in collaboration with the European Hematology Association (EHA), the European Society for Therapeutic Radiology and Oncology (ESTRO) and the International Cardio-Oncology Society (IC-OS): Developed by the task force on cardio-oncology of the European Society of Cardiology (ESC). *Eur. Heart J.* **2022**, *43*, 4229–4361. [CrossRef] [PubMed]
20. Oikonomou, E.K.; Kokkinidis, D.G.; Kampaktsis, P.N.; Amir, E.A.; Marwick, T.H.; Gupta, D.; Thavendiranathan, P. Assessment of Prognostic Value of Left Ventricular Global Longitudinal Strain for Early Prediction of Chemotherapy-Induced Cardiotoxicity: A Systematic Review and Meta-analysis. *JAMA Cardiol.* **2019**, *4*, 1007–1018. [CrossRef]
21. Muckiene, G.; Vaitiekus, D.; Zaliaduonyte, D.; Zabiela, V.; Verseckaite-Costa, R.; Vaiciuliene, D.; Juozaityte, E. Prognostic Impact of Global Longitudinal Strain and NT-proBNP on Early Development of Cardiotoxicity in Breast Cancer Patients Treated with Anthracycline-Based Chemotherapy. *Medicina* **2023**, *59*, 953. [CrossRef]
22. Zhou, F.; Yuan, H.; Sun, J.; Ran, H.; Pan, H.; Wu, P.; Yang, Q. Two-dimensional speckle tracking imaging cardiac motion-based quantitative evaluation of global longitudinal strain among patients with coronary Heart Disease and functions of left ventricular ischemic myocardial segment. *Int. J. Cardiovasc. Imaging.* **2024**, *40*, 351–359. [CrossRef]
23. Yu, Z.; Pan, H.; Cheng, Z.; Lu, K.; Hu, H. Evaluation of Left Ventricular Systolic Function in Patients with Coronary Microvascular Dysfunction by Three-Dimensional Speckle-Tracking Imaging. *Braz. J. Cardiovasc. Surg.* **2022**, *37*, 321–327. [CrossRef]
24. Yehia, A.; Zaki, A.; Sadaka, M.; Azeem, A.M.A.E. Incremental prognostic value of speckle tracking echocardiography and early follow-up echo assessment in predicting left ventricular recovery after reperfusion for ST-segment elevation myocardial infarction (STEMI). *Echocardiography* **2024**, *41*, e15725. [CrossRef]
25. Chang, W.-T.; Lin, C.H.; Hong, C.-S.; Liao, C.T.; Liu, Y.W.; Chen, Z.C.; Shih, J.Y. The predictive value of global longitudinal strain in patients with heart failure mid-range ejection fraction. *J. Cardiol.* **2021**, *77*, 509–516. [CrossRef]
26. Ashish, K.; Faisaluddin, M.; Bandyopadhyay, D.; Hajra, A.; Herzog, E. Prognostic value of global longitudinal strain in heart failure subjects: A recent prototype. *Int. J. Cardiol. Heart Vasc.* **2019**, *22*, 48–49. [CrossRef]
27. Di Salvo, G.; Pacileo, G.; Limongelli, G.; Baldini, L.; Rea, A.; Verrengia, M.; D'Andrea, A.; Russo, M.G.; Calabrò, R. Non sustained ventricular tachycardia in hypertrophic cardiomyopathy and new ultrasonic derived parameters. *J. Am. Soc. Echocardiogr. Off. Publ. Am. Soc. Echocardiogr.* **2010**, *23*, 581–590. [CrossRef]
28. Tower-Rader, A.; Betancor, J.; Popovic, Z.B.; Sato, K.; Thamilarasan, M.; Smedira, N.G.; Lever, H.M.; Desai, M.Y. Incremental Prognostic Utility of Left Ventricular Global Longitudinal Strain in Hypertrophic Obstructive Cardiomyopathy Patients and Preserved Left Ventricular Ejection Fraction. *J. Am. Heart Assoc.* **2017**, *6*, e006514. [CrossRef] [PubMed]
29. Zhuang, H.; Yang, K.; Zhao, S.; Wu, J.; Xu, N.; Zhang, L.; Qi, X.; Zhang, M.; Song, L.; Pang, K. Incremental value of myocardial global longitudinal strain in predicting major adverse cardiac events among patients with hypertrophic cardiomyopathy. *Echocardiography* **2024**, *41*, e15834. [CrossRef] [PubMed]

30. Chen, P.; Aurich, M.; Greiner, S.; Maliandi, G.; Müller-Hennessen, M.; Giannitsis, E.; Meder, B.; Frey, N.; Pleger, S.; Mereles, D. Prognostic relevance of global work index and global constructive work in patients with non-ischemic dilated cardiomyopathy. *Int. J. Cardiovasc. Imaging* **2024**, *40*, 1575–1584. [CrossRef] [PubMed]
31. Dorbala, S.; Ando, Y.; Bokhari, S.; Dispenzieri, A.; Falk, R.H.; Ferrari, V.A.; Fontana, M.; Gheysens, O.; Gillmore, J.D.; Glaudemans, A.W.J.M.; et al. ASNC/AHA/ASE/EANM/HFSA/ISA/SCMR/SNMMI Expert Consensus Recommendations for Multimodality Imaging in Cardiac Amyloidosis: Part 2 of 2-Diagnostic Criteria and Appropriate Utilization. *J. Card. Fail.* **2019**, *25*, 854–865. [CrossRef]
32. Garcia-Pavia, P.; Rapezzi, C.; Adler, Y.; Arad, M.; Basso, C.; Brucato, A.; Burazor, I.; Caforio, A.L.P.; Damy, T.; Eriksson, U.; et al. Diagnosis and treatment of cardiac amyloidosis: A position statement of the ESC Working Group on Myocardial and Pericardial Diseases. *Eur. Heart J.* **2021**, *42*, 1554–1568. [CrossRef]
33. Behar, J.M.; Claridge, S.; Jackson, T.; Sieniewicz, B.; Porter, B.; Webb, J.; Rajani, R.; Kapetanakis, S.; Carr-White, G.; Rinaldi, C.A. The role of multi modality imaging in selecting patients and guiding lead placement for the delivery of cardiac resynchronization therapy. *Expert Rev. Cardiovasc. Ther.* **2017**, *15*, 93–107. [CrossRef]
34. Antoniou, N.; Kalaitzoglou, M.; Tsigkriki, L.; Baroutidou, A.; Tsaousidis, A.; Koulaouzidis, G.; Giannakoulas, G.; Charisopoulou, D. Speckle Tracking Echocardiography in Patients with Non-Ischemic Dilated Cardiomyopathy Who Undergo Cardiac Resynchronization Therapy: A Narrative Review. *Diagnostics* **2024**, *14*, 1178. [CrossRef] [PubMed]
35. Glikson, M.; Nielsen, J.C.; Kronborg, M.B.; Michowitz, Y.; Auricchio, A.; Barbash, I.M.; Barrabés, J.A.; Boriani, G.; Braunschweig, F.; Brignole, M.; et al. 2021 ESC Guidelines on cardiac pacing and cardiac resynchronization therapy: Developed by the Task Force on cardiac pacing and cardiac resynchronization therapy of the European Society of Cardiology (ESC) with the special contribution of the European Hear. *Eur. Heart J.* **2021**, *42*, 3427–3520. [CrossRef]
36. Smiseth, O.A.; Torp, H.; Opdahl, A.; Haugaa, K.H.; Urheim, S. Myocardial strain imaging: How useful is it in clinical decision making? *Eur. Heart J.* **2016**, *37*, 1196–1207. [CrossRef]
37. Khan, F.Z.; Virdee, M.S.; Palmer, C.R.; Pugh, P.J.; O'Halloran, D.; Elsik, M.; Read, P.A.; Begley, D.; Fynn, S.P.; Dutka, D.P. Targeted left ventricular lead placement to guide cardiac resynchronization therapy: The TARGET study: A randomized, controlled trial. *J. Am. Coll. Cardiol.* **2012**, *59*, 1509–1518. [CrossRef]
38. Alahdab, F.; Ahmed, A.I.; Nayfeh, M.; Han, Y.; Abdelkarim, O.; Alfawara, M.S.; Little, S.H.; Reardon, M.J.; Faza, N.N.; Goel, S.S.; et al. Myocardial Blood Flow Reserve, Microvascular Coronary Health, and Myocardial Remodeling in Patients with Aortic Stenosis. *J. Am. Heart Assoc.* **2024**, *13*, e033447. [CrossRef]
39. Le, T.-T.; Huang, W.; Singh, G.K.; Toh, D.F.; Ewe, S.H.; Tang, H.C.; Loo, G.; Bryant, J.A.; Ang, B.; Tay, E.L.; et al. Echocardiographic Global Longitudinal Strain Is Associated with Myocardial Fibrosis and Predicts Outcomes in Aortic Stenosis. *Front. Cardiovasc. Med.* **2021**, *8*, 750016. [CrossRef]
40. Daios, S.; Anastasiou, V.; Bazmpani, M.-A.; Angelopoulou, S.M.; Karamitsos, T.; Zegkos, T.; Didagelos, M.; Savopoulos, C.; Ziakas, A.; Kamperidis, V. Moving from left ventricular ejection fraction to deformation imaging in mitral valve regurgitation. *Curr. Probl. Cardiol.* **2024**, *49*, 102432. [CrossRef] [PubMed]
41. Sonaglioni, A.; Fagiani, V.; Nicolosi, G.L.; Lombardo, M. Echocardiographic assessment of left ventricular mechanics in individuals with mitral valve prolapse: A systematic review and meta-analysis. *Int. J. Cardiovasc. Imaging* **2024**, *40*, 1617–1629. [CrossRef]
42. Egbe, A.C.; Miranda, W.R.; Anderson, J.H.; Pellikka, P.A.; Connolly, H.M. Prognostic Value of Left Ventricular Global Longitudinal Strain in Patients With Congenital Heart Disease. *Circ. Cardiovasc. Imaging* **2022**, *15*, e014865. [CrossRef]
43. Dorobantu, D.M.; Amir, N.H.; Wadey, C.A.; Sharma, C.; Stuart, A.G.; Williams, C.A.; Pieles, G.E. The Role of Speckle-Tracking Echocardiography in Predicting Mortality and Morbidity in Patients with Congenital Heart Disease: A Systematic Review and Meta-analysis. *J. Am. Soc. Echocardiogr.* **2024**, *37*, 216–225. [CrossRef] [PubMed]
44. Di Salvo, G.; Pergola, V.; Fadel, B.; Bulbul, Z.A.; Caso, P. Strain Echocardiography and Myocardial Mechanics: From Basics to Clinical Applications. *J. Cardiovasc. Echogr.* **2015**, *25*, 1–8. [CrossRef] [PubMed] [PubMed Central]
45. Borrelli, N.; Di Salvo, G.; Sabatino, J.; Ibrahim, A.; Avesani, M.; Sirico, D.; Josen, M.; Penco, M.; Fraisse, A.; Michielon, G. Serial changes in longitudinal strain are associated with outcome in children with hypoplastic left heart syndrome. *Int. J. Cardiol.* **2020**, *317*, 56–62. [CrossRef] [PubMed]
46. Festa, P.; Lovato, L.; Bianco, F.; Alaimo, A.; Angeli, E.; Baccano, G.; Barbi, E.; Bennati, E.; Bonhoeffer, P.; Bucciarelli, V.; et al. Recommendations for cardiovascular magnetic resonance and computed tomography in congenital heart disease: A consensus paper from the CMR/CCT Working Group of the Italian Society of Pediatric Cardiology and the Italian College of Cardiac Radiology endorsed by the Italian Society of Medical and Interventional Radiology (Part II). *J. Cardiovasc. Med.* **2024**, *25*, 473–487. [CrossRef] [PubMed]
47. Di Salvo, G.; Pacileo, G.; Limongelli, G.; Verrengia, M.; Rea, A.; Santoro, G.; Gala, S.; Castaldi, B.; D'Andrea, A.; Caso, P.; et al. Abnormal regional myocardial deformation properties and increased aortic stiffness in normotensive patients with aortic coarctation despite successful correction: An ABPM, standard echocardiography and strain rate imaging study. *Clin. Sci.* **2007**, *113*, 259–266. [CrossRef] [PubMed]
48. Egbe, A.C.; Miranda, W.R.; Ahmed, M.; Burchill, L.J.; Jain, C.C.; Karnakoti, S.; Kandlakunta, S.; Connolly, H.M. Diagnostic and Prognostic Role of Left Ventricular Strain Imaging in Adults with Coarctation of aorta. *Am. J. Cardiol.* **2024**, *211*, 98–105. [CrossRef] [PubMed]

49. Kheradvar, A.; Houle, H.; Pedrizzetti, G.; Tonti, G.; Belcik, T.; Ashraf, M.; Lindner, J.R.; Gharib, M.; Sahn, D. Echocardiographic particle image velocimetry: A novel technique for quantification of left ventricular blood vorticity pattern. *J. Am. Soc. Echocardiogr. Off. Publ. Am. Soc. Echocardiogr.* **2010**, *23*, 86–94. [CrossRef]
50. Mele, D.; Smarrazzo, V.; Pedrizzetti, G.; Capasso, F.; Pepe, M.; Severino, S.; Luisi, G.A.; Maglione, M.; Ferrari, R. Intracardiac Flow Analysis: Techniques and Potential Clinical Applications. *J. Am. Soc. Echocardiogr. Off. Publ. Am. Soc. Echocardiogr.* **2019**, *32*, 319–332. [CrossRef]
51. Kim, W.Y.; Walker, P.G.; Pedersen, E.M.; Poulsen, J.K.; Oyre, S.; Houlind, K.; Yoganathan, A.P. Left ventricular blood flow patterns in normal subjects: A quantitative analysis by three-dimensional magnetic resonance velocity mapping. *J. Am. Coll. Cardiol.* **1995**, *26*, 224–238. [CrossRef]
52. Stugaard, M.; Koriyama, H.; Katsuki, K.; Masuda, K.; Asanuma, T.; Takeda, Y.; Sakata, Y.; Itatani, K.; Nakatani, S. Energy loss in the left ventricle obtained by vector flow mapping as a new quantitative measure of severity of aortic regurgitation: A combined experimental and clinical study. *Eur. Heart J.—Cardiovasc. Imaging* **2015**, *16*, 723–730. [CrossRef]
53. Uejima, T.; Koike, A.; Sawada, H.; Aizawa, T.; Ohtsuki, S.; Tanaka, M.; Furukawa, T.; Fraser, A.G. A new echocardiographic method for identifying vortex flow in the left ventricle: Numerical validation. *Ultrasound Med. Biol.* **2010**, *36*, 772–788. [CrossRef]
54. Fiorencis, A.; Pepe, M.; Smarrazzo, V.; Martini, M.; Severino, S.; Pergola, V.; Evangelista, M.; Incarnato, P.; Previtero, M.; Maglione, M.; et al. Noninvasive Evaluation of Intraventricular Flow Dynamics by the HyperDoppler Technique: First Application to Normal Subjects, Athletes, and Patients with Heart Failure. *J. Clin. Med.* **2022**, *11*, 2216. [CrossRef] [PubMed]
55. Kilner, P.J.; Yang, G.Z.; Wilkes, A.J.; Mohiaddin, R.H.; Firmin, D.N.; Yacoub, M.H. Asymmetric redirection of flow through the heart. *Nature* **2000**, *404*, 759–761. [CrossRef] [PubMed]
56. Rodríguez Muñoz, D.; Moya Mur, J.L.; Fernández-Golfín, C.; Becker Filho, D.C.; González Gómez, A.; Fernández Santos, S.; Lázaro Rivera, C.; Rincón Díaz, L.M.; Casas Rojo, E.; Zamorano Gómez, J.L. Left ventricular vortices as observed by vector flow mapping: Main determinants and their relation to left ventricular filling. *Echocardiography* **2015**, *32*, 96–105. [CrossRef]
57. Poh, K.K.; Lee, L.C.; Shen, L.; Chong, E.; Tan, Y.L.; Chai, P.; Yeo, T.C.; Wood, M.J. Left ventricular fluid dynamics in heart failure: Echocardiographic measurement and utilities of vortex formation time. *Eur. Heart J. Cardiovasc. Imaging* **2012**, *13*, 385–393. [CrossRef]
58. Gharib, M.; Rambod, E.; Kheradvar, A.; Sahn, D.J.; Dabiri, J.O. Optimal vortex formation as an index of cardiac health. *Proc. Natl. Acad. Sci. USA* **2006**, *103*, 6305–6308. [CrossRef]
59. Pugliese, N.R.; Colli, A.; Falcetta, G.; Del Punta, L.; Puccinelli, C.; Fiocco, A.; Petronio, A.S.; Taddei, S.; Masi, S.; Besola, L. Flow dynamic assessment of native mitral valve, mitral valve repair and mitral valve replacement using vector flow mapping intracardiac flow dynamic in mitral valve regurgitation. *Front. Cardiovasc. Med.* **2023**, *10*, 1047244. [CrossRef]
60. Kheradvar, A.; Rickers, C.; Morisawa, D.; Kim, M.; Hong, G.-R.; Pedrizzetti, G. Diagnostic and prognostic significance of cardiovascular vortex formation. *J. Cardiol.* **2019**, *74*, 403–411. [CrossRef]
61. Pagel, P.S.; Hudetz, J.A. Chronic pressure-overload hypertrophy attenuates vortex formation time in patients with severe aortic stenosis and preserved left ventricular systolic function undergoing aortic valve replacement. *J. Cardiothorac. Vasc. Anesth.* **2013**, *27*, 660–664. [CrossRef] [PubMed]
62. Pagel, P.S.; Boettcher, B.T.; De Vry, D.J.; Freed, J.K.; Iqbal, Z. Moderate Aortic Valvular Insufficiency Invalidates Vortex Formation Time as an Index of Left Ventricular Filling Efficiency in Patients with Severe Degenerative Calcific Aortic Stenosis Undergoing Aortic Valve Replacement. *J. Cardiothorac. Vasc. Anesth.* **2016**, *30*, 1260–1265. [CrossRef]
63. Borrelli, N.; Avesani, M.; Sabatino, J.; Ibrahim, A.; Josen, M.; Paredes, J.; Di Salvo, G. Blood speckle imaging: A new echocardiographic approach to study fluid dynamics in congenital heart disease. *Int. J. Cardiol. Congenit. Heart Dis.* **2021**, *2*, 100079. [CrossRef]
64. Goliasch, G.; Goscinska-Bis, K.; Caracciolo, G.; Nakabo, A.; Smolka, G.; Pedrizzetti, G.; Narula, J.; Sengupta, P.P. CRT improves LV filling dynamics: Insights from echocardiographic particle imaging velocimetry. *JACC Cardiovasc. Imaging* **2013**, *6*, 704–713. [CrossRef]
65. Mangual, J.O.; Kraigher-Krainer, E.; De Luca, A.; Toncelli, L.; Shah, A.; Solomon, S.; Galanti, G.; Domenichini, F. Comparative numerical study on left ventricular fluid dynamics after dilated cardiomyopathy. *J. Biomech.* **2013**, *46*, 1611–1617. [CrossRef]
66. Ouyang, D.; He, B.; Ghorbani, A.; Yuan, N.; Ebinger, J.; Langlotz, C.P.; Heidenreich, P.A.; Harrington, R.A.; Liang, D.H.; Ashley, E.A.; et al. Video-based AI for beat-to-beat assessment of cardiac function. *Nature* **2020**, *580*, 252–256. [CrossRef]
67. Marchese, P.; Cantinotti, M.; Van den Eynde, J.; Assanta, N.; Franchi, E.; Pak, V.; Santoro, G.; Koestenberger, M.; Kutty, S. Left ventricular vortex analysis by high-frame rate blood speckle tracking echocardiography in healthy children and in congenital heart disease. *Int. J. Cardiol. Heart Vasc.* **2021**, *37*, 100897. [CrossRef]

Journal of
Clinical Medicine

MDPI

Article

The Sub-Pulmonary Left Ventricle in Patients with Systemic Right Ventricle, the Paradoxical Neglected Chamber: A Cardiac Magnetic Resonance Feature Tracking Study

Sofia Piana [1,†], Alice Pozza [1,†], Annachiara Cavaliere [2], Anna Molinaroli [1], Irene Cattapan [1], Jennifer Fumanelli [1], Martina Avesani [1], Elena Reffo [1] and Giovanni Di Salvo [1,*]

[1] Paediatric Cardiology Unit, Department of Women and Children's Health, University Hospital of Padua, 35128 Padua, Italy; sofia.piana@studenti.unipd.it (S.P.); alice.pozza@aopd.veneto.it (A.P.); anna.molinaroli@studenti.unipd.it (A.M.); irene.cattapan@aopd.veneto.it (I.C.); jennifer.fumanelli@aopd.veneto.it (J.F.); martina.avesani@aopd.veneto.it (M.A.); elena.reffo@aopd.veneto.it (E.R.)

[2] Pediatric Radiology, Neuroradiology Unit, University Hospital of Padua, 35128 Padua, Italy; annachiara.cavaliere@aopd.veneto.it

* Correspondence: giovanni.disalvo@unipd.it; Tel.: +39-049-821-3550

† These authors contributed equally to this work.

Abstract: Background/Objective: The impact of subpulmonary left ventricle (LV) dysfunction in patients with a systemic right ventricle (SRV) is insufficiently characterized, with only a few studies suggesting its prognostic significance. Additionally, its evaluation through imaging techniques is a challenge. To assess the correlation between quantitative cardiac magnetic resonance-feature tracking (CMR-FT) data and the risk of clinical events related to the natural history of SRV failure. **Methods**: In this cross-sectional study, 21 patients with a diagnosis of transposition of the great arteries (TGA) and atrial switch operation (AtSO) or congenitally corrected transposition (ccTGA) were recruited. All participants underwent CMR-FT analysis. Considered clinical events included NYHA class deterioration (from I-II to III-IV), increased diuretic therapy, arrhythmias, sudden cardiac death, and hospitalizations. **Results**: The cohort consisted of 52.4% males (mean age: 25.4 ± 11.9 years). Eleven patients were diagnosed with ccTGA. Of the 10 patients with TGA post-AtSO, 50% had undergone Mustard repair. Clinical events occurred in 11 patients, with 47.6% experiencing hospitalizations and 28.6% developing arrhythmias. Left ventricular global longitudinal strain (LV GLS) was significantly associated with event-risk in both univariate and multivariate analyses ($p = 0.011$; $p = 0.025$). A cut-off value of LV GLS > −19.24 was proposed to stratify high-risk patients ($p = 0.001$). **Conclusions**: Our study confirms the role of subpulmonary LV function in determining outcomes of SRV patients. The assessment of LV GLS by using CMR-FT could significantly enhance clinical management during follow-up.

Keywords: subpulmonary left ventricle; systemic right ventricle; global longitudinal strain; cardiac magnetic resonance; feature tracking

1. Introduction

Patients with a systemic right ventricle (SRV) and biventricular physiology, like those with congenitally corrected transposition of great arteries (ccTGA) or transposition of the great arteries (TGA) following an atrial switch operation (AtSO), such as a Mustard or Senning operation, represent ≈10% of all congenital heart diseases (CHDs), and their prognosis remains inadequately understood [1–3].

While the role of SRV function in the outcome and exercise capacity is well established, the impact of subpulmonary left ventricular (LV) dysfunction is less clear, with only a few studies suggesting a possible role in the outcome of these patients [4,5]. In addition, because of geometrical distortion, reduced afterload and ventricular interactions, the method of evaluating subpulmonic LV function in patients with SRV is not fully established.

Cardiac magnetic resonance (CMR) is considered the gold standard for volume quantification and ejection fraction (EF) for both left and right ventricles in CHDs [6].

Feature tracking (FT) techniques allow for the measuring of myocardial strain in CMR images. Myocardial strain is a geometry independent index that is not affected by tethering from adjacent segments or ventricular interaction and less affected by loading conditions compared with EF [7,8].

The primary objective of this study was to calculate CMR-FT derived strain of both the systemic right ventricle and sub-pulmonary left ventricle in patients with SRV and biventricular physiology. The secondary objective was to assess the correlation between these data and the risk of clinical events related to the natural history of SRV failure.

2. Materials and Methods

2.1. Study Population

This cross-sectional study was conducted on 21 patients with SRV and biventricular physiology, who were regularly followed at the Pediatric Cardiology Unit of the University Hospital of Padua (Department of Women's and Children's Health). They were invited to participate in the study and provided their informed consent. Data collection occurred consecutively between November 2022 and May 2024.

Patients were considered eligible for this study in the presence of SRV and biventricular physiology (TGA post-atrial switch operation and ccTGA). Only patients who underwent a CMR study with feature tracking analysis were included in the study.

Patients with pacemakers (PM), implantable cardioverter defibrillators (ICD), or any other devices incompatible with CMR were excluded from the study. Patients suffering from claustrophobia were excluded. Patients who had never undergone CMR due to compliance issues were also excluded from the study.

Patients' records were reviewed from the medical platform of Padua University Hospital. Clinical data extracted from medical records included height, weight, body surface area (BSA) according to the Mosteller formula, body mass index (BMI), New York Heart Association (NYHA) class, history of previous clinical events (as will be defined in Section 2.2), and pharmacological treatment, including β-blockers, ACE inhibitors, sartans, diuretics, sacubitril/valsartan, gliflozins, antiarrhythmics, anticoagulants, and antiplatelets.

All data were collected while maintaining confidentiality and were anonymized for statistical analysis. All the information collected was part of routine care. The study was submitted to the attention of the HIT Research Centre Ethical Committee of the University of Padua (Protocol No. 2024_247, 2 May 2024).

2.2. Clinical Events

Considered clinical events related to SRV failure were defined as follows: (a) hospitalizations; (b) arrhythmic events (detected either as clinical events requiring hospitalization or during routine Holter ECG monitoring); (c) worsening of NYHA class to III-IV; (d) implementation of diuretic therapy [9–11]; (e) sudden cardiac death.

2.3. CMR Imaging

Each examination was conducted by a pediatric cardiologist specialized in CMR imaging (ER) and a pediatric radiologist (AC); the investigation was carried out at the Pediatric Neuroradiology Unit of the University Hospital of Padua.

The images were acquired using the same MRI machine (Achieva 1.5T, Philips Healthcare Medical System; Best, The Netherlands).

The standard CMR protocol for evaluating patients with SRV and biventricular physiology includes the following sequences: real-time localization imaging in three axes, non-ECG-gated and free-breathing; cine steady-state free precession (SSFP) sequences, ECG- and respiratory-gated; phase contrast; whole-heart isotropic 3D SSFP imaging; magnetic resonance angiography sequences. Moreover, all patients were administered gadolinium at a dose of 0.2 mmol/kg to detect ventricular wall fibrosis using LGE in both 4-chamber long-axis (4C BTFE) and short-axis views (SA BTFE) [12,13].

The analysis of volumes and biventricular ejection fraction was performed using Philips Intellispace Cardiovascular software (Version 7.0). The endocardial and epicardial borders of the SRV and the sub-pulmonary left ventricle (LV) were manually traced in the cineSSFP short-axis sequences, in both the end-diastole and end-systole. Trabeculations and papillary muscles were excluded from the calculation (Figure 1). Measurements were conducted by the same operator (ER) to ensure data consistency.

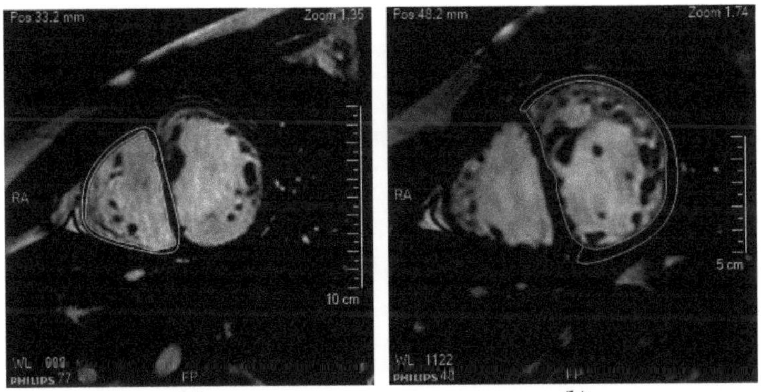

(a) (b)

Figure 1. Quantification of the volumes of the sub-pulmonary left ventricle (**a**) and systemic right ventricle (**b**). Calculation of end-diastolic volumes (EDV) and myocardial mass in short axis view (SA BTFE). Trabeculae and papillary muscles were excluded from the calculation. Green line: endocardial border LV; Yellow line: epicardial border LV; Orange line: endocardial border sRV; Blue line: epicardial border sRV.

The following parameters were calculated for both SRV and LV: end-diastolic volume (EDV), end-diastolic volume indexed to BSA (EDVi), end-systolic volume (ESV), end-systolic volume indexed to BSA (ESVi), ejection fraction (EF), stroke volume (calculated as the difference between end-diastolic and end-systolic volume), stroke index (calculated as the difference between indexed end-diastolic and end-systolic volumes), cardiac index ((stroke volume × heart rate/BSA)/1000), and the ratio between SRV and LV EDV.

Additionally, the presence of systemic tricuspid regurgitation (TR) was evaluated in cineSSFP short-axis sequences. The severity of TR was quantified based on the percentage of regurgitant fraction (RF): mild TR for RF $< 20\%$; moderate TR for RF 20–40%; severe TR for RF $> 40\%$.

For both ventricles, myocardial strain was assessed using feature tracking (FT) applied to SSFP cine images during post-processing with dedicated software (Qstrain, Medis Suite Version 4.0.38.4, Leiden, The Netherlands). All calculations were performed by the same operator (SP) to enhance data consistency.

Global longitudinal strains were assessed in 4C BTFE, while global circumferential and radial strains were assessed in SA BTFE.

Images where the walls of both ventricles were clearly delineated were selected to ensure accurate myocardial strain calculation.

The endocardial and epicardial borders were manually traced in end-diastole and then applied to all cardiac cycle phases using an automatic detection algorithm. The accuracy of the borders was checked in all cardiac phases and manually adjusted if necessary. Trabeculations and papillary muscles were excluded.

2.4. Statistical Analysis

Normally distributed continuous variables are reported as mean ± standard deviation, while non-normally distributed variables are expressed as the median and interquartile range (IQR). The Shapiro–Wilk test was used to assess the normality of continuous variables. Categorical variables were expressed as percentages.

Initially, a linear regression model was employed. Subsequently, a univariate analysis was conducted. Student's t-test for independent samples was used if normality and homogeneity of variances (tested with Levene's test) were confirmed, Welch's test when normality was confirmed but homogeneity of variances was not, and the Mann–Whitney U test when normality was not confirmed. Fisher's exact test was employed to analyze categorical variables.

Significant variables from the univariate analysis were subjected to a multivariate analysis using the MANCOVA test.

The level of statistical significance for all tests was set at $p \leq 0.050$.

Data were analyzed using the statistical software Jamovi Version 2.5.5 (2024).

Significant parameters from both the univariate and multivariate MANCOVA tests were used for binary logistic regression. Then, ROC curves were generated to determine the optimal cut-off values. The cut-off point was calculated according to the Youden index to optimize sensitivity (Se) and specificity (Sp); subsequently, the AUC (Area Under the Curve) value and the corresponding real cut-off values were calculated using automated software. This part of the analysis was performed using MedCalc software (MedCalc Software Ltd., version 22.023, Ostend, Belgium).

3. Results

3.1. Population

According to our selection criteria, we identified 31 patients with SRV and biventricular physiology. Of these, 10 were excluded: five patients because they did not undergo CMR; four patients had complete atrioventricular block and were fitted with non-CMR-compatible pacemakers; one patient was lost to follow-up.

Consequently, the study population comprised 21 patients.

Feature tracking (CMR-FT) was technically feasible in all 21 patients for both the systemic right ventricle and the subpulmonary left ventricle.

3.2. Clinical Data

In our cohort, 11 patients were male (52.4%) and 10 female (47.6%).

Ten patients were diagnosed with TGA at birth and underwent AtSO (47.6%, 5 Mustard and 5 Senning), while 11 were affected by ccTGA (52.4%). The median age at which the AtSO was performed was 5.5 months (IQR 4.3–11.3).

At the last visit, the mean age was 25.4 ± 11.9 years. The median age of patients with ccTGA was lower compared to those who underwent the AtSO (19 years (IQR 16.0–30.0) vs. 30 years (IQR 22.5–35.8)). Furthermore, a significant percentage of the patients in the study (n = 15, 71.4%) were aged between their second and third–fourth decades of life at the last visit.

Nine patients were found to be overweight (42.9%), defined as having a BMI between 25 and 30 kg/m^2, while one patient suffered from mild to moderate obesity (4.8%).

Anamnestic and clinical features of the patients are summarized in Table 1.

Thirteen patients (61.9%) were on pharmacological therapy at the last visit. The most frequently used medications were beta-blockers (n = 5, 23.8%), ACE inhibitors (n = 6, 28.6%) and angiotensin II receptor blockers (n = 4, 19.0%). In our cohort, two patients were on diuretic therapy (9.5%). Two patients (9.5%) included in the study were treated with sacubitril/valsartan. Two patients (9.5%) were on antiarrhythmic therapy, both with cordarone, for complex ventricular arrhythmias. Two patients (9.5%) were on anticoagulant therapy and two patients (9.5%) were on antiplatelet therapy.

Table 1. Anamnestic and clinical features of the population.

Anamnestic and Clinical Data	Sample Size (n = 21)
Age at last visit (years)	25.4 ± 11.9
Gender, n (%)	
Male	11 (52.4%)
Female	10 (47.6%)
Primary cardiac diagnosis	
ccTGA, n (%)	11 (52.4%)
TGA, n (%)	10 (47.6%)
s/p Mustard	5 (23.8%)
s/p Senning	5 (23.8%)
Age at operation (months)	5.5 (IQR 4.3–11.3)
Associated cardiac abnormalities	
ASD at birth, n (%)	2 (9.5%)
VSD at birth, n (%)	9 (42.9%)
Pulmonary stenosis at birth, n (%)	7 (33.3%)
Pulmonary atresia at birth, n (%)	3 (14.3%)
DORV, n (%)	1 (4.8%)
Ebstein's anomaly, n (%)	2 (9.5%)
Straddling tricuspid valve, n (%)	1 (4.8%)
Cardiac situs, n (%)	
Levocardia	17 (81.0%)
Dextrocardia	4 (19.0%)
Anthropometric measurements	
Height (m)	1.7 (IQR 0.9–1.8)
Weight (kg)	66.6 ± 21.7
BSA (m^2)	1.8 (IQR 0.6–2.3)
BMI (kg/m^2)	24.4 ± 0.4

Pharmacological treatments at the last visit are summarized in Table 2.

Table 2. Pharmacological therapies administered at the last visit.

Pharmacological Therapies	Sample Size (n = 21)
Ongoing therapy, n (%)	13 (61.9%)
Beta-blockers	5 (23.8%)
ACE-inhibitors	6 (28.6%)
Sartans	4 (19.0%)
Diuretics	2 (9.5%)
Sacubitril/valsartan	2 (9.5%)
SGLT2 inhibitors	0 (0%)
Antiarrhythmics	2 (9.5%)
Anticoagulants	2 (9.5%)
Antiplatelets	2 (9.5%)

3.3. Clinical Events

Eleven out of twenty-one patients (52.4%) had clinical events, and seven patients experienced multiple events.

Hospitalizations (n = 10, 47.6%) and arrhythmic episodes (n = 6, 28.6%) comprised most of the clinical events.

The reasons for hospitalization included arrhythmic episodes (n = 7), post-AtSO complications (n = 2), and heart failure (n = 1). Among the patients with post-AtSO complications, one experienced an occlusion of the pulmonary venous baffle, while the other had a minor baffle leak in association with pulmonary arterial hypertension with a mixed pre- and post-capillary component.

The main arrhythmic events recorded included atrial flutter (n = 3) and ventricular arrhythmias (n = 3). Additionally, one patient had an episode of paroxysmal supraventricular tachycardia, one patient had atrial fibrillation, and one patient had a complete atrioventricular block.

No patients were classified in NYHA class III or IV. Ten patients were classified as NYHA I (47.6%) and eleven patients as NYHA II (52.4%).

One patient had an episode of sudden cardiac arrest, after which an ICD was implanted.

Three patients adjusted their heart failure therapy by either increasing the dose of diuretics (n = 1) or adding HF medications (n = 2).

The clinical events are summarized in Table 3.

Table 3. Clinical events related to SRV failure in our cohort.

Clinical Events	Sample Size (n = 21)
Events, n (%)	11 (52.4%)
Hospitalizations	10 (47.6%)
Arrhythmias	6 (28.6%)
Sudden cardiac death	1 (4.8%)
Implementation of anti-failure therapy	3 (14.3%)
NYHA III-IV	0 (0%)

3.4. CMR Imaging Data

All patients (n = 21) underwent CMR imaging between May 2019 and November 2023. The mean age of the participants at the time of the examination was 25.1 years ± 11.7. Quantitative CMR imaging data are summarized in Table 4.

Table 4. Quantitative CMR imaging data: mean values and univariate analysis. The first column reports the mean values of the following parameters in the study population. The second and third columns display the mean values for the subpopulations with and without events, respectively. The fourth column presents the p-value associated with the univariate analysis.

	All (n = 21)	Patients with Previous Events (n = 11)	Patients without Previous Events (n = 10)	p-Value * ($p \leq 0.050$)
SRV EDV (mL)	183.0 ± 59.1	192.0 ± 58.5	173.8 ± 61.5	0.496
SRV EDVi (mL/m^2)	105.0 ± 20.3	110.7 ± 20.1	98.4 ± 19.4	0.169
SRV ESV (mL)	93.2 ± 37.8	102.9 ± 38.9	82.4 ± 35.4	0.223
SRV ESVi (mL/m^2)	52.7 ± 14.9	58.7 ± 15.5	46.1 ± 11.7	**0.050**
SRV EF (%)	50.2 ± 7.61	47.4 ± 7.4	53.4 ± 6.9	0.068
SRV stroke index (mL/m^2)	52.1 ± 11.0	52.0 ± 9.4	52.3 ± 13.0	0.952
SRV stroke volume (mL)	90.2 ± 27.1	89.0 ± 24.1	91.4 ± 31.5	0.847
SRV cardiac index (L/min/m^2)	3.7 ± 0.9	3.0 ± 0.6	4.0 ± 1.0	0.077
LV EDV (mL)	122.0 ± 46.5	119.4 ± 47.6	124.4 ± 47.7	0.812
LV EDVi (mL/m^2)	69.3 ± 20.9	68.3 ± 25.0	70.4 ± 16.4	0.822
LV ESV (mL)	47.1 ± 24.7	44.0 ± 26.3	50.5 ± 23.6	0.559
LV ESVi (mL/m^2)	26.5 ± 12.3	26.8 ± 14.3	29.6 ± 8.7	0.587
LV EF (%)	62.9 ± 7.9	65.0 ± 7.4	60.6 ± 8.1	0.210
LV stroke index (mL/m^2)	42.8 ± 10.7	45.7 ± 8.5	43.3 ± 10.6	0.853
LV stroke volume (mL)	74.7 ± 25.3	75.4 ± 23.6	73.9 ± 28.4	0.896
LV cardiac index (L/min/m^2)	3.0 ± 0.9	2.8 ± 0.8	3.3 ± 1.0	0.207
SRV EDV/LV EDV	1.5 (IQR 0.8–3.4)	1.6 (IQR 1.5–1.9)	1.4 (IQR 1.2–1.6)	0.173

* Bold p-value indicates statistically significant.

Patients with previous clinical events had larger SRV EDV and ESV and lower EF compared to patients without events (SRV EDV 192.0 mL ± 58.5 vs. 173.8 mL ± 61.5,

p = 0.496; SRV ESV 102.9 mL ± 38.9 vs. 82.4 mL ± 35.4, p = 0.223; SRV EF 47.4% ± 7.4 vs. 53.4% ± 6.9, p = 0.068). This finding aligns with the natural history of the SRV.

The only significant parameter in the univariate analysis was SRV ESVi (p = 0.050). It can be observed that patients who experienced clinical events appear to have a higher SRV ESVi compared to patients without events (58.7 mL/m^2 ± 15.5 vs. 46.1 mL/m^2 ± 11.7).

LV EDV and LV ESV values were reduced in patients who had experienced previous clinical events compared to those who had not (LV EDV 119.4 mL ± 47.6 vs. 124.4 ± 47.7, p = 0.812; LV ESV 44.0 mL ± 26.3 vs. 50.5 ± 23.6, p = 0.559).

Moreover, patients with events had a higher LV EF compared to the group without events (LV EF 65% ± 7.4 vs. 60.6% ± 8.1, p = 0.210).

Comparisons of stroke volume, stroke index, and cardiac index for both the systemic right ventricle and the left ventricle among the groups did not yield statistically significant results. Similarly, there were no significant differences in the SRV EDV/LV EDV ratio.

The study did not reveal any correlation between the presence of fibrosis in the systemic right ventricle (p = 0.696) and/or left ventricle (p = 0.835) and the risk of major events. However, a higher presence of LV fibrosis was observed in both patient groups.

Additionally, no significant correlation between moderate and severe tricuspid regurgitation (RF > 20%) and the risk of major events was demonstrated (p = 1.000).

Qualitative CMR imaging data are summarized in Table 5.

Table 5. Qualitative CMR imaging data: absolute frequencies and univariate analysis. The first column reports the absolute frequency and the relative percentage of the following qualitative data in the study population. The second and third columns display the absolute frequencies and relative percentages in the subpopulations with and without events, respectively. The fourth column presents the p-value associated with the univariate analysis.

	All (n = 21)	Patients with Previous Events (n = 11)	Patients without Previous Events (n = 10)	p-Value ($p \leq 0.050$)
SRV fibrosis, n (%)	5 (23.8%)	3 (27.3%)	2 (10.0%)	0.696
LV fibrosis, n (%)	10 (47.6%)	5 (45.5%)	5 (50.0%)	0.835
TR, n (%) Mild Moderate Severe	13 (61.9%) 7 (33.3%) 4 (19.0%) 2 (9.5%)	8 (72.7%) 5 (45.5%) 3 (27.3%) 0 (0%)	5 (50.0%) 2 (20.0%) 1 (10.0%) 2 (20.0%)	0.284
Moderate-severe TR, n (%)	6 (28.6%)	3 (27.3%)	3 (27.3%)	1.000

3.5. Feature Tracking Data

Results of the analysis are reported in Table 6.

Table 6. Feature tracking data. Mean values in the study population and in the subpopulations with and without events, respectively. Univariate analysis and p-values.

	All (n = 21)	Patients with Previous Events (n = 11)	Patients without Previous Events (n = 10)	p-Value * ($p \leq 0.050$)
SRV GLS (%)	−20.2 ± 5.3	−18.6 ± 5.6	−22.0 ± 4.5	0.145
SRV GCS (%)	−22.0 ± 4.3	−21.6 ± 5.3	−22.4 ± 3.1	0.655
SRV GRS (%)	80.2 (IQR 60.1–134.0)	69.0 (IQR 58.7–116.0)	109.1 (IQR 69.2–138.4)	0.605
LV GLS (%)	−21.1 ± 6.8	−17.7 ± 6.3	−24.9 ± 5.3	**0.011**
LV GCS (%)	−24.8 ± 5.4	−26.5 ± 6.2	−23.1 ± 3.9	0.156
LV GRS (%)	60.1 ± 27.6	51.2 ± 20.3	69.9 ± 32.1	0.137

* Bold p-value indicates statistically significant.

Data analysis indicates that the only parameter significantly associated with the risk of events in the univariate analysis is left ventricle global longitudinal strain (LV GLS).

In the studied population (n = 21), the mean LV GLS value was −21.1 ± 6.8, and patients who experienced clinical events related to SRV failure had a less negative LV GLS value compared to those without events (−17.7 ± 6.3 vs. −24.9 ± 5.3, p = 0.011).

In Figure 2a,b, two distinct LV GLS measurements and their associated strain curves are presented.

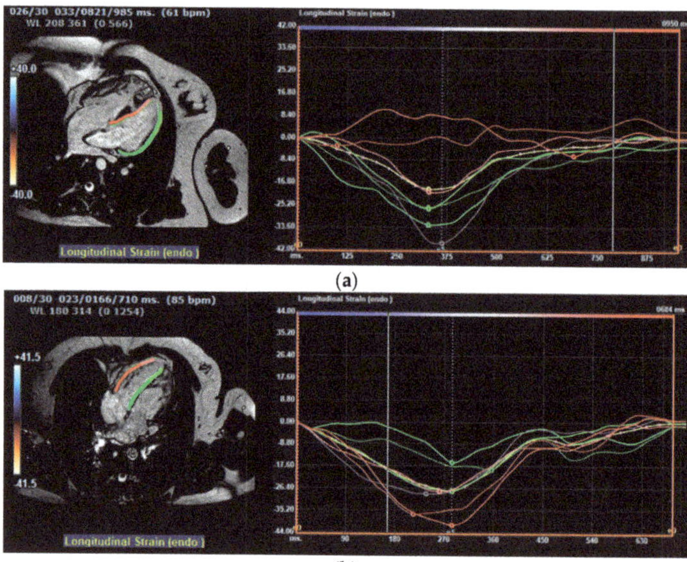

Figure 2. (**a**) LV GLS measurement obtained from a 4C BTFE view is presented for a patient who has undergone AtSO, along with the corresponding strain curve. This patient experienced clinical events: atrial flutter and subsequent hospitalization. (**b**) LV GLS measurement obtained from a 4C BTFE view is presented for a with ccTGA, along with the corresponding strain curve. The patient did not experience clinical events. In both figures (**a**,**b**), the curve representing the mean LV GLS value is depicted in white. The analysis included the average peak strain value of all curves.

3.6. Multivariate Analysis

SR ESVi and LV GLS were found to be significant in the univariate analysis. These variables were then used to perform the MANCOVA test, which yielded a p-value of 0.025 from the multivariate analyses. Given the borderline significance for SRV ESVi, the decision was made to focus the analysis on LV GLS. In Table 7, a comparison of values in the univariate and MANCOVA multivariate analyses is presented.

Table 7. Comparison of values in univariate and MANCOVA multivariate analyses. The results are statistically significant, with a borderline significance noted for SRV ESVi (p = 0.050).

Univariate Analysis	Dependent Variables	p-Value
Events	SRV ESVi	0.050
	LV GLS	0.011
Multivariate Analysis	**Dependent Variables**	**p-Value**
Events	SRV ESVi, LV GLS	0.025

3.7. ROC Curve and Interactive Dot Diagram

For LV GLS, a cut-off value of >−19.24% is proposed. Patients with LV GLS values less negative than this cut-off are at a higher risk for clinical events associated with SRV failure. This threshold demonstrates a Youden's index of 0.6364, with a sensitivity (Se) of 63.64% (95% CI 30.8–89.1), a specificity (Sp) of 100% (95% CI 69.2–100.0), and an Area Under the Curve (AUC) of 0.818 (p = 0.001). These results are reported in Figure 3.

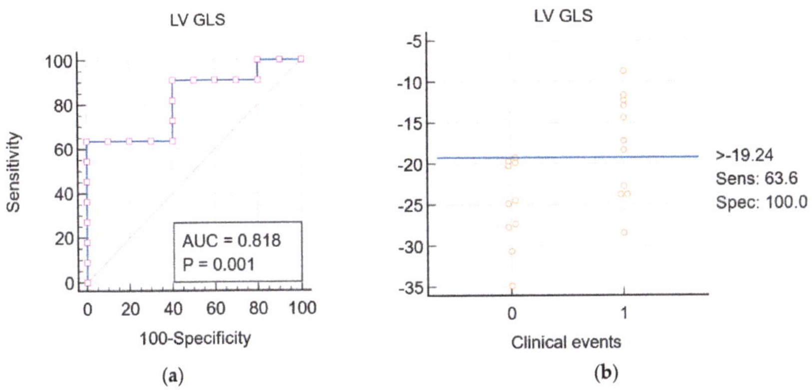

Figure 3. (**a**) LV GLS ROC curve; (**b**) LV GLS interactive dot diagram: the values above the horizontal line are suggested to be associated with a higher risk of clinical events.

4. Discussion

This study is the first to use CMR-FT to analyze the myocardial function of the subpulmonary LV in patients with SRV.

To the best of our knowledge, only a few studies have focused on the subpulmonary LV in patients with SRV and these have primarily used echocardiographic results. In 2021, Surkova et al. (n = 157) observed that subpulmonary LV dysfunction detected by echocardiography is associated with increased severity of SRV dysfunction and worsening of the NYHA class [5]. In 2023 (n = 180), the same group demonstrated that echocardiographic parameters of the left ventricle (LV-ESDi, LV-FAC) can predict mortality risk and need for transplantation [4]. These studies appear to inaugurate a new perspective on the role of the subpulmonary LV, which has been largely neglected. In detail, these findings raise important questions about the role of the subpulmonary left ventricle and whether its assessment should be included in routine follow-up care.

However, the assessment of subpulmonic LV by using those echo parameters may be limited by geometrical assumption and poor visualization of the morphologically left ventricle. In addition, the used echo parameters are affected by tethering from adjacent segments and ventricular–ventricular interaction. Thus, they may just reflect on the subpulmonic LV and the SRV dysfunction, rather than measure an objective subpulmonic LV dysfunction. Thus, an approach that is not limited by poor visualization, is not affected by geometrical confounder, independent from ventricular interaction, and not affected by loading conditions, may be of value to fully assess the role of the subpulmonic LV. To overcome all these limitations, we used CMR, which is not affected by poor image quality, and we used an FT-derived strain, a parameter that is not affected by geometry, load conditions or ventricular interactions.

Both univariate and multivariate analyses demonstrated a statistical significance of LV GLS (p = 0.011; p = 0.025) in predicting the risk of clinical events.

Our findings indicate that, even with preserved ejection fraction, a LV GLS > −19.24 could identify latent left ventricle dysfunction. This may be due to the load dependency and influence of geometry in the assessment of EF even by CMR, the gold standard. Santens et al. (2022) have also noted that standard follow-up parameters often fail to detect preclinical dysfunction and deterioration [14]. Our data suggest incorporating the evaluation of the subpulmonary LV in the routine follow-up of these patients, including an evaluation of LV GLS by CMR-FT or by echo in the presence of a good acoustic window.

Our results showed that SRV patients with clinical events had smaller LV EDV and ESV (119.4 ± 47.6 mL vs. 124.4 ± 47.7 mL). This finding is in contrast with the results of Santens et al. In their study (n = 33), higher values of LV EDVi and LV ESVi (assessed by CMR both at rest and under stress) were associated with an increased risk of SRV failure, arrhythmias, and death [14]. However, compared with our study, Santens' group included a larger proportion of patients with Mustard/Senning repairs (58%), older age (37 ± 8 years) and a higher number of cases with moderate/severe tricuspid regurgitation (63%). Thus, the results from Santens et al. reflect a more advanced stage of the disease compared to our study. In this regard, our data suggest that subpulmonary LV dysfunction is associated with events even in an earlier stage of the disease and thus plays an important role in risk stratification.

Moreover, we noted that patients with events had a higher LV EF compared to the group without events (65.0 ± 7.4% vs. 60.6 ± 8.1%). It is known that ejection fraction may not be a sufficiently sensitive parameter to detect changes in ventricular function, being affected by afterload and geometry [15]. For this reason, myocardial strain has been introduced as an intrinsic index of myocardial contractility and function, and our data confirm the higher sensitivity of myocardial strain in detecting early subclinical abnormalities [16–18].

Limitations

The primary limitation of this study is the relatively small sample size of the studied cohort. However, this reflects the prevalence of the disease (10% of all CHDs) and the selection criteria that were applied.

The calculation of myocardial strain using feature tracking software can be relatively time-consuming. However, this process can be significantly expedited with experience.

Furthermore, these results require both intra-operator and inter-operator evaluations to assess data concordance. Therefore, we call for multicenter studies with larger sample sizes to pool expertise and compare results. Such studies will clarify the reproducibility of this parameter and further validate these findings. Additionally, long-term follow-up is necessary to confirm the prognostic significance of this parameter.

5. Conclusions

This study has identified an important parameter, the left ventricular global longitudinal strain (LV GLS), which may have significant prognostic value for patients with a systemic right ventricle (SRV). Feature tracking software may overcome some structural limitations often associated with echocardiography in assessing subpulmonary left ventricle function, so its use could be suggested as part of routine follow-ups.

The proposed cut-off value of LV GLS > −19.24 provides a promising reference threshold to identify patients at high risk of SRV failure-related events. Early recognition of LV dysfunction could lead to improved therapeutic strategies, thereby optimizing clinical management and outcomes in this population.

Author Contributions: S.P., A.P. and G.D.S. reviewed the literature and drafted and edited the work; A.P. and G.D.S. revised the work critically; G.D.S. and S.P. worked on statistical analysis; E.R. and A.C. analyzed cardiac magnetic resonance; S.P., A.M., A.P., E.R., M.A., I.C. and J.F. collected clinical data; G.D.S. proposed the topic, designed the work, and reviewed the final version. All authors have read and agreed to the published version of the manuscript.

Funding: This research received no external funding.

Institutional Review Board Statement: The study was conducted in accordance with the Declaration of Helsinki and submitted to the HIT Research Centre Ethical Committee of the University of Padua (Protocol No. 2024_247, 2 May 2024).

Informed Consent Statement: Informed consent was obtained from all subjects involved in the study. All the information being collected was part of the routine care.

Data Availability Statement: Data sharing is not applicable to this article.

Conflicts of Interest: The authors declare no conflicts of interest.

Abbreviations

CHDs	congenital heart diseases
SRV	systemic right ventricle
LV	left ventricle
ccTGA	congenitally corrected transposition of the great arteries
TGA	transposition of the great arteries
AtSO	atrial switch operation
ASD	atrial septal defect
VSD	ventricular septal defect
DORV	double outlet right ventricle
CMR	cardiac magnetic resonance
CMR-FT	cardiac magnetic resonance-feature tracking
LGE	late gadolinium enhancement
SRV EDV	systemic right ventricle end-diastolic volume
SRV EDVi	systemic right ventricle end-diastolic volume indexed to BSA
SRV ESV	systemic right ventricle end-systolic volume
SRV ESVi	systemic right ventricle end-systolic volume indexed to BSA
SRV EF	systemic right ventricle ejection fraction
LV EDV	left ventricle end-diastolic volume
LV EDVi	left ventricle end-diastolic volume indexed to BSA
LV ESV	left ventricle end-systolic volume
LV ESVi	left ventricle end-systolic volume indexed to BSA
LV EF	left ventricle ejection fraction
TR	tricuspid regurgitation
SRV GLS	systemic right ventricle global longitudinal strain
SRV GCS	systemic right ventricle global circumferential strain
SRV GRS	systemic right ventricle global radial strain
LV GLS	left ventricle global longitudinal strain
LV GCS	left ventricle global circumferential strain
LV GRS	left ventricle global radial strain

References

1. Samánek, M.; Slavík, Z.; Zborilová, B.; Hrobonová, V.; Vorísková, M.; Skovránek, J. Prevalence, treatment, and outcome of heart disease in live-born children: A prospective analysis of 91,823 live-born children. *Pediatr. Cardiol.* **1989**, *10*, 205–211. [CrossRef] [PubMed]
2. Spadotto, V.; Frescura, C.; Ho, S.Y.; Thiene, G. The concept of double inlet-double outlet right ventricle: A distinct congenital heart disease. *Cardiovasc. Pathol.* **2017**, *26*, 39–44. [CrossRef] [PubMed]
3. Nartowicz, S.A.; Jakielska, E.; Ratajczak, P.; Lesiak, M.; Trojnarska, O. Clinical Factors Affecting Survival in Patients with Congenitally Corrected Transposition of the Great Arteries: A Systematic Review and Meta-Analysis. *J. Clin. Med.* **2024**, *13*, 3127. [CrossRef] [PubMed]
4. Surkova, E.; Constantine, A.; Xu, Z.; Segura de la Cal, T.; Bispo, D.; West, C.; Senior, R.; Dimopoulos, K.; Li, W. Prognostic significance of subpulmonary left ventricular size and function in patients with a systemic right ventricle. *Eur. Heart J.-Cardiovasc. Imaging* **2023**, *25*, 58–65. [CrossRef] [PubMed]
5. Surkova, E.; Segura, T.; Dimopoulos, K.; Bispo, D.; Flick, C.; West, C.; Babu-Narayan, S.V.; Senior, R.; Gatzoulis, M.A.; Li, W. Systolic dysfunction of the subpulmonary left ventricle is associated with the severity of heart failure in patients with a systemic right ventricle. *Int. J. Cardiol.* **2021**, *324*, 66–71. [CrossRef] [PubMed]
6. Di Salvo, G.; Miller, O.; Babu Narayan, S.; Li, W.; Budts, W.; Valsangiacomo Buechel, E.R.; Frigiola, A.; Bosch, A.E.V.D.; Bonello, B.; Mertens, L.; et al. Imaging the adult with congenital heart disease: A multimodality imaging approach—Position paper from the EACVI. *Eur. Heart J.-Cardiovasc. Imaging* **2018**, *19*, 1077–1098. [CrossRef] [PubMed]
7. Sutherland, G.R.; Di Salvo, G.; Claus, P.; D'hooge, J.; Bijnens, B. Strain and strain rate imaging: A new clinical approach to quantifying regional myocardial function. *J. Am. Soc. Echocardiogr.* **2004**, *17*, 788–802. [CrossRef] [PubMed]

8. Stokke, T.M.; Hasselberg, N.E.; Smedsrud, M.K.; Sarvari, S.I.; Haugaa, K.H.; Smiseth, O.A.; Edvardsen, T.; Remme, E.W. Geometry as a Confounder When Assessing Ventricular Systolic Function: Comparison Between Ejection Fraction and Strain. *J. Am. Coll. Cardiol.* **2017**, *70*, 942–954. [CrossRef] [PubMed]
9. Chaix, M.A.; Dore, A.; Mondésert, B.; Mongeon, F.P.; Roy, V.; Desrosiers-Gagnon, C.; Guertin, M.-C.; White, M.; Ibrahim, R.; O'meara, E.; et al. Angiotensin receptor-neprilysin inhibitor vs. placebo in congenital systemic right ventricular heart failure: The PARACYS-RV trial. *Eur. Heart J.* **2024**, *45*, 1481–1483. [CrossRef]
10. Fusco, F.; Scognamiglio, G.; Merola, A.; Iannuzzi, A.; Palma, M.; Grimaldi, N.; Sarubbi, B. Safety and Efficacy of Sacubitril/Valsartan in Patients with a Failing Systemic Right Ventricle: A Prospective Single-Center Study. *Circ. Heart Fail.* **2023**, *16*, e009848. [CrossRef] [PubMed]
11. Nederend, M.; Kiès, P.; Regeer, M.V.; Vliegen, H.W.; Mertens, B.J.; Robbers-Visser, D.; Bouma, B.J.; Tops, L.F.; Schalij, M.J.; Jongbloed, M.R.M.; et al. Tolerability and beneficial effects of sacubitril/valsartan on systemic right ventricular failure. *Heart* **2023**, *109*, 1525–1532. [CrossRef] [PubMed]
12. Fogel, M.A.; Anwar, S.; Broberg, C.; Browne, L.; Chung, T.; Johnson, T.; Muthurangu, V.; Taylor, M.; Valsangiacomo-Buechel, E.; Wilhelm, C. Society for Cardiovascular Magnetic Resonance/European Society of Cardiovascular Imaging/American Society of Echocardiography/Society for Pediatric Radiology/North American Society for Cardiovascular Imaging Guidelines for the Use of Cardiac Magnetic Resonance in Pediatric Congenital and Acquired Heart Disease: Endorsed by The American Heart Association. *Circ. Cardiovasc. Imaging* **2022**, *15*, e014415. [CrossRef] [PubMed]
13. Canan, A.; Ashwath, R.; Agarwal, P.P.; François, C.; Rajiah, P. Multimodality Imaging of Transposition of the Great Arteries. *RadioGraphics* **2021**, *41*, 338–360. [CrossRef] [PubMed]
14. Santens, B.; Helsen, F.; Van De Bruaene, A.; De Meester, P.; Budts, A.L.; Troost, E.; Moons, P.; Claus, P.; Rega, F.; Bogaert, J.; et al. Adverse functional remodelling of the subpulmonary left ventricle in patients with a systemic right ventricle is associated with clinical outcome. *Eur. Heart J.-Cardiovasc. Imaging* **2022**, *23*, 680–688. [CrossRef] [PubMed]
15. Taylor, R.J.; Moody, W.E.; Umar, F.; Edwards, N.C.; Taylor, T.J.; Stegemann, B.; Townend, J.N.; Hor, K.N.; Steeds, R.P.; Mazur, W.; et al. Myocardial strain measurement with feature-tracking cardiovascular magnetic resonance: Normal values. *Eur. Heart J.-Cardiovasc. Imaging* **2015**, *16*, 871–881. [CrossRef] [PubMed]
16. Rajiah, P.S.; Kalisz, K.; Broncano, J.; Goerne, H.; Collins, J.D.; François, C.J.; Ibrahim, E.-S.; Agarwal, P.P. Myocardial Strain Evaluation with Cardiovascular MRI: Physics, Principles, and Clinical Applications. *RadioGraphics* **2022**, *42*, 968–990. [CrossRef] [PubMed]
17. Scatteia, A.; Baritussio, A.; Bucciarelli-Ducci, C. Strain imaging using cardiac magnetic resonance. *Heart Fail. Rev.* **2017**, *22*, 465–776. [CrossRef] [PubMed]
18. Sperlongano, S.; D'Andrea, A.; Mele, D.; Russo, V.; Pergola, V.; Carbone, A.; Ilardi, F.; Di Maio, M.; Bottino, R.; Giallauria, F.; et al. Left Ventricular Deformation and Vortex Analysis in Heart Failure: From Ultrasound Technique to Current Clinical Application. *Diagnostics* **2021**, *11*, 892. [CrossRef] [PubMed]

Journal of
Clinical Medicine

MDPI

Case Report

A Dynamic Multimodality Imaging Assessment of Right Ventricular Thrombosis in a Middle-Aged Man with Lymphocytic Interstitial Pneumonia: The Additive Role of Tissue Doppler Imaging

Andrea Sonaglioni [1,*], Alessandro Lucidi [2], Francesca Luisi [2], Antonella Caminati [2], Gian Luigi Nicolosi [3], Gaetana Anna Rispoli [4], Maurizio Zompatori [5], Michele Lombardo [1] and Sergio Harari [2,6]

1 Division of Cardiology, IRCCS MultiMedica, 20123 Milan, Italy; michele.lombardo@multimedica.it
2 Division of Pneumology, Semi-Intensive Care Unit, IRCCS MultiMedica, 20123 Milan, Italy; alessandro.lucidi@unimi.it (A.L.); francesca.luisi@multimedica.it (F.L.); antonella.caminati@multimedica.it (A.C.); sergio.harari@unimi.it (S.H.)
3 Division of Cardiology, Policlinico San Giorgio, 33170 Pordenone, Italy; gianluigi.nicolosi@gmail.com
4 Division of Radiology, IRCCS MultiMedica, 20123 Milan, Italy; gaetanaanna.rispoli@multimedica.it
5 DIMES Department, University of Bologna, 40126 Bologna, Italy; maurizio.zompatori@unibo.it
6 Department of Clinical Sciences and Community Health, Università di Milano, 20122 Milan, Italy
* Correspondence: andrea.sonaglioni@multimedica.it; Tel.: +39-0285994276

Abstract: Background: Right ventricular thrombosis (RVT) is rarely detected in clinical practice. Depending on its aetiology, RVT may originate from a deep venous thrombosis (type A) or in situ (type B). Type A is characterized by increased mobility and frequent pulmonary embolization, whereas type B is nonmobile and is associated with significant right ventricular (RV) dilatation and dysfunction. **Methods:** A type B RVT complicated by subsegmental pulmonary embolism (PE) was diagnosed in a 46-year-old man with acute-on-chronic respiratory failure secondary to acute exacerbation of interstitial lung disease. He underwent a multimodality imaging assessment of the RV mass that comprehensively incorporated TTE, TEE, contrast-enhanced chest CT, and LGE-CMR. **Results:** During the clinical course, a serial echocardiographic assessment of the RV mass allowed for a dynamic evaluation of its features and cardiac haemodynamics. Conventional TTE was implemented with colour tissue Doppler imaging (TDI) and pulsed wave (PW) TDI to improve the visualization of the RV mass and to objectively measure its mobility. The increased RVT mass peak antegrade velocity (>10 cm/s) was predictive of subsequent RVT fragmentation and PE. **Conclusions:** Colour TDI and PW-TDI may aid in the differential diagnosis of RV masses and may improve the prognostic risk stratification of patients with right-sided intracardiac masses.

Keywords: right ventricular thrombosis; pulmonary embolism; multimodality imaging assessment; tissue Doppler imaging; prognosis

1. Introduction

Right ventricular thrombosis (RVT) is a rare and frequently underdiagnosed life-threatening condition [1]. It can be detected in 2.6–18% of patients with pulmonary embolism (PE) [2–4].

The main risk factors for RVT are the following: a younger age, previous bleeding events, congestive heart failure, intracardiac procedures, cancer, episodes of syncope, a transient systolic blood pressure <100 mmHg, and arterial oxyhaemoglobin saturation

<90% [2]. Hypercoagulability, secondary to Factor 5 Leiden or antithrombin 3 mutations, is another factor that has been associated with RVT occurrence [5]. In certain cases, hypercoagulability may be secondary to occult malignancy [6]. Loeffler's endocarditis [7] and takotsubo cardiomyopathy, affecting the right ventricular (RV) apex [8], are other causes of RVT, which are rarely detected in clinical practice.

Most patients with RVT have significant RV dilatation and dysfunction. Cases of RVT have also been reported in patients with acute inferior-wall myocardial infarction complicated by RV infarction [9]. From a pathophysiological point of view, mechanisms for RVT formation in situ are related to the so-called "Virchow's triad", which consists of blood stasis, endothelial dysfunction, and concomitant hypercoagulability.

Based on its aetiology, RVT is classified in types A, B, and C. Type A is a highly mobile serpiginous thrombus, which is entrapped within the Chiari's network and/or in right heart cavities, that originates from the embolization of a deep venous thrombosis (DVT) and is commonly associated with PE. Type B is nonmobile, originates in situ, and is associated with cardiac abnormalities. Type C has intermediate characteristics between type A and B [10,11].

RVT is generally asymptomatic before the occurrence of complications such as PE or paradoxical stroke [12]. However, the mortality rate associated with RVT is high, ranging between 27% and 100% [1,2], especially if it is complicated by PE. Indeed, the prognosis of these patients is primarily related to the haemodynamic consequences of RVT rather than its characteristics.

Due to the severity of RVT occurrence and complications, immediate diagnosis and rapid prognostic risk stratification of RVT patients are mandatory.

Two-dimensional transthoracic echocardiography (TTE) and transoesophageal echocardiography (TEE) are the first-line imaging modalities for detecting and monitoring RVT [11]. It is noteworthy that both TTE and TEE have a higher sensitivity and specificity for detecting left ventricular thrombosis rather than RVT. The first assessment of RVT by TTE may be difficult in an emergency setting and in patients with tachy-arrhythmias, haemodynamic instability, or poor acoustic windows [13]. Additionally, approximately 50% of RV thrombi are identified by using off-axis echocardiographic sections [11]. Therefore, RVT presence may be considerably underestimated in clinical practice.

Given that the echogenicity of thrombotic formation may be indistinguishable from that of surrounding myocardium, TTE may provide limited information concerning the differential diagnosis of intracardiac masses [14]. In the setting of poor acoustic windows and/or suboptimal TTE imaging, contrast echocardiography may considerably improve the endocardial definition by enhancing the blood pool–myocardial interface, thus facilitating RVT detection and characterization [15].

Due to its unique capability in providing an accurate and reproducible assessment of RV structure, function, and tissue characterization, cardiac magnetic resonance (CMR) with late gadolinium enhancement (LGE) has shown higher sensitivity and specificity than TTE and/or TEE for detecting RVT [16,17].

Finally, contrast-enhanced chest computed tomography (CT) represents another useful technique for evaluating RVT, due to its rapid acquisition and high spatial and temporal resolution [18–20].

Herein, we present a challenging case of type B RVT that was diagnosed by a multimodality imaging approach in a 46-year-old man with acute-on-chronic respiratory failure secondary to acute exacerbation of interstitial lung disease.

2. Clinical Course

A 46-year-old man (BSA 1.92 m^2; BMI 24.5 Kg/m^2) without previous cardiovascular events, who was affected by anti-Mi2 dermatomyositis and lymphocytic interstitial pneumonia (LIP) with chronic respiratory failure and was treated with 50 mg of azathioprine daily, 25 mg prednisone daily, 700 mg of intravenous (IV) rituximab once weekly, and oxygen therapy (1 to 6 L per minute), was admitted to the Emergency Department (ED) of our institution due to ongoing dyspnoea, chest pain, and general malaise. At the hospital admission, the patient's arterial oxygen saturation (SaO2) in ambient air was 66%, their blood pressure was 110/70 mmHg, their heart rate was 102 b.p.m., and their body temperature was 36.3 °C. A blood gas analysis showed hypoxemia (PaO2 = 39.6 mmHg) and hypocapnia (PaCO2 = 27.2 mmHg), pH = 7.3, and a lactate level of 7.7 mmol/L (normal range: 0.36–1.25 mmol/L). Blood tests revealed a serum haemoglobin amount of 12.8 g/dL; a serum white blood cell count of 13,900 $\times$ 10^6/L (normal range: 4000–11,000 $\times$ 10^6/L); a serum Neutrophil–Lymphocyte Ratio (NLR) of 18.6; a serum creatinine level of 1.57 mg/dL; a serum troponin I level of 0.42 ng/mL (normal range 0.00–0.04 ng/mL); a serum C-reactive protein (CRP) amount of 58 mg/L (normal range: 0–5 mg/L); a serum D-dimer of 4215 microg/L (normal range: 1–500 microg/L); and a serum N-terminal pro-B-type natriuretic peptide (NT-proBNP) level of 6474 pg/mL (normal range: <125 pg/mL).

The ECG recorded in the ED showed a sinus rhythm with normal atrio-ventricular conduction, mild RV conduction delay, and deep T-wave inversion in right precordial leads and inferior leads, suggesting RV overload (Figure 1).

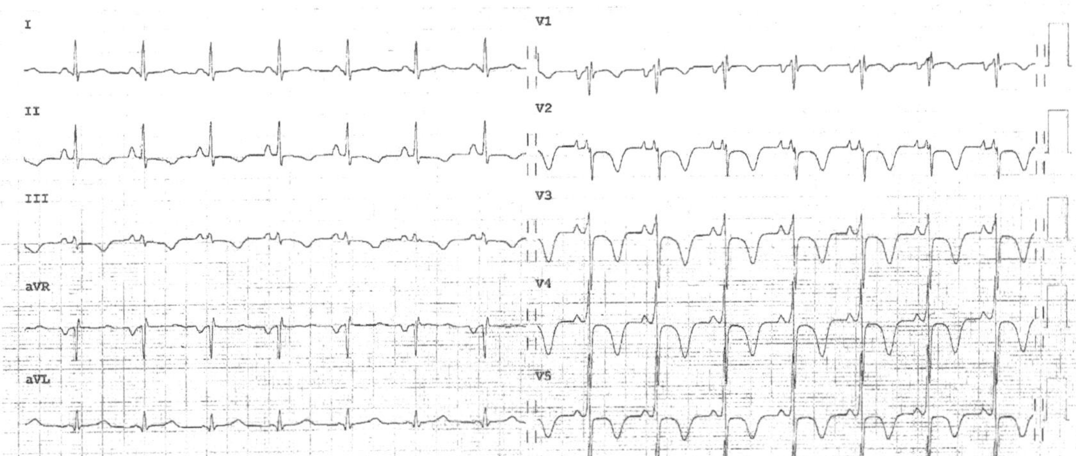

Figure 1. A 12-lead electrocardiogram showing a sinus rhythm with normal atrio-ventricular conduction, mild right ventricular conduction delay, and deep T-wave inversion in right precordial leads and inferior leads, suggesting right ventricular overload.

Chest X-rays showed diffuse fibrosing interstitial lung disease with multiple bilateral parenchymal opacities, with no clear evidence of inflammatory foci (Figure 2).

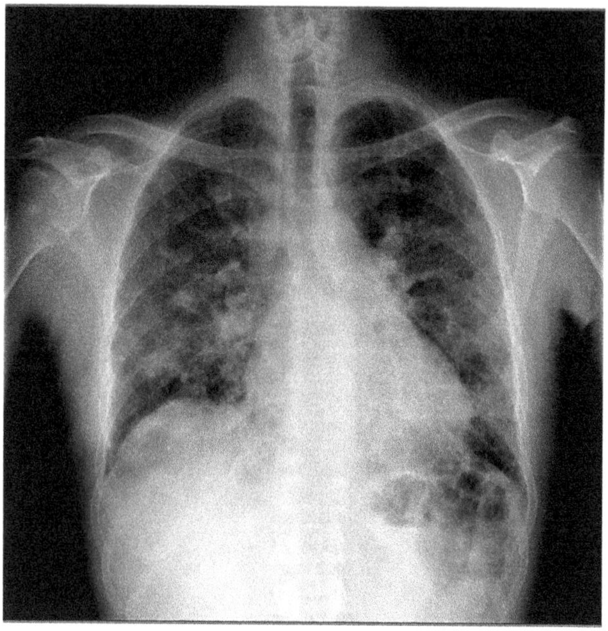

Figure 2. Chest X-rays revealing diffuse fibrosing interstitial lung disease with multiple bilateral parenchymal opacities, with no clear evidence of inflammatory foci.

An urgent bedside echocardiogram highlighted a significant dilatation of right-sided cardiac chambers (RV-to-left ventricular basal diameter ratio = 2.4; RV inflow tract diameter = 60 mm) and mild hypokinesia of the RV lateral wall, as assessed by tricuspid annular plane systolic excursion (TAPSE) magnitude (17 mm). A moderate tricuspid regurgitation was present. The peak tricuspid regurgitation velocity (TRV) was 3.4 m/s, indicating a high probability of pulmonary hypertension (PH). The inferior vena cava was significantly dilated (transverse diameter = 2.8 cm), with inspiratory excursions < 50%. Accordingly, the estimated systolic pulmonary artery pressure (sPAP) was 60 mmHg. From the RV-focused apical four-chamber view, a large sessile echogenic formation with hyperechoic edges (size: 3.9 cm × 2.6 cm), attached to the mid-apical portion of the RV free wall and protruding into the RV cavity, was detected (Figure 3A,B). By placing a 5 mm sample volume of pulsed wave (PW)-tissue Doppler imaging (TDI) at the level of the mobile portion of the RV mass, an RV mass peak antegrade velocity (Va) of 13 cm/s was obtained. Moreover, on PW-TDI, the RV mass showed a pattern of incoherent motion, totally discordant and independent from the surrounding myocardial tissue (Figure 3C).

Careful observation allowed for the detection of akinesia of the RV mid-apical wall. Therefore, McConnell's sign was excluded. Compared to the right-sided cardiac chambers, the left-sided cavity chambers' size was reduced. The left ventricle showed a D-shaped left ventricular configuration due to the flattening of the interventricular septum caused by the significant RV overload. The left ventricular ejection fraction (assessed by a modified Simpson's biplane method) was preserved (estimated value = 60%). A first degree of diastolic dysfunction (E/A ratio < 1 on transmitral PW Doppler) was diagnosed in the presence of normal left ventricular filling pressure, as measured by the E/average e' ratio (estimated value = 5.2). The mitral and aortic valves were normal, whereas a mid-systolic notch of the RV outflow tract PW-Doppler envelope, compatible with PH, was detected. The urgent TTE was compared with a previous one, performed electively three months earlier, which showed normal biventricular cavity sizes, normal biventricular systolic function, and normal sPAP (estimated value: 27 mmHg). Accordingly, the actual TTE findings were considered to be suggestive of acute RV overload due to PH, complicated by the RV mass of nonunivocal interpretation.

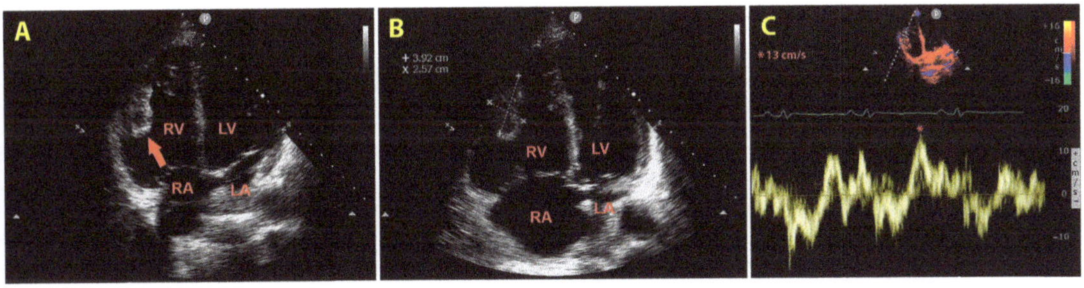

Figure 3. Transthoracic echocardiography. Right-ventricular-focused apical four-chamber view. (**A**) Large sessile echogenic formation with hyperechoic edges (red arrow), attached to the mid-apical portion of the right ventricular free wall and protruding into the RV cavity. (**B**) Measurement of the right ventricular mass size. (**C**) Assessment of the right ventricular mass peak antegrade velocity by pulsed wave tissue Doppler imaging. The right ventricular mass showed a pattern of incoherent motion, totally discordant and independent from the surrounding myocardial tissue. LA, left atrium; LV, left ventricle; RA, right atrium; RV, right ventricle. The symbol * indicates the right ventricular mass peak antegrade velocity.

Based on the ECG and echocardiographic findings and the patient's complex history, the pulmonologist suggested a diagnostic study with a contrast-enhanced chest CT. The examination confirmed severe RV dilatation with a large filling defect involving the mid-apical region of the right ventricle (Figure 4).

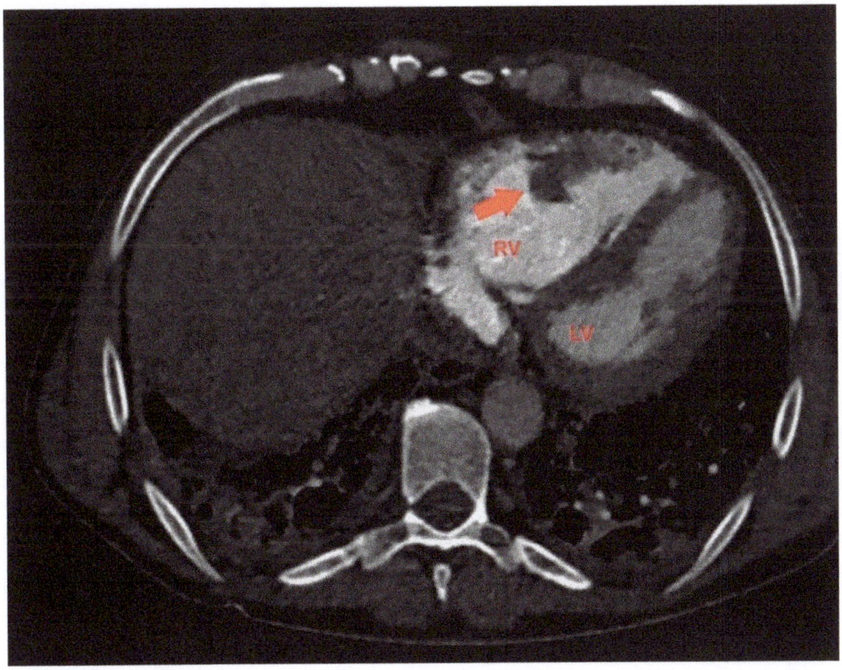

Figure 4. Axial contrast-enhanced chest computed tomography showing a large filling defect (red arrow) involving the mid-apical region of the right ventricle. LV, left ventricle; RV, right ventricle.

A CT scan also confirmed severe interstitial pulmonary fibrosis with diffuse ground glass opacities and thin-walled cysts and excluded PE.

A venous Doppler ultrasound of the lower extremities excluded concomitant DVT.

The patient was admitted to the Intensive Care Unit (ICU) and underwent high-flow oxygen therapy (reservoir mask with 10–15 L/min) and medical treatment with anticoagulants (enoxaparin sodium: 6000 I.U. twice daily by subcutaneous injection), IV antibiotics (Piperacillin/Tazobactam: 4 g/0.5 g three times daily), IV corticosteroids (methylprednisolone: 40 mg three times daily), IV antibiotics (ceftriaxone: 2 g daily) and IV diuretics (furosemide: 40 mg daily).

Even if the patient did not have a fever during hospitalization, aerobic and anaerobic blood cultures were performed to exclude the infectious origin of the RV mass. However, blood cultures yielded negative results.

A repeated TTE during the stay in the ICU demonstrated a slight reduction in RV mass size (3 cm × 2 cm) that changed its echogenicity, being characterized by an anechoic central space and a hyperechoic border (Figure 5A). The same echocardiographic findings of the RV mass were confirmed from an RV-focused mid-oesophageal section obtained during TEE (Figure 5B).

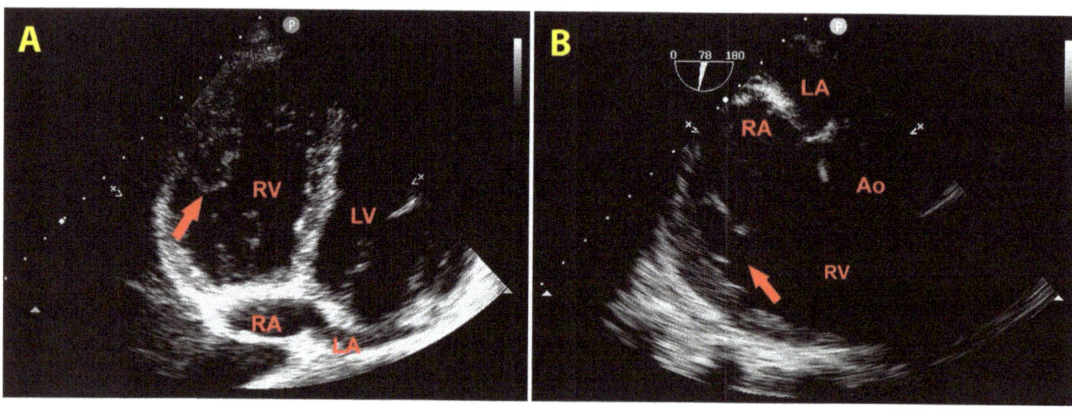

Figure 5. (**A**) Transthoracic echocardiography. Right-ventricular-focused apical four-chamber view demonstrating a slight reduction in right ventricular mass size (red arrow), characterized by an anechoic central space and a hyperechoic border. (**B**) Right-ventricular-focused mid-oesophageal section showing the same echocardiographic features of the right ventricular mass (red arrow), observed from the transthoracic approach. Ao, aorta; LA, left atrium; LV, left ventricle; RA, right atrium; RV, right ventricle.

A further contrast-enhanced chest CT scan revealed segmental and subsegmental filling defects in the right upper lobe (Figure 6) and a concomitant mild reduction in RV mid-apical filling defect.

After a multidisciplinary discussion, late gadolinium enhancement (LGE) cardiac magnetic resonance (CMR) was performed. LGE-CMR allowed for the detection of an RV mass with inhomogeneous peripheral enhancement (Figure 7).

After seven days of ICU monitoring, the patient's clinical conditions gradually improved, and he was transferred to the Division of Pneumology. On the 10th day of hospitalization, an echocardiographic control showed the total disappearance of the RV mass (Figure 8) and concomitantly improved TRV (estimated value: 2.5 m/s).

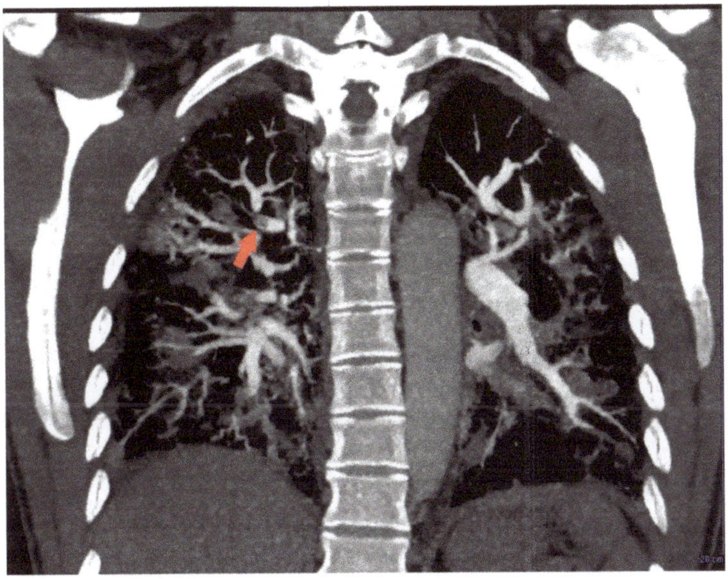

Figure 6. Coronal contrast-enhanced chest computed tomography revealing segmental and subsegmental filling defects (red arrow) in the right upper lobe.

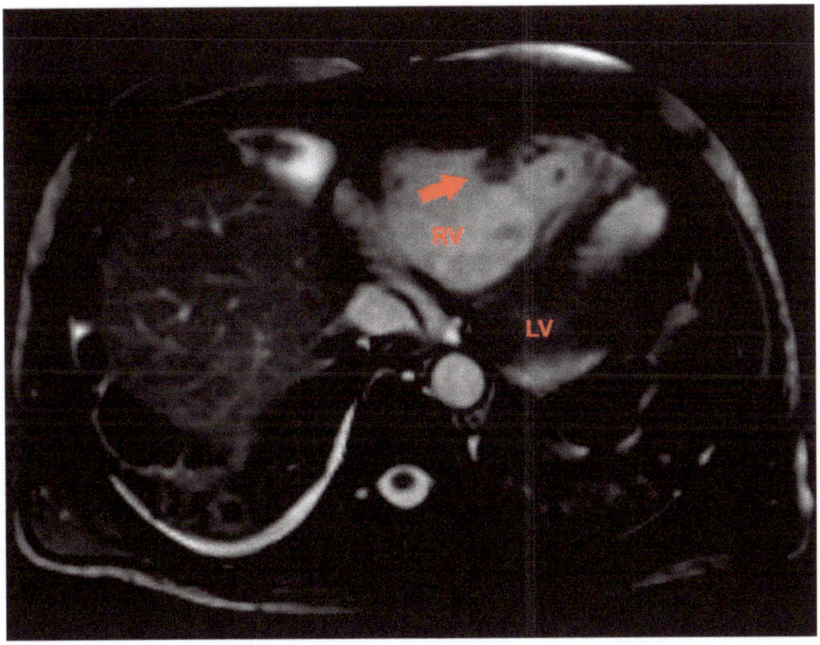

Figure 7. Axial late gadolinium enhancement cardiac magnetic resonance showing a right ventricular mass (red arrow) with inhomogeneous peripheral enhancement. LV, left ventricle; RV, right ventricle.

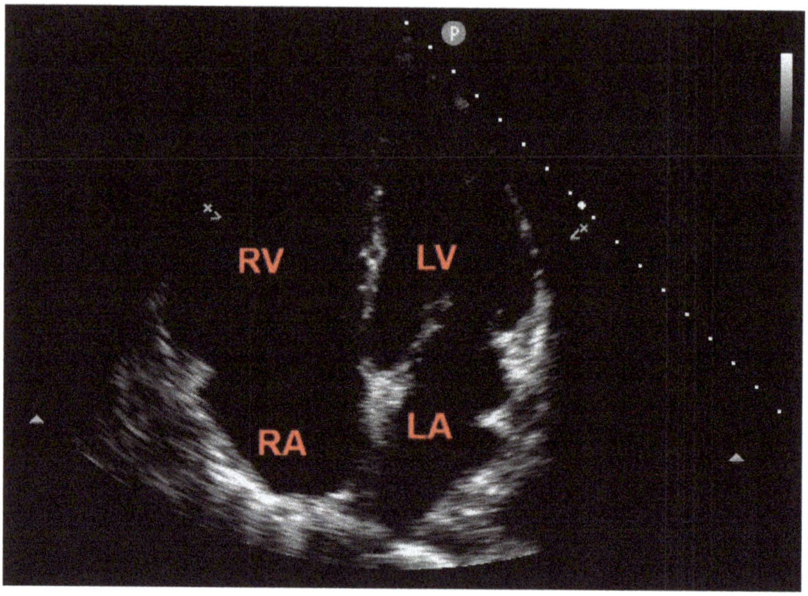

Figure 8. Transthoracic echocardiography. Apical four chamber view demonstrating the total disappearance of the right ventricular mass. LA, left atrium; LV, left ventricle; RA, right atrium; RV, right ventricle.

In light of the favourable echocardiographic evolution, the RV mass was more appropriately considered as a thrombotic formation with peripheral organization and liquefactive central necrosis, originating in situ, at the level of a significantly dilated and dysfunctional right ventricle, causing subsegmental PE, which was completely resolved after anti-coagulant treatment.

Repeated blood tests demonstrated the normalization of serum levels of CRP (2.8 mg/L) and troponin I (0.02 ng/mL) and a significant reduction in serum levels of both D-dimer (430 microg/L) and NT-proBNP (69 pg/mL). From a repeated blood gas analysis in ambient air, SaO2 was 91.4%, PaO2 was 59 mmHg, PaCO2 was 43 mmHg, pH was 7.41, and the lactate level was 1.01 mmol/L. During the hospital stay, the patient also underwent thrombophilia screening, which produced a negative result. The haematology consultant recommended anticoagulant therapy at discharge with 5 mg of apixaban twice daily lifelong.

On the 14th day of hospitalization, the patient was discharged with the diagnosis of acute-on-chronic respiratory failure secondary to acute exacerbation of interstitial lung disease, leading to acute RV overload with akinesia of the RV mid-apical segments, complicated by RV thrombosis in situ, causing subsegmental PE. The suggested discharge medical treatment included 5 mg of apixaban twice daily, oxygen therapy via the nasal cannula of 1 L/min at rest and 6 L/min on effort, 50 mg of azathioprine daily, and 25 mg of prednisone daily.

3. Discussion

This challenging clinical case highlights the complexity of the differential diagnosis of RV masses, involving tumours, vegetations, and thrombi.

3.1. Right Ventricular Tumors

RV neoplastic lesions may be benign or malignant. The most common benign cardiac tumours are myxomas, but those originating from the RV free wall are extremely rare, representing only 5% of cases [21,22]. RV myxomas may have obstructive features, potentially leading to right heart failure with systemic congestion or causing arrhythmias, syncope, and even sudden death [23]. Depending on their mobility, RV myxomas may be complicated by PE [24,25]. Rhabdomyomas represent another type of benign RV neoplastic lesion, predominantly detected in children and commonly associated with tuberous sclerosis complex; they are multiple lesions, that generally regress spontaneously [26].

Primary malignant cardiac tumours are generally right atrial masses that rapidly infiltrate valves or chamber walls destroy the primary structure of hearts [27]. Other characteristics of malignant tumours are the wide point of attachment, a size of >5 cm, pericardial effusion, and extracardiac extension [28]. Among the malignant cardiac tumours, the most frequent ones are cardiac sarcomas [29], particularly angiosarcomas, representing 30% to 45% of sarcomas [30]. Lymphomas are rare, accounting for 1% to 2% of primary malignant cardiac tumours, involving the right atrium or the right ventricle. Lymphomas are more frequently non-Hodgkin type, associated with immunodeficiency syndromes [28].

Distinctive features of primary malignant cardiac tumours assessed by CMR are heterogeneous enhancement, tumour necrosis, and multiple foci of calcification [31]. Compared with benign tumours, malignant masses have generally non-left localization, have a greater diameter, are sessile, are polylobate, have an inhomogeneous appearance, are infiltrating, and are accompanied by pericardial effusion. As opposed to the avascular nature of thrombi, cardiac tumours have a vascular supply. At LGE, malignant masses are more frequently hyperintense compared with benign ones [32].

Due to its high spatial and temporal resolution, fast acquisition times, and multiplanar image reconstruction capabilities, cardiac CT with ECG gating represents a valid alternative to CMR in many patients, particularly in those with contraindications to CMR. CT may precisely assess lesion margins, may define the cardiovascular extent of the mass, and exclude concomitant obstructive coronary artery disease [33]. Additionally, when combined with 18 F-fluorodeoxyglucose (FDG) positron emission tomography (PET), cardiac CT is also useful for detecting primary malignant cardiac tumours and metastasis, which generally show a significantly higher glucose uptake than primary benign cardiac tumours [34].

3.2. Right Ventricular Endocarditis

Right-sided infective endocarditis (IE), accounting for 5% to 10% of all IE cases, are generally associated with intravenous drug use, intracardiac devices, and central venous catheters, primarily involving the tricuspid valve and rarely, the pulmonary valve [35,36]. On the other hand, isolated RV mural endocarditis is very rare and generally arises from the RV moderator band, where trabeculations could act as a facilitating location for infection [37–39]. RV mural endocarditis may be suspected in patients with prolonged fever and RV endocardial masses, particularly attached to the RV moderator band, even when blood cultures are persistently negative. Cases of RV mural endocarditis involving the RV free wall have been reported in individuals who regular used intravenous drugs. These cases have been ascribed to the coarse trabeculae of the RV acting as a nidus for infection, similar to the RV moderator band [40,41].

The differential diagnosis between right-sided vegetations and thrombi may be difficult, because both are generally masses without gadolinium contrast enhancement [42]. However, a number of CMR findings may be suggestive of IE, particularly, delayed enhancement involving the cardiovascular structures, indicating endothelial inflammation, irreversible myocardial damage or fibrosis [43,44], LGE of the endothelial lining, or a perivalvular abscess [45]. Multislice CT may contribute to the diagnosis of right-sided IE, by providing a high-resolution anatomical assessment of vegetations, valvular and peri-valvular lesions, and also extra-cardiac lesions [46,47].

3.3. *Right Ventricular Thrombosis*

Given its higher sensitivity and specificity over echocardiographic techniques, CMR may facilitate the differential diagnosis between intracardiac thrombi and tumours, as demonstrated in various case reports and case series [13,14,48]. On CMR, first-pass perfusion imaging, early gadolinium enhancement, and delayed gadolinium enhancement with a prolonged inversion time are commonly used to assess the thrombotic nature of cardiac masses [49]. RVT is generally visualized as a homogeneously dark mass with no contrast uptake, characteristics that are consistent with a homogeneous, avascular mass [50]. However, peripheral enhancement may be occasionally observed in chronic organic thrombotic formations due to fibrotic components [51].

Another imaging technique commonly employed for the diagnostic study of RV masses is a chest CT scan, where RVT generally appears as a hypodense mass within enhanced RV cavity [52].

In the present case, a multidisciplinary evaluation and a dynamic multimodality imaging approach allowed for the correct differential diagnosis between RVT and both RV tumours and vegetation. Notably, an RV neoplastic lesion was excluded due to the absence of pericardial effusion and extracardiac extension and the rapid response to the anticoagulant treatment. Moreover, the infectious or inflammatory origin of the RV mass was not considered as a plausible hypothesis for the absence of a septic syndrome, for the negativity of blood cultures, and for the RV mass location, without any relation with the RV coarse trabeculae and/or the moderator band, which are generally considered possible sites for infection.

In our findings, the serial echocardiographic monitoring performed during hospitalization appeared to be more effective than contrast-enhanced chest CT and CMR for clarifying the real nature of the RV mass. During the acute phase, the bedside TTE raised the suspicion of severe PH complicated by mid-apical RV akinesia and a superimposed RV mass. The implementation of conventional TTE with PW-TDI provided a precise measurement of the RV mass's mobility and embolic potential. In the sub-acute phase, TTE showed a slight reduction in RV mass size and identified a central anechoic area, confirmed by TEE examination. The subsequent contrast-enhanced chest CT confirmed the diagnosis of segmental and subsegmental PE, indicating that the reduction in RV mass size and central echogenicity were likely related to its fragmentation with consequent pulmonary embolization. The increased RV mass peak Va, assessed by PW-TDI in the acute phase, predicted its subsequent embolization early. Finally, after 10 days of hospitalization, TTE demonstrated the total disappearance of the RV mass, thus confirming its thrombotic nature.

In the present case, the thrombotic nature of the RV mass might have been suspected by the echocardiographic evidence of the underlying RV mid-apical free wall akinesia (similar to what has been observed for left ventricular apical aneurysms complicated by thrombosis) and by its gradual regression after the initiation of anticoagulant treatment. In light of our findings, the RVT we detected was a type B RVT, originating in situ and associated with significant RV dilatation and dysfunction.

For improving RV mass detection, we used colour PW-TDI rather than contrast echocardiography. As has been previously demonstrated [53], colour TDI may improve the visualization of intracardiac masses characterized by a pattern of motion that is totally different from that of surrounding myocardial structures. Indeed, these intracardiac masses are codified with different colours compared to the adjacent myocardium. Additionally, as was recently demonstrated by our study group [54], PW-TDI sampling of the free mobile portion of intracardiac pathological masses allows for the identification of their typical pattern of incoherent motion (totally asynchronous with respect to the cardiac walls) and the precise measurement of the mass peak Va. The higher the mass peak Va, the higher the risk of embolic complications [54]. In the present case, the patient was diagnosed with a mass peak Va >10 cm/s, thus confirming that this simple PW-TDI-derived parameter may represent an innovative important predictor of the embolic risk associated with mobile intracardiac masses.

3.4. Implications for Clinical Practice

PW-TDI is commonly employed for assessing the left ventricular filling pressures and/or the longitudinal systolic function of both ventricles. For this reason, the sample volume of PW-TDI is placed in the ventricular myocardium immediately adjacent to the mitral and/or tricuspid annulus [55]. Moreover, PW-TDI may be used for distinguishing between right atrial masses, characterized by uncoordinated motion, and pseudomasses, characterized by concordant motion with the surrounding myocardial tissue [56].

The assessment of cardiac masses' mobility by PW-TDI is an innovative application of this imaging modality. To measure the mass peak Va, the sample volume of PW-TDI should be placed on the free mobile portion of the intracardiac mass. Even if it has not still been validated by multicentric studies, a mass peak Va > 10 cm/s may represent an adjunctive marker of the increased risk of systemic or pulmonary embolization, depending on the cardiac mass location. Accordingly, by analogy with what was demonstrated in patients with left ventricular apical thrombi [54], the echocardiographic detection of an RV mass peak Va > 10 cm/s may represent an important marker of increased embolic risk, thus strengthening the indication for prompt anticoagulant treatment.

4. Conclusions

The differential diagnosis of RV masses is complex, involving thrombi, tumours, and vegetations.

RVT should always be suspected in young patients with dilated and dysfunctional right ventricles and with systemic disorders associated with hypercoagulability.

A dynamic multimodality imaging approach, comprehensively incorporating colour and PW-TDI, may improve the visualization of RV masses, allowing clinicians to identify, among RV masses, those with an increased embolic potential.

Author Contributions: Conceptualization, A.S., A.L., F.L. and A.C.; methodology, A.S., G.A.R. and M.Z.; software, A.S.; validation, G.L.N., M.Z., M.L. and S.H.; formal analysis, A.S.; investigation, A.S., G.A.R. and M.Z.; resources, S.H.; data curation, A.S., G.A.R. and M.Z.; writing—original draft preparation, A.S.; writing—review and editing, G.L.N. and S.H.; visualization, G.L.N., M.Z., M.L. and S.H.; supervision, M.L. and S.H.; project administration, S.H.; funding acquisition, A.S. All authors have read and agreed to the published version of the manuscript.

Funding: This research was funded by the Italian Ministry of Health, Ricerca Corrente IRCCS MultiMedica.

Institutional Review Board Statement: In accordance with the guidelines by the Comitato Etico Territoriale Lombardia 5, ethical review and approval were not required for this case report.

Informed Consent Statement: Informed consent was obtained from the individual included in the present case report.

Data Availability Statement: Data extracted from the present case report are publicly available on Zenodo (https://zenodo.org) (accessed on 15 February 2025).

Acknowledgments: The authors wish to thank Monica Fumagalli for her graphical support.

Conflicts of Interest: The authors declare no conflicts of interest.

References

1. Chartier, L.; Béra, J.; Delomez, M.; Asseman, P.; Beregi, J.P.; Bauchart, J.J.; Warembourg, H.; Théry, C. Free-floating thrombi in the right heart: Diagnosis, management, and prognostic indexes in 38 consecutive patients. *Circulation* **1999**, *99*, 2779–2783. [CrossRef] [PubMed]
2. Barrios, D.; Rosa-Salazar, V.; Jiménez, D.; Morillo, R.; Muriel, A.; Del Toro, J.; López-Jiménez, L.; Farge-Bancel, D.; Yusen, R.; Monreal, M.; et al. Right heart thrombi in pulmonary embolism. *Eur. Respir. J.* **2016**, *48*, 1377–1385. [CrossRef]
3. Nkoke, C.; Faucher, O.; Camus, L.; Flork, L. Free Floating Right Heart Thrombus Associated with Acute Pulmonary Embolism: An Unsettled Therapeutic Difficulty. *Case Rep. Cardiol.* **2015**, *2015*, 364780. [CrossRef]
4. Ferrari, E.; Benhamou, M.; Berthier, F.; Baudouy, M. Mobile thrombi of the right heart in pulmonary embolism: Delayed disappearance after thrombolytic treatment. *Chest* **2005**, *127*, 1051–1053. [CrossRef]
5. Dinesh Kumar, U.S.; Nareppa, U.; Shetty, S.P.; Wali, M. Right ventricular thrombus in case of atrial septal defect with massive pulmonary embolism: A diagnostic dilemma. *Ann. Card. Anaesth.* **2016**, *19*, 173–176. [CrossRef] [PubMed]
6. Varki, A. Trousseau's syndrome: Multiple definitions and multiple mechanisms. *Blood* **2007**, *110*, 1723–1729. [CrossRef]
7. Muñiz, M.T.; Eiras, M.; Selas, S.; Garcia, J. Loeffler endocarditis associated with a massive right intraventricular thrombus. *Intensive Care Med.* **2018**, *44*, 2296–2297. [CrossRef] [PubMed]
8. Robaei, D.; Buchholz, S.; Feneley, M. Biventricular stress-induced (Tako-tsubo) cardiomyopathy complicated by right ventricular thrombus. *J. Echocardiogr.* **2012**, *10*, 104–105. [CrossRef]
9. Iga, K.; Konishi, T.; Kusukawa, R. Intracardiac thrombi in both the right atrium and right ventricle after acute inferior-wall myocardial infarction. *Int. J. Cardiol.* **1994**, *46*, 169–171. [CrossRef]
10. Charif, F.; Mansour, M.J.; Hamdan, R.; Najjar, C.; Nassar, P.; Issa, M.; Chammas, E.; Saab, M. Free-Floating Right Heart Thrombus with Acute Massive Pulmonary Embolism: A Case Report and Review of the Literature. *J. Cardiovasc. Echogr.* **2018**, *28*, 146–149. [CrossRef]
11. Roy, R.; Guile, B.; Sun, D.; Szasz, T.; Singulane, C.C.; Nguyen, D.; Abutaleb, A.; Lang, R.M.; Addetia, K. Right Ventricular Thrombus on Echocardiography. *Am. J. Cardiol.* **2024**, *211*, 64–68. [CrossRef]
12. Goh, F.Q.; Leow, A.S.; Ho, J.S.; Ho, A.F.; Tan, B.Y.; Yeo, L.L.; Li, T.Y.; Galupo, M.J.; Chan, M.Y.; Yeo, T.C.; et al. Clinical characteristics, treatment and long-term outcomes of patients with right-sided cardiac thrombus. *Hell. J. Cardiol.* **2022**, *68*, 1–8. [CrossRef] [PubMed]
13. Tsang, B.K.; Platts, D.G.; Javorsky, G.; Brown, M.R. Right ventricular thrombus detection and multimodality imaging using contrast echocardiography and cardiac magnetic resonance imaging. *Heart Lung Circ.* **2012**, *21*, 185–188. [CrossRef] [PubMed]
14. Barbagallo, M.; Naef, D.; Köpfli, P.; Hufschmid, U.; Niemann, T.; Gebker, R.; Beer, J.H.; Hireche-Chiakoui, H. Right ventricular thrombus, a challenge in imaging diagnostics: A case series. *Eur. Heart J. Case Rep.* **2021**, *5*, ytab340. [CrossRef] [PubMed]
15. Kurt, M.; Shaikh, K.A.; Peterson, L.; Kurrelmeyer, K.M.; Shah, G.; Nagueh, S.F.; Fromm, R.; Quinones, M.A.; Zoghbi, W.A. Impact of contrast echocardiography on evaluation of ventricular function and clinical management in a large prospective cohort. *J. Am. Coll. Cardiol.* **2009**, *53*, 802–810. [CrossRef]
16. Marcu, C.B.; Beek, A.M.; Van Rossum, A.C. Cardiovascular magnetic resonance imaging for the assessment of right heart involvement in cardiac and pulmonary disease. *Heart Lung Circ.* **2006**, *15*, 362–370. [CrossRef]
17. Galea, N.; Carbone, I.; Cannata, D.; Cannavale, G.; Conti, B.; Galea, R.; Frustaci, A.; Catalano, C.; Francone, M. Right ventricular cardiovascular magnetic resonance imaging: Normal anatomy and spectrum of pathological findings. *Insights Imaging* **2013**, *4*, 213–223. [CrossRef]
18. Syed, I.S.; Motiei, A.; Connolly, H.M.; Dearani, J.A. Pulmonary embolism, right ventricular strain, and intracardiac thrombus-in-transit: Evaluation using comprehensive cardiothoracic computed tomography. *J. Cardiovasc. Comput. Tomogr.* **2009**, *3*, 184–186. [CrossRef]
19. Kusume, T.; Kubokawa, S.; Kaname, N.; Nakaoka, Y.; Kotani, T.; Imai, R.; Nishida, K.; Seki, S.; Kawai, K.; Hamashige, N.; et al. Right ventricular mobile thrombus in end-stage hypertrophic cardiomyopathy. *J. Cardiol. Cases* **2017**, *15*, 173–175. [CrossRef]
20. Artico, J.; Belgrano, M.; Bussani, R.; Sinagra, G. The curious case of a massive right heart thrombosis: A case report. *Eur. Heart J. Case Rep.* **2021**, *5*, ytab156. [CrossRef]
21. Hirota, J.; Akiyama, K.; Taniyasu, N.; Maisawa, K.; Kobayashi, Y.; Sakamoto, N.; Komatsu, N. Injury to the tricuspid valve and membranous atrioventricular septum caused by huge calcified right ventricular myxoma: Report of a case. *Circ. J.* **2004**, *68*, 799–801. [CrossRef]
22. Karagöz, A.; Keskin, B.; Karaduman, A.; Tanyeri, S.; Adademir, T. Multidisciplinary Approach to Right Ventricular Myxoma. *Braz. J. Cardiovasc. Surg.* **2021**, *36*, 257–260. [CrossRef] [PubMed]

23. Singh, V.; Singh, S.K.; Devenraj, V.; Kumar, S. Giant right ventricular myxoma obstructing both inflow and outflow tract. *Indian J. Thorac. Cardiovasc. Surg.* **2019**, *35*, 499–501. [CrossRef]
24. Singhal, P.; Luk, A.; Rao, V.; Butany, J. Molecular basis of cardiac myxomas. *Int. J. Mol. Sci.* **2014**, *15*, 1315–1337. [CrossRef] [PubMed]
25. Lu, C.; Yang, P.; Hu, J. Giant right ventricular myxoma presenting as right heart failure with systemic congestion: A rare case report. *BMC Surg.* **2021**, *21*, 64. [CrossRef]
26. Sciacca, P.; Giacchi, V.; Mattia, C.; Greco, F.; Smilari, P.; Betta, P.; Distefano, G. Rhabdomyomas and tuberous sclerosis complex: Our experience in 33 cases. *BMC Cardiovasc. Disord.* **2014**, *14*, 66. [CrossRef] [PubMed]
27. Mondal, S.; Jubar, J.; Kostibas, M.P. Near Total Occlusion of Right Ventricle by Cardiac Mass. *J. Cardiothorac. Vasc. Anesth.* **2019**, *33*, 2085–2090. [CrossRef]
28. Burazor, I.; Aviel-Ronen, S.; Imazio, M.; Markel, G.; Grossman, Y.; Yosepovich, A.; Adler, Y. Primary malignancies of the heart and pericardium. *Clin. Cardiol.* **2014**, *37*, 582–588. [CrossRef]
29. Leja, M.J.; Shah, D.J.; Reardon, M.J. Primary cardiac tumors. *Tex. Heart Inst. J.* **2011**, *38*, 261–262.
30. Llombart-Cussac, A.; Pivot, X.; Contesso, G.; Rhor-Alvarado, A.; Delord, J.P.; Spielmann, M.; Türsz, T.; Le Cesne, A. Adjuvant chemotherapy for primary cardiac sarcomas: The IGR experience. *Br. J. Cancer* **1998**, *78*, 1624–1628. [CrossRef]
31. Puppala, S.; Hoey, E.T.; Mankad, K.; Wood, A.M. Primary cardiac angiosarcoma arising from the interatrial septum: Magnetic resonance imaging appearances. *Br. J. Radiol.* **2010**, *83*, e230–e234. [CrossRef] [PubMed]
32. Paolisso, P.; Bergamaschi, L.; Angeli, F.; Belmonte, M.; Foà, A.; Canton, L.; Fedele, D.; Armillotta, M.; Sansonetti, A.; Bodega, F.; et al. Cardiac Magnetic Resonance to Predict Cardiac Mass Malignancy: The CMR Mass Score. *Circ. Cardiovasc. Imaging* **2024**, *17*, e016115. [CrossRef]
33. Kassop, D.; Donovan, M.S.; Cheezum, M.K.; Nguyen, B.T.; Gambill, N.B.; Blankstein, R.; Villines, T.C. Cardiac Masses on Cardiac CT: A Review. *Curr. Cardiovasc. Imaging Rep.* **2014**, *7*, 9281. [CrossRef]
34. Rahbar, K.; Seifarth, H.; Schäfers, M.; Stegger, L.; Hoffmeier, A.; Spieker, T.; Tiemann, K.; Maintz, D.; Scheld, H.H.; Schober, O.; et al. Differentiation of malignant and benign cardiac tumors using 18F-FDG PET/CT. *J. Nucl. Med.* **2012**, *53*, 856–863. [CrossRef] [PubMed]
35. Shmueli, H.; Thomas, F.; Flint, N.; Setia, G.; Janjic, A.; Siegel, R.J. Right-Sided Infective Endocarditis 2020: Challenges and Updates in Diagnosis and Treatment. *J. Am. Heart Assoc.* **2020**, *9*, e017293. [CrossRef]
36. Sonaglioni, A.; Binda, G.; Rigamonti, E.; Vincenti, A.; Trevisan, R.; Nicolosi, G.L.; Zompatori, M.; Lombardo, M.; Anzà, C. A rare case of native pulmonary valve infective endocarditis complicated by septic pulmonary embolism. *J. Cardiovasc. Med.* **2019**, *20*, 152–155. [CrossRef] [PubMed]
37. Vinod, G.V.; Kanjirakadavath, B.; Krishnan, M.N. Large mural vegetation from right ventricle, accompanying tricuspid valve endocarditis. *Heart Asia* **2013**, *5*, 82–83. [CrossRef]
38. Koshy, A.G.; Kanjirakadavath, B.; Velayudhan, R.V.; Kunju, M.S.; Francis, P.K.; Haneefa, A.R.; Rajagopalan, R.V.; Krishnan, S. Images in cardiovascular medicine. Right ventricular mural bacterial endocarditis: Vegetations over moderator band. *Circulation* **2009**, *119*, 899–901. [CrossRef]
39. Diaz-Navarro, R.A.; Kerkhof, P.L.M. Case report on right ventricular mural endocarditis, not diagnosed clinically, but histopathologically after cardiac surgery. *Eur. Heart J. Case Rep.* **2022**, *6*, ytac376. [CrossRef]
40. Tomaszuk Kazberuk, A.; Sobkowicz, B.; Hirnle, T.; Lewczuk, A.; Sawicki, R.; Musiał, W. Giant right ventricular mural vegetation mimicking a cardiac tumour. *Kardiol. Pol.* **2011**, *69*, 587–589.
41. Mandelkern, T.F.; Sultan, I.; Levenson, J.E. Righting on the Wall: A Case of Medically Managed Right Ventricular Mural Endocarditis. *Circ. Cardiovasc. Imaging* **2023**, *16*, 591–593. [CrossRef] [PubMed]
42. Sparrow, P.J.; Kurian, J.B.; Jones, T.R.; Sivananthan, M.U. MR imaging of cardiac tumors. *Radiographics* **2005**, *25*, 1255–1276. [CrossRef] [PubMed]
43. Dursun, M.; Yılmaz, S.; Yılmaz, E.; Yılmaz, R.; Onur, İ.; Oflaz, H.; Dindar, A. The utility of cardiac MRI in diagnosis of infective endocarditis: Preliminary results. *Diagn. Interv. Radiol.* **2015**, *21*, 28–33. [CrossRef]
44. Dursun, M.; Yilmaz, S.; Ali Sayin, O.; Olgar, S.; Dursun, F.; Yekeler, E.; Tunaci, A. A rare cause of delayed contrast enhancement on cardiac magnetic resonance imaging: Infective endocarditis. *J. Comput. Assist. Tomogr.* **2005**, *29*, 709–711. [CrossRef] [PubMed]
45. Sverdlov, A.L.; Taylor, K.; Elkington, A.G.; Zeitz, C.J.; Beltrame, J.F. Images in cardiovascular medicine. Cardiac magnetic resonance imaging identifies the elusive perivalvular abscess. *Circulation* **2008**, *118*, e1–e3. [CrossRef] [PubMed]
46. Thuny, F.; Grisoli, D.; Cautela, J.; Riberi, A.; Raoult, D.; Habib, G. Infective endocarditis: Prevention, diagnosis, and management. *Can. J. Cardiol.* **2014**, *30*, 1046–1057. [CrossRef]
47. Grob, A.; Thuny, F.; Villacampa, C.; Flavian, A.; Gaubert, J.Y.; Raoult, D.; Casalta, J.P.; Habib, G.; Moulin, G.; Jacquier, A. Cardiac multidetector computed tomography in infective endocarditis: A pictorial essay. *Insights Imaging* **2014**, *5*, 559–570. [CrossRef]
48. Mitsis, A.; Alexi, A.; Constantinides, T.; Chatzantonis, G.; Avraamides, P. A Case of Right Ventricular Thrombus in a Patient With Recent COVID-19 Infection. *Cureus* **2022**, *14*, e25150. [CrossRef]

49. Angeli, F.; Bodega, F.; Bergamaschi, L.; Armillotta, M.; Amicone, S.; Canton, L.; Fedele, D.; Suma, N.; Cavallo, D.; Foà, A.; et a Multimodality Imaging in the Diagnostic Work-Up of Patients With Cardiac Masses: *JACC: CardioOncology* State-of-the-Ar Review. *JACC Cardio Oncol.* **2024**, *6*, 847–862. [CrossRef]
50. Shenoy, C.; Grizzard, J.D.; Shah, D.J.; Kassi, M.; Reardon, M.J.; Zagurovskaya, M.; Kim, H.W.; Parker, M.A.; Kim, R.J. Cardic vascular magnetic resonance imaging in suspected cardiac tumour: A multicentre outcomes study. *Eur. Heart J.* **2021**, *43*, 71–8([CrossRef]
51. Li, X.; Chen, Y.; Liu, J.; Xu, L.; Li, Y.; Liu, D.; Sun, Z.; Wen, Z. Cardiac magnetic resonance imaging of primary cardiac tumor *Quant. Imaging Med. Surg.* **2020**, *10*, 294–313. [CrossRef]
52. Achuthanandan, S.; Harris, C.L.; Farooqui, A.A.; Hollander, G. Right Ventricular Thrombus Masquerading as a Tumor. *Cureu* **2022**, *14*, e26014. [CrossRef] [PubMed]
53. Hiemetzberger, R.; Müller, S.; Bartel, T. Incremental use of tissue Doppler imaging and three-dimensional echocardiography fo optimal assessment of intracardiac masses. *Echocardiography* **2008**, *25*, 446–447. [CrossRef] [PubMed]
54. Sonaglioni, A.; Nicolosi, G.L.; Lombardo, M.; Anzà, C.; Ambrosio, G. Prognostic Relevance of Left Ventricular Thrombus Motility Assessment by Pulsed Wave Tissue Doppler Imaging. *Angiology* **2021**, *72*, 355–363. [CrossRef] [PubMed]
55. Ho, C.Y.; Solomon, S.D. A clinician's guide to tissue Doppler imaging. *Circulation* **2006**, *113*, e396–e398. [CrossRef]
56. Sonaglioni, A.; Nicolosi, G.L.; Muti-Schünemann, G.E.U.; Lombardo, M.; Muti, P. Could Pulsed Wave Tissue Doppler Imaging Solve the Diagnostic Dilemma of Right Atrial Masses and Pseudomasses? A Case Series and Literature Review. *J. Clin. Med.* **2024** *14*, 86. [CrossRef]

MDPI AG
Grosspeteranlage 5
4052 Basel
Switzerland
Tel.: +41 61 683 77 34

Journal of Clinical Medicine Editorial Office
E-mail: jcm@mdpi.com
www.mdpi.com/journal/jcm

www.ingramcontent.com/pod-product-compliance
Lightning Source LLC
Chambersburg PA
CBHW062034220926
51850CB00010B/2548
* 9 7 8 3 7 2 5 8 5 8 1 1 8 *